Oesophageal Atresia

During the years 1948—1988, 584 patients with oesophageal atresia and/or tracheo-oesophageal fistula were admitted to the Royal Children's Hospital, Melbourne.

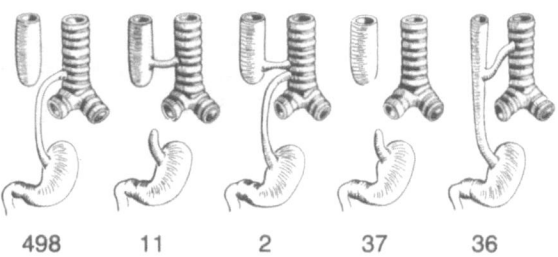

498   11   2   37   36

Oesophageal Atresia

Edited by

S.W. Beasley,
Consultant Paediatric Surgeon,
Royal Children's Hospital, Melbourne, Australia

N.A, Myers
Honorary Senior Consultant Surgeon
Royal Children's Hospital, Melbourne, Australia

and

A.W. Auldist
Chief, Department General Surgery
Royal Children's Hospital, Melbourne, Australia

 Springer-Science+Business Media, B.V.

First edition 1991

© 1991 Springer Science+Business Media Dordrecht
Originally published by Chapman & Hall in 1991
Softcover reprint of the hardcover 1st edition 1991

Typeset in 10/12 Palatino by
Acorn Bookwork, Salisbury, Wiltshire

ISBN 978-0-412-34820-4   ISBN 978-1-4899-3079-8 (eBook)
DOI 10.1007/978-1-4899-3079-8

British Library Cataloguing in Publication Data
Oesophageal atresia.
   1. Newborn babies. Congenital abnormalities
   I. Beasley, Spencer W.   II. Myers, N.A.   III. Auldist, A.W.
   618.920043
ISBN 978-0-412-34820-4

Library of Congress Cataloging-in-Publication Data

available

TO ALL BABIES WITH OESOPHAGEAL
ATRESIA
– BORN AND UNBORN –
AND THE STAFF WHO CARE FOR THEM

Contents

viii *Contents*

Contributors

Alex W. Auldist, MBBS, FRACS, Chief of General Pediatric Surgery, Royal Children's Hospital, Melbourne, Australia.

Agnes Bankier, MBBS, FRACP, Medical Geneticist, Royal Children's Hospital, Australia.

Spencer W. Beasley, MS, FRACS, Consultant Paediatric Surgeon, Royal Children's Hospital, Melbourne; Senior Lecturer in Paediatric Surgery, Department of Paediatrics, University of Melbourne, Australia.

Jocelyn Brady, Registered Medical Record Administrator; Research Assistant, Long-term follow-up oesophageal atresia study.

T. C. Kester Brown, MD, FFARACS, Director of Anaesthesia, Royal Children's Hospital, Melbourne, Australia.

Neil Campbell, MBBS, FRACP, Director of Department of Neonatology, Royal Children's Hospital, Melbourne, Australia.

Philip A. J. Chetcuti, MBBS, MRCP, Research Fellow, Department of Paediatrics, Royal Children's Hospital, University of Melbourne; Current appointment: Senior Registrar in Paediatrics, Royal Children's Hospital, Bristol, England.

D. Robert V. Dickens, FRACS, Orthopaedic Surgeon, Royal Children's Hospital, Melbourne, Australia.

Robert L. Eyres, FFARACS, FFARCS, Staff Anaesthetist, Royal Children's Hospital, Melbourne, Australia.

John H. Graham, MA, Vice President, Royal Children's Hospital Auxiliaries, Melbourne, Australia, Past President Oesophageal Atresia Research Auxiliary.

Dale G. Johnson, MD, Surgeon-in-Chief, Primary Children's Medical Center; Professor of Surgery, University of Utah College of Medicine; Professor of Pediatrics, University of Utah College of Medicine.

Justin H. Kelly, FRACS, Chief of Surgery, Royal Children's Hospital, Melbourne, Australia.

Maxwell Kent, FRACS, Consultant Paediatric Surgeon, Royal Children's Hospital, Melbourne, Australia.

Geraldine E. McDonnell, SRN, DC, Charge Nurse, Neonatal Unit, Royal Children's Hospital, Melbourne, Australia.

Roger B. B. Mee, FRACS, Director, Victorian Paediatric Cardiac Unit, Royal Children's Hospital, Melbourne, Australia.

N. A. Myers, AM, MD, FRCS, FRACS, Senior Consultant Surgeon, Royal Children's Hospital, Melbourne; Previous Professorial Associate, University of Melbourne, Australia.

Ethna Phelan, MB, ChB (NUI), FRCR, Staff Radiologist, Royal Children's Hospital, Melbourne, Australia.

Peter D. Phelan, BSc, MD, FRACP, Stevenson Professor and Chairman, Department of Paediatrics, University of Melbourne; Chief Thoracic Physician, Royal Children's Hospital, Melbourne, Australia.

R. Neil D. Roy, MBBS, FRACP, Director, Newborn Emergency Transport Service and Senior Paediatrician, Royal Women's Hospital, Melbourne, Australia.

Hazel Speirs, ADWS, RNTC, Neonatal Social Worker, Royal Children's Hospital, Melbourne, Australia.

Lewis Spitz, MBChB, PhD, FRCS (Edin), FRCS (Eng) FAAP (Hon), Nuffield Professor of Paediatric Surgery. Institute of Child Health, University of London; Consultant Paediatric Surgeon, Hospital for Sick Children, Great Ormond Street, London.

Keith B. Stokes, MBBS, FRACS, Consultant Surgeon, Department of Paediatric Surgery, Royal Children's Hospital, Melbourne, Australia.

Heather M. Telfer, RN, BEd, Formerly Deputy Head (Clinical) Mackinnon School of Nursing, Royal Children's Hospital, Melbourne, Australia.

Acknowledgements

It is a pleasure to record our thanks to the many people who have contributed to this book.

We would particularly like to thank Mrs Elizabeth Vorrath, ably assisted by Mrs Judith Hayes, for their enormous commitment and effort in typing the manuscript.

We also wish to thank Miss Anne Esposito, Medical Artist, and the photographic department of the Royal Children's Hospital Educational Resources Centre for their help with the figures. We acknowledge the help of Mr Peter Borzi and Dr Koenraad Schwaghten, Surgical Registrars, in retrieving information, and Mr Wyn Beasley for reading the manuscript. We are indebted to Miss Jocelyn Brady, Research Assistant, for her dedication over several years in tracing the patients whom we reviewed. Our thanks are expressed also to Professor R. McMahon of Monash Medical Centre, and to the Chairman and Secretary of the Consultative Council on Obstetric and Paediatric Mortality, Professor Beischer and Mr Peter Gardner. Throughout, assistance has been given freely by the staff of the Royal Children's Hospital Library.

Our families have shown admirable patience and tolerance.

We are very grateful to Dr Peter Altman of Chapman and Hall who has provided us with considerable support and encouragement throughout; his patience has been appreciated.

Preface

This book on oesophageal atresia and tracheo-oesophageal fistula sets out to describe all aspects of a congenital anomaly which has been described as 'the epitome of modern surgery' and 'the raison d'etre of paediatric surgery'. Although the literature contains references to the survival of one baby with oesophageal atresia (without fistula) who was born in 1935, the major component of the oesophageal atresia story concerns the most frequent anomaly, namely oesophageal atresia with a distal tracheo-oesophageal fistula. The first long-term survivals of babies born with this anomaly were in 1939; it is appropriate therefore that this book should be compiled 50 years later. Surgery and neonatal care have made striking advances during this half century, and nowhere is this more obvious than in the field of neonatal surgery. But the care of the baby with oesophageal atresia requires more than a surgeon and a neonatologist, and our experience has shown the need for a multidisciplinary approach involving anaesthetists, intensive care therapists, thoracic physicians, general paediatricians, cardiologists and cardiac surgeons, orthopaedic surgeons, radiologists, nephrologists and geneticists. The involvement of representatives of all of these disciplines is evident in the pages that follow and in the list of contributors; however, a central theme in the care of patients with oesophageal atresia is that they, and their families, are able to identify with one doctor who has the ultimate responsibility for patient care and the counselling of the family.

Our experience with the definitive surgical treatment of oesophageal atresia commenced in 1948 and during the period 1948–88 we managed 584 patients with atresia and/or fistula. A unique feature of this series, which has provided background information for many of the chapters which follow, is that only eight surgeons have had the clinical responsibility for the patients. Of these eight, three are editors of the book and two others have contributed to it. To provide some balance, particularly where we felt that our own experience was limited, we invited contributions from two esteemed colleagues – Lewis Spitz of London and Dale Johnson of Utah, USA. In addition to contributions from members of the medical staff of the Royal Children's Hospital, Melbourne, we also invited contributions from nursing staff, from a medical social worker, from a Past President of our Oesophageal Atresia Research Auxiliary (he is also a parent of one of our patients) and from the Director of the Victorian Neonatal Emergency Transport Service. We hope that this has given balance to the book as well as permitting all areas of the subject to be covered with authority.

The book is presented in eight parts, commencing with a summary of the historical events of significance. In Part Two attention is directed to the basic sciences: epidemiology and genetics, embryology, anatomy and pathophysiology. The clinical aspects commence in Part Three where chapters deal with diagnosis, transport, anaesthesia and intensive care. This is followed by a section which addresses the surgical aspects of the specific variants of the anomaly.

A major problem in a baby with oesophageal atresia is the associated anomalies which are present in over 50% of the patients; therefore Part Five is devoted to the consideration of these anomalies with emphasis on the most important specific anomalies.

We thought it logical to consider the overall care of the child and family and to complete the book by describing the management of specific problems and complications, and the long-term results of surgery.

This book is presented in the hope that it will be of help to all concerned with the care of the baby with oesophageal atresia and its family, recognizing that the field is wide, involving as it does representatives of many medical and paramedical disciplines.

Foreword

In a newborn baby the oesophagus is as exquisite as the slender rose vase which it resembles, yet simultaneously as treacherous as a writhing viper; which its shape and muscle action suggest. Surgeons; Beasley, Myers, and Auldist have provided a careful record of enormous experience with anomalies of the oesophagus. All who struggle with reconstruction of the malformed oesophagus will be helped by the insight and instruction recorded here; moving as they do from formation, to form, to malfunction, thence to function, the sections and chapters are as logical and orderly as a bolus of food passing down the normal gullet. The authors have generously included the work of others before stating their own conclusions, which have been formulated by comprehensive evaluation of 584 babies born with oesophageal atresia or one of its variants. These patients have been treated over a 40 year span in the same operating theatre by a sturdy band of only eight surgeons related collegially or as pupils. What an encyclopaedic reference compendium! We will mine this rich lode for years to come. Do you need to know the incidence in patients born with oesophageal atresia, of radial club hand, renal hypoplasia, the changing impact of congenital heart disease on survival, or most importantly, what is to be done when a planned surgical effort goes awry? It is all here.

The authors have drafted a thoughtful essay on the distress of the entire family constellation when the long awaited baby turns out to have oesophageal atresia. Their gentle perceptions stimulate all who render surgical care to neonates to reach for the sensitivity evinced in these pages. There is a frank discussion of the consequences of withholding surgical treatment from patients with concomitant limiting anomalies such as renal agenesis or trisomy 18. Clear guidelines for this arduous course of action and the necessary support for the family and the health care team have not previously been so courageously described. The late study of adults treated for oesophageal atresia is undoubtedly the greatest boon to surgeons trying to comprehend the long-term impact of an oesophageal malformation. Over 100 patients greater than 18 years of age have undergone clinical analysis. The fullness of this perspective has been achieved through lifetime experiences of both the surgeons and their patients. For younger surgeons who may require their own lifetime to achieve such understanding and proficiency, time has been compacted in this volume. The authors have dedicated their book 'to babies born and unborn with oesophageal malformation'. They have presented a great gift to babies so afflicted and to those who care for them.

Judson Randolph, M.D.
Washington DC

PART ONE
History

1 The early history of oesophageal atresia and tracheo-oesophageal fistula

N. A. MYERS

He who cannot take part in the friendly meal is half shut out from the society of man. W. Thomson (1878)

The history of oesophageal atresia extends over three centuries and contains many fascinating accounts of the anomaly. Initially, these accounts described the clinical presentation and pathology, but as time passed, an increasing interest in the surgical management developed. The critical year was 1888, the year in which Charles Steele made the first surgical attempt at correction of the anomaly. Significant events in the understanding and management of oesophageal atresia before and after that date are summarized in Tables 1.1 and 1.2.

Table 1.1 Early descriptions and contributions: 1670–1888

Year	Author	Contribution
1670:	Durston	Description of 'A Monstrous Birth in Plymouth'
1697:	Gibson	First description of oesophageal atresia with distal fistula (the commonly encountered anomaly)
1793:	Hunter	Described use of eel skin as a gavage tube
1821:	Martin	Reported the second known case of oesophageal atresia with a distal fistula
1840:	Hill	First report of oesophageal atresia combined with an anorectal anomaly
1861:	Hirschsprung	Ten cases in the literature, added four of his own
1869:	Holmes	First suggestion of surgical treatment
1873:	Lamb	Described 'H' fistula
1880:	Morell Mackenzie	Article on 'Malformations of the Oesophagus'
1888:	Steele	First operation on oesophageal atresia in London

Table 1.2 Early surgical contributions: 1888–1949

1888	Surgical era commences (Steele)	
1898	Hoffman	First gastrostomy for oesophageal atresia
1913	Richter	Division of tracheo-oesophageal fistula
1923	Smith	Ligation of oesophagus (at cardia)
1928	Scott	Gastrostomy; divided oesophagus (at cardia)
1936	Gage and Oschner	Cervical oesophagostomy
		Ligation of oesophagus
		Gastrostomy
1938	Shaw	Attempted primary anastomosis
1938	Gamble	Cervical oesophagostomy; division of stomach
1939	Ladd	First survival (OA with distal fistula)
1939	Leven	Second survival (OA with distal fistula)
1940	Lanman	'A Study of 32 Cases'
1941	Haight	First successful primary anastomosis
1947	Franklin	First survival in United Kingdom
1949	Howard	First survival in Australia

1.1 Early descriptions

The documented history of oesophageal atresia begins with Durston in 1670, during the reign of Charles II. In that year William Durston, doctor in Physick, described oesophageal atresia in a conjoined twin. His description (Durston, 1670) (Figure 1.1) commences: 'One Grace Batter'd, the wife of a shoemaker of honest repute and mother of five children, now came to the full time to be delivered of a sixth birth, about twelve o'clock at night began to have travelling pains.' Later in the description, it became clear that Durston delivered a thoracopagus monster and when he performed a necropsy, having with some difficulty 'obtained the father's leave to dissect it', he found 'one navilvein, and one liver . . . and one stomach with the oesophagus from the mouth of no lower than a little above half an inch off the midriff, and there it ended'.

Ashcraft and Holder (1969) held that pride of place should be given to the description by Thomas Gibson of the most commonly encountered anomaly. In his *Anatomy of Humane Bodies Epitomized* he wrote:

About November 1696 I was sent for to an infant that would not swallow. The child seem'd very desirous of food, and took what was offer'd it in a spoon with greediness; but when it went to swallow it, it was like to be choked, and what should have gone down returned by the mouth and nose, and it fell into a struggling convulsive sort of fit;

A Narrative of a Monstrous Birth in Plymouth, *Octob. 22. 1670; together with the Anatomical Observations, taken thereupon by* William Durston *Doctor. in Physick, and communicated to Dr.* Tim. Clerk.

ONE, *Grace Batter'd*, the wife of a shoemaker, of honest Repute, and mother of five Children, now come to the full time to be delivered of a sixth Birth, about twelve a Clock at night began to have travelling pains; and near four a Clock in the morning the Head of a Child came to the Birth: When the Midwife, putting her hand to help off this, felt another, (by its heat and motion) alive; and therefore made all possible speed to deliver her of this.

'Tis observable, that in three of her former five travels she was so quick, as that she was deliver'd before the Midwife came; but now she could not so speedily effect her desire, in regard that not only the first child was suffocated by its stay in the Birth; but also the Head of the second turning aside from the inner orifice of the *Uterus* towards the groine, and the Twins being joyn'd together (as afterwards appeared) made it a different Birth. But the Midwife doing her part exceeding well, and the Mother having nimble travel, was delivered of those prodigious Twins, the *effigies* of which is here sent you inclosed, (See *Table 2. Figure 1.*) together with an Accompt of what we thought further worth observation.

This Birth, as you see, had two Heads, and two Necks; as also the Eyes, Mouths, and Ears, sutably double. Four Arms with Hands, and as many Leggs and Feet. There was to both but one Trunk; but two Back-bones, from the *Clavicles* to the *Hypogastrium*, and from the shoulders down to the bottom of the Loins they were not distinct, but cemented and concorporated, after this manner: The right *Clavicle* or Channel-bone of the Right-hand-Child (being long) joyned with the left *Clavicle* of the Left-hand-Child. The Ribbs on the face-side of both of them, by the Cartilages or Gristles were united without any intervening *Sternum* or Brest-bone;
and

Figure 1.1 From William Durston (1670) 'A Monstrous Birth in Plymouth'. The first documented case of oesophageal atresia occurred in one of conjoined twins.

but the next day died. The parents being willing to have it opened, I took two physicians and a surgeon with me . . . We blew a pipe down the gullet, but found no passage for the wind into the stomach. Then we made a slit in the stomach, and put a pipe into its upper orifice, and blowing, we found the wind had a vent, but not by the top of the gullet. Then we carefully slit open the back side of the gullet from the stomach upwards, and when we were gone a little above half way towards the pharynx we found it hollow no further. Then we began to slit it open from the pharynx downward, and it was hollow till within an inch of the other slit, and in the imperforate part of was narrower than in the hollowed. This isthmus (as it were) did not seem ever to have been hollow, for in the bottom of the upper, and the top of the lower cavity, there was not the least print of any such thing, but the parts were here as smooth as the bottom of an acorn-cup. Then searching what way the wind had passed when we blow from the stomach upwards, we found an oval hole (half an inch long) on the fore-side of the gullet opening into the aspera arteria a little above its first division, just under the lower part of the isthmus above mentioned.

Gibson's contribution in 1697 was followed by a barren period and it was not until the first quarter of the nineteenth century that further references to oesophageal atresia by Martin and Mondiere are found.

In 1840 Thomas Hill wrote an interesting account of oesophageal atresia in the *Boston Medical and Surgical Journal* and, as pointed out by Ashcraft and Holder, it would appear most unlikely that he had previously heard of the condition, which adds greater interest to his description. His patient also had rectal agenesis, such that Hill must be given credit for the first description of the combination of anomalies with which we are now so familiar. Hill observed the infant 'to salivate excessively since birth, and with each feeding it would cough, become cyanotic and regurgitate all its food'.

In the same year, 1840, Thomas Mellor of Charlton-upon-Medlock, near Manchester, UK further described the clinical features in the *London Medical Gazette*: 'I am induced to transmit the accompanying case for insertion into your excellent journal, in consequence of its extreme rarity, and under the conviction it may prove interesting to your numerous readers, should you deem it worthy of publication.

Among others whose names are associated with the history of oesophageal atresia in the nineteenth century are Hirschsprung and Morell Mackenie. Although Hirschsprung's name is most frequently associated with the disease which bears his name, he did write a thesis which included comments on oesophageal atresia. He had been able to find ten cases in the literature and added four of his own.

Morell Mackenzie was another well-known medical figure in the nineteenth century and his involvement with the ultimately fatal illness of the Crown Prince, subsequently Kaiser of Germany, was to lead to much vitriolic discussion. In an unrelated contribution in 1880 Mackenzie suggested that:

> Malformations of the oesophagus in all probability are an extremely rare occurrence. All the recorded cases which I have been able to collect do not number more than 56, and I am only able to add one from my own observation, making altogether 57 examples. These facts are especially significant when we remember that the presence of the affection, in viable infants at least, is attended by such striking symptoms, that it is hardly possible for it to escape notice, whilst its inevitably fatal result affords an invariable opportunity of investigating its cause.

1.2 From observation to intervention

By the second half of the nineteenth century, oesophageal atresia was a well-recognized entity, but considered to have a hopeless prognosis with no prospect of survival. Operative treatment of the anomaly had not been attempted, although Timothy Holmes had suggested its possibility. Perhaps the most significant comment reflecting the mood of the time was his comment in 1869 that '. . . in any case the attempt ought not, I think, be made.'

In the same year (1869) Thomas Annandale, a lecturer on surgery in Edinburgh resigned himself to the opinion: 'Examples of this form of congenital malformation cannot be considered to be of much practical importance to the surgeon owing to their extreme rarity and also to the fact that they do not admit of operative interference.' Even the remarks attributed by Annandale to Sedillot reveal a certain pessimism:

> In any case where the oesophagus is simply obliterated, withered or interrupted, gastrostomy would give the hope of saving the child without other accidents, save those related to the operation itself. If there were a communication between the inferior tip of the oesophagus and the trachea, one could fear that the substances carried into the stomach would be regurgitated into the respiratory tract; but the narrowness of the abnormal orifice and its natural tendency to close because there is no reason for it to exist should reassure against the eventuality of this problem, which it is not possible a priori to suspect.

It was not until 1888 that Charles Steele of London attempted to alter the natural history of the condition by surgical intervention. He reported in *The Lancet* of 20 October 1888:

> I was lately asked to see in consultation an infant twenty-four hours
> old who, shortly after being given nourishment, a little of which was
> taken readily, became very livid, had difficulty in breathing, and then
> returned the food and appeared to worsen. The gentleman in attend-
> ance wisely introduced a sound, and found that it passed about five
> inches and encountered an impassable obstruction. He then asked me
> to see the child, and I repeated the sounding with the same conclu-
> sion. We diagnosed that there was either a membrane across the
> oesophagus or that it ended in blind terminations; and I advised that
> through the night enemata of dessertspoonfuls of peptonised milk
> should be given every two hours and that by daylight the stomach
> should be opened and the oesophagus explored; if a membrane could
> be made out across a continuous canal, that it should be perforated in
> order to give a hope of life; and that, if we found any distance existed
> between the extremities, we could do no more; the parents, however,
> might feel that every possible endeavour had been made to save their
> child's life. This was agreed upon, and the father willingly acceded.
> On the following afternoon I was asked to perform an operation. The
> infant took chloroform well. I opened the abdomen above the umbili-
> cus in the middle line, exposed the stomach, and stitched it at four
> points to the skin, having some difficulty to keep the liver from
> protruding. The stomach was then opened, which was perfectly
> healthy, and of course empty. A bougie was passed down the
> oesophagus as before, and another upwards from the stomach for a
> short distance; but, they did not approach each other by what we
> judged to be an inch and a half. I then cut a gum-elastic catheter in
> half, and passed it from below, introducing up it a long slender steel
> probe and pressed it upwards as much as was justifiable, in case the
> lower part of the tube might be twisted or narrowed, and capable of
> being rendered pervious. All was of no avail, however; so the stomach
> wound was closed with sutures, also the abdominal wound, and we
> felt sure that the oesophagus was deficient for about an inch and a
> half. The infant slept for some time, and died twenty-four hours
> afterwards. The next afternoon, we made an examination, and found
> the oesophagus terminated above and below in blind rounded ends
> an inch and a half apart, and there was no cord or connexion between
> the parts. All the wound portions were quite healthy, and the appear-
> ance led to the conclusion that had there been a membranous occlu-
> sion a happy result might well have been hoped for. (Figure 1.2)

Despite the unsuccessful outcome, he had broken new ground and
shown that in some patients, survival might be possible. He has been

Clinical Notes:

MEDICAL, SURGICAL, OBSTETRICAL, AND THERAPEUTICAL.

CASE OF DEFICIENT ŒSOPHAGUS.
By CHARLES STEELE, M.D., F.R.C.S.

THE following case appears to me to be of interest from both a surgical and an anatomical point of view.

I was lately asked to see in consultation an infant twenty-four hours old, who, shortly after being given nourishment, a little of which was taken readily, became very livid, had difficulty in breathing, and then returned the food and appeared no worse. The gentleman in attendance wisely introduced a sound, and found that it passed about five inches and encountered an impassable obstruction. He then asked me to see the child, and I repeated the sounding with the same conclusion. We diagnosed that there was either a membrane across the œsophagus, or that it ended in blind terminations; and I advised that through the night enemata of dessertspoonfuls of peptonised milk should be given every two hours, and that by daylight the stomach should be opened and the œsophagus explored; if a membrane could be made out across a continuous canal, that it should be perforated in order to give a hope of life; and that, if we found any distance existed between the extremities, we could do no more; the parents, however, might feel that every possible endeavour had been made to save their child's life. This was agreed upon, and the father willingly acceded. On the following afternoon I was asked to perform the operation. The infant took chloroform well. I opened the abdomen above the umbilicus in the middle line, exposed the stomach, and stitched it at four points to the skin, having some difficulty to keep the liver from protruding. The stomach was then opened, which was perfectly healthy, and of course empty. A bougie was passed down the œsophagus as before, and another upwards from the stomach for a short distance; but they did not approach each other by what we judged to be an inch and a half. I then cut a gum-elastic catheter in half, and passed it from below, introduced up it a long slender steel probe, and pressed it upwards as much as was justifiable, in case the lower part of the tube might be twisted or narrowed, and capable of being rendered pervious. All was of no avail, however; so the stomach wound was closed with sutures, also the abdominal wound, and we felt sure that the œsophagus was deficient for about an inch and a half. The infant slept for some time, and died twenty-four hours afterwards. The next afternoon we made an examination, and found that the œsophagus terminated above and below in blind rounded ends an inch and a half apart, and there was no cord or connexion between the parts. All the wounded portions were quite healthy, and the appearances led to the conclusion that had there been only a membranous occlusion a happy result might well have been hoped for.

Figure 1.2   The first operation on oesophageal atresia, Charles Steele (1888).

credited by some writers as being the first surgeon to perform gastrostomy for oesophageal atresia. In fact, he performed a gastrotomy not a gastrostomy: the first gastrostomy for oesophageal atresia was performed by Hoffman in 1898.

During the early part of the twentieth century there were a few surgical contributions, and then a flood of reports in the 1930s culminated in the classic contributions of Leven, Ladd and Haight. Leven and Ladd were to achieve the first survivals in babies with oesophageal atresia and distal fistula utilizing a multistage approach, whereas Haight became the first surgeon successfully to perform end-to-end oesophageal anastomosis with survival.

1.3 Definitive surgery for oesophageal atresia

In 1913, long before Leven, Ladd and Haight achieved their milestones, Richter identified those factors which were later to dictate the surgical management of oesophageal atresia, and offered a plan of management which would enable survival until the technical difficulties of an oesophageal anastomosis had been overcome. His clarity of thought, at a time when thoracic surgery had barely entered its infancy and neonatal surgery was even younger, is shown by the following paragraph:

> Direct anastomosis of the ends, with closure of the trachea, in an infant less than a week old is certainly a hazardous proceeding. I am not certain however, that it may not prove impossible, and, if so, would be the ideal operation. I do not wish to dismiss the idea of immediate union of the two segments of the oesophagus. The technical difficulties would be rather greater than that of the operation here suggested. The greatest obstacle would be the danger of infection: however, I expect to attempt it at the first favourable opportunity . . . The present problem seems to be to close the communication with the trachea, do a gastrostomy, and so feed the child. The recent development of thoracic surgery justifies the hope that later in life a means of utilizing the gullet may be found.

Later, in 1923, Smith suggested ligation of the oesophagus at the cardia combined with gastrostomy.

The contributions of Richter and Smith were a necessary precursor to the approach advocated by Cameron Haight (Figure 1.3):

> In the surgical management of congenital atresia of the esophagus associated with tracheoesophageal fistula, two general plans of treatment can be used. One plan, the indirect attack, aims to circum-

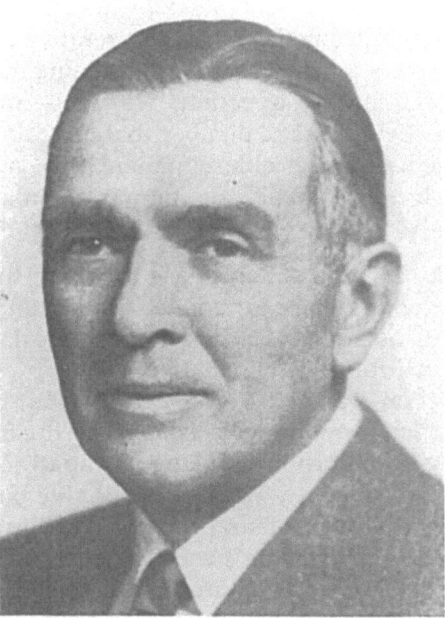

Figure 1.3 Cameron Haight (reproduced with permission from Ashcraft and Holder (1969)).

vent the anomaly by the use of staged operations. In principle, the indirect plan consists of gastrostomy for permanent feedings, ligation or exteriorization of the distal esophageal segment to prevent the regurgitation of gastric contents into the trachea and bronchi and exteriorization of the upper esophageal segment to allow for drainage of pharyngeal secretions onto the skin . . . The other plan of attack is the direct one whereby the contuinuity of the esophagus is restored.

The literature contains many references to the indirect approach and contributions were made by Mixter, Ravdin, Tucker and Pendergrass, Gage and Oschner and Scott (described in more detail by Myers, 1986). For example, Scott, as early as 1928, divided the oesophagus at the cardia and on at least one occasion combined this with exteriorization of the distal oesophagus.

Historically, the indirect approach was to give way to the direct approach and T. H. Lanman performed the first primary anastomosis of the oesophagus in 1936 and similar attempts were recorded at about the same time by Shaw. Lanman summarized the situation as follows:

> In spite of the fatal outcome in all the 30 operative cases, it is felt that considerable progress along rational lines is being made. The successful operative treatment of a patient with this anomaly is only a question of time. One must remember that an exterior esophagus as a palliative procedure for an elderly patient with cancer is justifiable and endurable, but one dreads to commit an infant to the sort of existence it entails.

Lanman predicted: 'Given a suitable case in which the patient is seen early, it is felt that, with greater experience, improved technic and good luck, the successful outcome to a direct anastomosis can and will be reported in the near future.'

Lanman's prediction was to become a reality, but before then Ladd and Leven were to achieve long-term survival by the indirect approach. Their patients were both born in 1939 one day apart. In Leven's patient gastrostomy was performed on the third day of life but it was not until several weeks later that extrapleural ligation of the oesophagus at its fistulous communication with the trachea was carried out. At a much later stage Leven interposed jejunum completing the replacement in 1951. Ladd reported his experience in 1944 and a particular feature was the courtesy he accorded Leven. Thus, Ladd wrote as follows:

> It is interesting to note that Leven at almost the identical time came to the same conclusion about methods of attacking this problem and adopted principles identical with ours with only minor variations of technique. So far as I know he has the oldest living patient with oesophageal atresia and a tracheo-oesophageal fistula, his patient being 24 hours older than our oldest living one. In a recent personal communication, he states that he has 4 additional patients living who have been operated on according to principles similar to those about to be described.

It is clear from Ladd's article that he performed gastrostomy on his patient on 28 November 1939, but did not divide the tracheo-oesophageal fistula until March the next year. Later he was to perform cervical oesophagostomy and antethoracic oesophagoplasty. Ladd wrote:

> From our experience and that of others, it seems fair to conclude that atresia of the esophagus with or without tracheoesophageal fistula should no longer be considered as a hopeless condition carrying with it a 100% mortality. It also seems justifiable to predict that if obstetricians and pediatricians are on the alert for making an early diagnosis, the mortality will be further lowered.

It should also be stated that the surgical methods for combating this condition are subject to change. At the present time, however, primary anastomosis of the esophagus appears to be the operation of choice when the two ends of the esophagus can be approximated without too much tension. In other cases, where the ends of the esophagus are far apart, the three-stage operation with the ultimate construction of an anterior thoracic esophagus is a safer operation.

As has been stated, Ladd's prediction was to become a reality and Haight's success occurred in March 1941 to be reported by Haight and Towsley in 1943. After 10 unsuccessful attempts to obtain a primary anastomosis, Haight reported:

> On the day following the admission [day 12], the patient's tracheo-esophageal fistula was ligated and divided through a left extrapleural approach; an end-to-end anastomosis was performed, employing a single layer of interrupted sutures of fine silk. Local anaesthesia was administered until construction of the anastomosis was begun, when ether by drip method was required so that enough relaxation could be achieved to allow approximation of the esophageal segments. The wound was closed around a narrow rubber drain. . . . the only anti-microbial agent used post-operatively was sulfathiazole, administered rectally. Fortunately, the patient survived in spite of the fact that generalized edema had appeared . . . and leakage of the anastomosis into the extrapleural wound had occurred on the seventh day after the operation. The parietal pleura had not been injured, however, at the time of operation, and the esophagocutaneous fistula remained localized and had healed by the twentieth post-operative day. In the interim, a gastrostomy to make feedings possible was performed on the tenth post-operative day . . . A stricture developed at the site of the anastomosis. Eventually, a single dilatation of the stricture was performed 17 months after the operation, and the patient was allowed to return home 20 months following the operation. She continued to improve and has developed normally.

Consistent with the respect that paediatric surgeons have always shown for each other, Haight acknowledged the pioneering efforts of many surgeons and gave credit to Richter, Ladd and Leven, Lanman and Shaw.

1.4 The Australian history

At the Royal Children's Hospital, Melbourne, the definitive surgery for oesophageal atresia commenced in 1948. Prior to that there were few

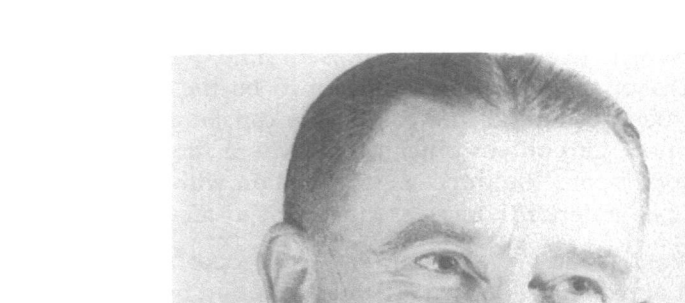

Figure 1.4   Russell Howard.

surgical endeavours and surgery was limited to gastrostomy. This was in keeping with the feeling of despondency reflected by a post-mortem report on a baby who died in 1936: 'At post mortem the baby has oesophageal atresia and a tracheo-oesophageal fistula. The condition is completely incompatible with life.'

However, with reports of a new approach and success from North America and the UK, Russell Howard (Figure 1.4) commenced operating on babies with oesophageal atresia in a definitive manner. He first achieved survival in 1949 and in that year two further survivals were obtained. The early experience was reported in the *Medical Journal of Australia* (Howard, 1950). Since then, the Royal Children's Hospital has admitted 584 infants with oesophageal atresia and/or tracheo-oesophageal fistula, an experience described more fully later in this book.

1.5   Oesophageal atresia without fistula

The history of oesophageal atresia, not surprisingly, contains many more references to atresia with a distal fistula than to the less frequently encountered anomalies. However, it is interesting to note that in 1928, Abel reported a patient with oesophageal atresia without fistula who survived following his endoscopic manipulations; and although there may be some doubt regarding the exact diagnosis of Abel's patient, there is no doubt regarding a patient described by Humphreys and Ferrer in 1964, who was born with oesophageal atresia without fistula in 1935. Ashcraft and Holder (1969) have summarized the case:

> . . . Contrast x-rays had demonstrated a blind proximal pouch. Gastrostomy was performed the next day . . . Ten days later barium placed through the gastrostomy tube demonstrated a distal blind esophagus extending about 4 cm above the diaphragm. The tube gastrostomy was converted to a more permanent mucosal-tube gastrostomy when the child was 2 years of age . . . At eleven years he was normally developed and well nourished. On August 14th, 1946, a long segment of jejunum was mobilized for interposition. The jejuno-gastrostomy was completed and the upper end closed and attached to the mediastinal pleura near the apex of the chest pending later oesophagojejunostomy. The upper 3 to 4 inches appeared dusky but viable at the end of closure. Nearly 4 weeks later, the child underwent operation for completion of the upper anastomosis. Dr Humphreys wrote – 'To our great disappointment it was found that although there was no evidence of pleural infection, the upper 4 inches of jejunum was necrotic, and that viable jejunum could not be mobilized. The necrotic jejunum was excised and the chest closed with drainage . . . He went home to Marlboro and resumed his former way of life.' For 5 years more he took all food through the gastrostomy . . . In 1951, Humphreys anastomosed (jejunum) to the cervical oesophageal stump. Thus, the first patient to survive with esophageal atresia was able to take oral feedings at 16 years of age.

1.6 The 'H' fistula

The initial description of tracheo-oesophageal fistula without atresia is attributed to Lamb in 1873 and the first operative success was reported by Imperatori in 1939. In his 'Atlas of Oesophageal Atresia', Kluth (1976) also mentions Pinard in 1873 and illustrated examples of double and triple fistulae as described by Hubner in 1943 and Leven in 1952. By 1969 Kappelman was able to report that approximately 125 cases of H-fistula had been recorded in the 'pediatric, surgical and otolaryngological literature'.

1.7   The contribution of radiology

Radiology has played a vital role in the evolution of the management of oesophageal atresia: a role which has included diagnosis, preoperative evaluation and recognition of associated anomalies. Perhaps the most significant contribution to the literature by a radiologist was by Vogt in 1929, who described the various anatomical types seen and suggested a simple classification using numbers and letters. This facilitated recognition of the difficult diagnostic and therapeutic requirements of each anatomical variant and as such was important at the time, although the modern tendency is to avoid numbers and letters and instead to use descriptive terms as suggested by El Shafie, Klippel and Blakemore in 1978.

References

Ashcraft, K. W. and Holder, T. M. (1969) The story of esophageal atresia and tracheo-esophageal fistula. *Surgery*, **65**, 332–40.

Durston, W. (1670) A narrative of a monstrous birth in Plymouth, October 22, 1670: together with the anatomical observations taken thereupon. *Philos. Trans. R. Soc.*, **V**, 2096.

El Shafie, M., Klippel, C. H. and Blakemore, W. S. (1978) Congenital esophageal anomalies: a plea for using anatomic description rather than classification. *J. Pediatr. Surg.*, **13**, 355.

Haight, C. and Towsley, H. A. (1943) Congenital atresia of the esophagus with tracheo-esophageal fistula. Extrapleural ligation of fistula and end-to-end anastomosis of esophageal segments. *Surg. Gynecol. Obstet.*, **76**, 672–88.

Howard, R. (1950) Oesophageal atresia with tracheo-oesophageal fistula: report of six cases with two successful oesophageal anastomoses. *Med. J. Aust.*, **i**, 401–4.

Kluth, D. (1976) Atlas of esophageal atresia. *J. Pediatr. Surg.*, **11**, 901–19.

Myers, N. A. (1986) The history of oesophageal atresia and tracheo-oesophageal fistula – 1670–1984. *Progr. Pediatr. Surg.*, **20**, 106–57.

PART TWO
Basic Sciences

2 *Epidemiology and genetics*

A. BANKIER, J. BRADY and N. A. MYERS

2.1 Introduction

Although oesophageal atresia and tracheo-oesophageal fistula are relatively common birth defects, little is known of their genetics and epidemiology. Most cases have been sporadic with occasional reports of familial occurrence. On the basis of the familial reports, some authors have concluded that genetic factors are important (Il'ina and Lurie, 1984; Pfeiffer, 1986). Other reports based on retrospective studies have suggested environmental and teratogenic factors (Warkany *et al.*, 1948; Ingalls and Prindle, 1949) with no conclusive evidence for any specific aetiological agent. Reports on the experience of various centres have concentrated on the outcome of the surgical management of indexed cases. Population and family studies have been lacking.

Before 1950, there were few survivors of oesophageal atresia. Only two follow-up studies have examined the occurrence of oesophageal atresia in offspring of affected individuals: in one, the incidence was low (Warren *et al.*, 1979) and in the other, there was no recurrence (Chetcuti *et al.*, 1988). The follow-up information was incomplete (80% and 86% respectively) and therefore does not directly indicate the risk of recurrence in offspring.

In this chapter, the available epidemiological information from the literature and our yet unpublished pedigree data are presented.

In an attempt to clarify genetic and epidemiological data, perinatal and pedigree information on patients born in the ten-year period, 1975–1984, was gathered. Cases were ascertained by personal search of hospital and pathology records. Patients who died were checked against the perinatal mortality register. In the State of Victoria, the Consultative Council of the Maternal and Perinatal Mortality established a compulsory register of neonatal deaths in 1962, and of stillbirths from 1968. By the 1970s, 98% of perinatal deaths were reported to the Council and the necropsy rate reached 80%. Repair of oesophageal atresia in the State was performed in one of two centres, with over 80% being performed at the Royal Children's Hospital by one of four surgeons. Surviving patients have been reviewed on a regular basis and therefore it was thought that this period was most likely to provide a complete ascertainment and follow-up. Good ascertainment was achieved, with pedigree information available in 84% of cases. Further studies are in progress.

2.2   Incidence

The documented incidence of oesophageal atresia (and of tracheo-oesophageal fistula) varies from 1 : 3000 to 1 : 10 000 live births (Babbott and Ingalls, 1961; Leck *et al.*, 1968; Cudmore, 1978). Briard *et al.* (1985) observed that the incidence is notably increased when stillbirths and abortions are included, i.e. to 1 : 2000 and 1 : 68.5 respectively.

In Victoria, the incidence has been estimated to be 1 : 4500 live births (Myers, 1974, 1989), a figure similar to that quoted by Haight (1957).

In the more recent ten-year study, there were 175 index cases born in Victoria, including nine stillbirths, representing a total birth incidence of 1 : 3448 and a live birth incidence of 1 : 3570.

2.3   Perinatal data

The pregnancy information was unremarkable in the ten-year group. There was no consistent exposure to teratogens or infections recorded. Maternal polyhydramnios was present in all cases of oesophageal atresia alone and in oesophageal atresia with proximal fistula.

In the full series of 584 patients born with oesophageal atresia referred to the Royal Children's Hospital (1948–1988), 39% were 36 weeks' gestation or less (Figure 2.1). In the early years of study, some infants with extreme prematurity may not have been diagnosed and transferred for surgery. In the ten-year group (1975–1984), 32% of patients were premature, compared with an expected rate of 5% for Victoria (Annual Report of the Consultative Council, 1984), and in 39%, the birth weight was less than 2500 g.

2.4   Twins

The frequency of twinning has been found to be higher than expected. The twins have generally been discordant for oesophageal atresia and

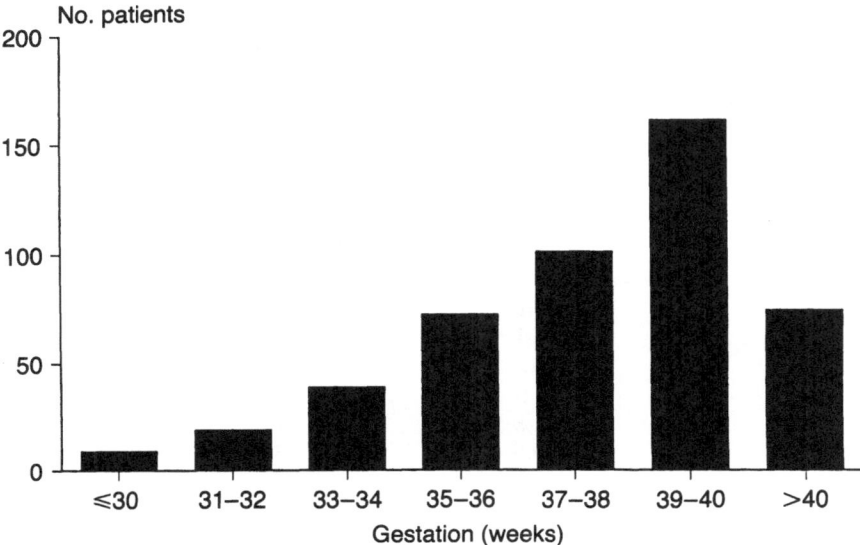

Figure 2.1 Gestation in oesophageal atresia.

tracheo-oesophageal fistula. There have also been reports of both twins affected (Woolley *et al.*, 1961; Blank *et al.*, 1967; Okhuma, 1978).

In the Royal Children's Hospital series (1948–1988) there were 23 twin pairs, and all were discordant for oesophageal atresia and tracheo-oesophageal fistula. In the ten-year subgroup, there were 11 twin pairs, a frequency of twinning of 7%, compared to the expected rate of 2.3% for our population. All twin pairs were discordant for oesophageal atresia.

2.5 Birth order

Current data on the place in the family of infants born with oesophageal atresia is contradictory. Warren *et al.* (1979) found an excess of first-borns and a deficit of later-borns, whereas Schimke *et al.* (1972) found that the infant with oesophageal atresia tended to be last-born twice as frequently as first-born.

In our ten-year series there were significantly more index cases born following the third and fourth pregnancy than expected (Table 2.1). The possible confounding factor of a maternal age effect remains to be clarified.

Table 2.1 Birth order in oesophageal atresia
and tracheo-oesophageal fistula (not corrected
for maternal age)

	Parity	
	1982 figures in Victoria (%)	*1975–1984 Oesophageal atresia* (%)
0	41	38.5
1	34	24.3
2	17	14.7
3	6	8.3
4	1.5	5.1
5	0.6	1.3
6	0.2	0.6

Chi-squared = 27.6 : significant at 1% level for parity $\geqslant$ 4.

2.6 Sex distribution

In all large series a male predominance of oesophageal atresia has been
reported (Jacobs and Papper, 1959; Wayson *et al.*, 1965; Romsdahl *et al.*,
1966; Holden and Wooler, 1970; Schimke *et al.*, 1972; Cozzi and Wilkinson, 1975; Strodel *et al.*, 1979; Ozimek *et al.*, 1982).

In our total series, 59% were male and 41% were female; the male
predominance applied equally to each anatomical variant. In the ten-
year series, 57% were male and 43% female; the sex distribution was not
significantly different when examined according to the type of associated birth defect. When compared to the expected sex ratio for our
population, the apparent male predominance did not reach statistical
significance (chi squared value 1.54).

There is no explanation for the recorded male predominance but there
is an analogy with other birth defects, such as Hirschsprung's disease
and pyloric stenosis. A male predominance has also been reported for
the VATER association (Czeizel and Ludanyi, 1985).

2.7 Associated birth defects

In our total series, over 50% of patients with oesophageal atresia had
one or more associated congenital anomalies (Chapters 14–17). In the

ten-year subgroup, 30% had isolated lesions, and 22% were associated with a known syndrome. The most common are the VATER (15 cases) and CHARGE (one case) associations; trisomy 21 (four cases) and trisomy 18 (five cases); duplication 4p (one case); Di George syndrome (three suspected cases); facio-auriculo-vertebral spectrum (two cases); Potter syndrome (four cases) and Fanconi syndrome (two cases). One or more associated birth defects were present in 48% of cases. It is of note that most of the associated defects were those lesions seen as part of the VATER association, an observation also noted by others.

Barry and Auldist (1974) studied a group of patients from the Royal Children's Hospital in a ten-year period (1963–1972) who presented with either oesophageal atresia, imperforate anus or radial aplasia. In groups other than radial aplasia, they found associated birth defects in the VATER spectrum in 50% of cases. They concluded, 'the VATER association should be regarded as part of a spectrum that ranges from the occurrence of any one of the defects singly to the full set of VATER anomalies plus congenital heart disease' (Chapter 14). Pfeiffer (1986) also suggested that isolated oesophageal atresia could be regarded as one end of the spectrum of the VATER association. These associations

Table 2.2 Syndromes for which oesophageal atresia has been reported

Acrorenal syndromes
CHARGE association
Chromosome B, trisomy 8 mosaicism
Chromosome 18, trisomy 18
Chromosome 21, trisomy 21
Chromosome d/u, triploidy 69XXX/XXY
Colobomata; tracheo-oesophageal fistula, heart defects
Di George sequence
Oesophageal atresia, coloboma, talipes
Facio-auriculo-vertebral dysplasia
Laryngotracheo-oesophageal cleft, unilateral pulmonary hypoplasia
Microcephaly, tracheo-oesophageal fistula, hand defect
Opitz–Frias syndrome
Potter sequence
Schisis association
Sirenomelia sequence
Tracheal agenesis association
Tracheo-oesophageal fistula, bat ears, symphalangism/fifth finger
VATER association

Source: Bankier *et al.*, 1988.

may tell us more about the timing of the insult in embryological development, rather than the cause, which is likely to be heterogeneous.

One theory is that an abnormality occurring in mesodermal development may result from single or multifactorial 'insults' to the embryo at the end of the third and beginning of fourth week of gestation (Stevenson, 1972). This may lead to oesophageal anomalies in isolation, or in combination with renal, radial, vertebral, anorectal and cardiovascular anomalies. In this context, Pfeiffer (1986) suggested that the incidence in relatives is increased because they share predisposing factors.

POSSUM (Pictures of Standard Syndromes and Undiagnosed Malformations) has identified many syndromes in which oesophageal atresia has been reported (Table 2.2).

2.8   Familial occurrence

Most cases of oesophageal atresia and tracheo-oesophageal fistula have been sporadic. There have been a number of reports of more than one affected person in the family (Grieve and McDermott, 1939; Lanman, 1940; Copleman *et al.*, 1952; Sloan and Haight, 1956; Engel *et al.*, 1970; Schimke *et al.*, 1972; McIntosh and Wright, 1986). Most familial reports have involved siblings or first-degree relatives, including parent/child involvement (Engel *et al.*, 1970; Dennis *et al.*, 1973; Warren *et al.*, 1979; Erichsen *et al.*, 1981) (Table 2.3).

In the Royal Children's Hospital series of 584 patients, 14 patients had a relative with oesophageal atresia or tracheo-oesophageal fistula. These involved nine families, five of which were ascertained in the series, while the other four had relatives with oesophageal atresia diagnosed elsewhere. These numbers may give the impression of higher than random occurrence.

In the 10-year subgroup, four of 146 families had more than one affected member. This included one pair of siblings, one first cousin, one second cousin pair and a twin (of like sex) discordant for oesophageal atresia with an affected uncle. The recurrence risk of oesophageal atresia for siblings based on our study is 0.9%.

Parent and child involvement has been reported. Of the 79 families studied by Warren *et al.* (1979), 15 parents had 28 children of whom one had oesophageal atresia. Of the 125 families studied by Chetcuti *et al.* (1988), 60 had 55 children, three of whom had other birth defects (duodenal atresia, pyloric stenosis, scimitar syndrome), but none had oesophageal atresia. They concluded that, on the evidence currently available, the risk for children was similar to the risk for siblings, and was of the order of 1%. Pfeiffer (1986) also calculated the risk of

Table 2.3 Familial occurrence of oesophageal atresia or tracheo-oesophageal fistula (excluding twins)

Author	Year	Details
Grieve and McDermott	1939	Brothers
Lanman	1949	Siblings (male and female)
Pilcher	1951	Cited by McIntosh and Wright (two females)
Copleman *et al.*	1952	Brothers
Sloan and Haight	1956	Brothers
Haight	1957	Two siblings (Male)
Hausmann *et al.*	1957	Three consecutive siblings
Engel *et al.*	1970	Mother and child
Forrester and Cohen	1970	Three siblings
Schimke *et al.*	1972	Two, possibly five, male children
Dennis *et al.*	1973	Three cases in two generations
Warren *et al.*	1979	Mother and son
Erichsen *et al.*	1981	Mother and daughter (and mother's second cousin)
McIntosh and Wright	1986	Siblings
Glasson	1990	Father and child
RCH Melbourne	1989	Nine families with 2nd involvement

oesophageal atresia in siblings to be about 1%. These numbers are based on small sample size and further studies are necessary to establish the true risk of recurrence.

From multivariate analysis, it has been estimated that for defects to have a genetic cause, the frequency of the birth defect in the first-degree relatives is the square root of the instance of the defect in the general population (Edwards, 1960). In our 157 patients, who had 282 siblings, the expected incidence would have been 1.6% and the actual incidence was 0.7%. Since the actual incidence is lower than expected, genetic aetiology is not supported. These figures are based on a small sample size, and for this reason the studies are being extended to clarify the actual risk of recurrence.

2.9 Other birth defects in family members

In the pedigree study (1975–1984) a higher than expected frequency of birth defects was not found in other family members. A total of 5.4% (32/591) of first-degree relatives, 2% (32/1567) of second-degree relatives, and 2.4% (38/1576) of first cousins were known to have a significant birth defect other than oesophageal atresia. It is of interest that none of the relatives (other than one family with three children who had the Fanconi syndrome) had distinct syndromes, but up to 50% had birth defects seen in the VATER spectrum.

2.10 Geographic clustering

Ozimek *et al.* (1982), in a study from the state of North Carolina, found no evidence for regional clustering of oesophageal atresia. Little other information is available regarding the demographic distribution. In the 10-year group, 69% were from the metropolitan area and the remainder from country districts, comparable to the overall population distribution in Victoria. However, these data do not take into account geographical factors relating to place of conception and address of the mother during pregnancy, and therefore have little epidemiological significance.

2.11 Temporal clustering

An increase in oesophageal atresia has been reported for the month of April (Babbott and Ingalls, 1961) and during the winter season (Knox, 1971). Ozimek *et al.* (1982) found no seasonal or monthly effect for birth or estimated conception date, but there was a clustering of cases over time (years) raising the possible effect of an infective agent. They observed that the incidence of oesophageal atresia without other anomalies shows the greatest cyclical variation over years, whereas oesophageal atresia with other documented malformations appeared to occur sporadically over time.

In our ten-year study group, there was neither significant seasonal nor monthly clustering, nor cyclical annual variations.

2.12 Conclusions

Little is known of the epidemiology and genetics of oesophageal atresia but the cause appears to be heterogeneous. It is known that about half the patients have associated birth defects and a distinct syndrome may be identified in as many as 20% of cases. There are at least 18 syndromes which may be associated with oesophageal atresia (Table 2.2). It is therefore important systematically to assess any baby for associated birth defects and if birth defects and dysmorphic features are present, to consider the possibility of a syndrome diagnosis and consult a geneticist. If a syndrome is identified, the chance of recurrence in siblings will be the risk of recurrence of the particular syndrome.

Reports of familial occurrence suggest some genetic predisposition. Our pedigree studies, and the accumulating information from follow-up of treated survivors, suggest that the risk of recurrence for oesophageal atresia in the family is small and is in the order of 1 : 100 (1%). (The risk of a birth defect from the VATER spectrum may also be in the order of 1 : 100.) It remains to be established by further family studies whether this small risk is related to a genetic susceptibility or is simply a reflection of the occurrence of a not uncommon birth defect.

The possible role of environmental factors remains to be explored. No such factors were apparent in our families. It is well known that retrospective enquiry is fraught with inaccuracies and prospective case studies will be needed to clarify whether there are possible environmental factors.

References

Babbott, J. G. and Ingalls, T. H. (1961) Tracheo-oesophageal fistula occurring in Pennsylvania. *Q. Rev. Pediatr.*, **16**, 86–92.

Bankier, A., McGill, J. J., Danks, J. J., McGill, J. A. and Danks, D. M. (1988) Dysmorphology: problems in nomenclature. *Dysmorphol. Clin. Gen.*, **2**, 24–50.

Barry, J. E. and Auldist, A. W. (1974) The VATER association. One end of a spectrum of anomalies. *Am. J. Dis. Child.*, **128**, 769–71.

Bianchine, J. W., Burney, N., Moore, R. *et al.* (1976) Esophageal atresia with tracheo-esophageal fistula in four male members of a kindred. *South. Med. J.*, **69**, 1098–9.

Blank, R. H., Prillaman, P. E. and Minor, G. R. (1967) Congenital esophageal atresia with tracheo-esophageal fistula occurring in identical twins. *J. Thor. Cardiovasc. Surg.*, **53**, 192–6.

Chetcuti, P., Myers, N. A., Phelan, P. D. *et al.* (1988) Adults who survived repair of congenital oesophageal atresia and tracheo-oesophageal fistula. *Br. Med. J.*, **297**, 344–6.

Copleman, B., Cannata, B. V. and London, W. (1952) Tracheo-esophageal anomaly in siblings. *J. Med. Soc. NJ.*, **47**, 415.

Cozzi, F. and Wilkinson, A. W. (1975) Low birth weight babies with oesophageal atresia or tracheo-oesophageal fistula. *Arch. Dis. Child.*, **50**, 791–5.

Cudmore, R. E. (1978) in *Neonatal Surgery* (eds P. P. Rickham, J. Listed and I. M. Irvine), Butterworths, London, pp. 191–2.

Czeizel, A. and Ludanyi, I. (1985) An aetiological study of the VACTERL-association. *Eur. J. Pediatr.*, **144**, 331–7.

Dennis, N. R., Nicholas, J. L. and Kovar, I. (1973) Oesophageal atresia: 3 cases in 2 generations. *Arch. Dis. Child.*, **48**, 980–2.

Edwards, J. H. (1960) The simulation of Mendelism. *Acta Genet.*, **10**, 63–70.

Engel, P. M. A., Vos, J. L. M., de Vries, J. A. *et al.* (1970) Esophageal atresia with tracheo-esophageal fistula in mother and child. *J. Pediatr. Surg.*, 5, 564–5.

Erichsen, G., Hauge, M., Madsen, C. M. *et al.* (1981) Two-generation transmission of oesophageal atresia with tracheo-oesophageal fistula. *Acta Paediatr. Scand.*, 70, 253–4.

Forrester, R. M. and Cohen, S. J. (1970) Esophageal atresia associated with an ano-rectal anomaly and probable laryngeal fissure in three siblings. *J. Pediatr. Surg.* 5, 674–5.

Fujimoto, S. and Manabe, A. (1962) Two cases, sister and brother, with esophageal atresia associated with tracheo-oesophageal fistula. *Adv. Obstet. Gynecol. (Osaka)*, 14, 155–8.

Glasson, M. (1990) Personal communication.

Grieve, J. E. and McDermott, J. E. (1939) Congenital atresia of the oesophagus in two brothers. *Can. Med. Assoc. J.*, 41, 185–6.

Haight, C. (1957) Some observations on esophageal atresias and tracheo-esophageal fistulas of congenital origin. *J. Thorac. Surg.*, 34, 141–72.

Hausmann, P. F., Close, A. S. and Williams, L. P. (1957) Occurrence of tracheo-esophageal fistula in 3 consecutive siblings. *Surgery*, 41, 542–3.

Holden, M. P. and Wooler, G. H. (1970) Tracheo-oesophageal and oesophageal atresia: results of 30 years' experience. *Thorax*, 25, 406–12.

Il' ina, E. G. and Lurie, I. V. (1984) Genetics of congenital esophageal defects. *Genetics*, 18, 463–4.

Ingalls, T. H. and Prindle, R. A. (1949) Esophageal atresia with tracheo-esophageal fistula. Epidemiologic and teratologic implications. *N. Engl. J. Med.*, 240, 987–95.

Jacobs, R. G. and Papper, E. M. (1959) Anaesthetic management of atresia of the esophagus and tracheo-esophageal fistula: a review of seven years' experience and 72 cases. *NY State J. Med.*, 59, 995–1002.

Knox, E. G. (1959) Secular pattern of congenital oesophageal atresia. *Br. J. Prev. Soc. Med.*, 13, 222–8.

Knox, E. G. (1971) Epidemics of rare diseases. *Br. Med. Bull.*, 27, 43–7.

Lanman, T. H. (1940) Congenital atresia of the esophagus. *Arch. Surg.*, 41, 1060–83.

Leck, I., Record, R. E., McKeown, T. *et al.* (1968) The incidence of malformations in Birmingham, England, 1950–1959. *Teratology*, 1, 263–80.

McIntosh, D. and Wright, J. E. (1986) Tracheo-oesophageal fistula in siblings. *Pediatr. Surg. Int.*, 1, 246–8.

Myers, N. A. (1974) Oesophageal atresia: the epitome of modern surgery. *Ann. R. Coll. Surg.*, 54, 277–87.

Myers, N. A. (1989) *Oesophageal Atresia and Tracheo-oesophageal Fistula: Changing Trends in Management*, MD Thesis, University of Melbourne.

Okhuma, R. (1978) Congenital esophageal atresia with tracheo-esophageal fistula in identical twins. *J. Pediatr. Surg.*, 13, 361–2.

Ozimek, C. D., Grimson, R. C. and Aylsworth, A. S. (1982) An epidemiological study of tracheo-esophageal fistula and esophageal atresia in North Carolina. *Teratology*, 25, 53–9.

Pfeiffer, R. A. (1986) Survey of genetic and epidemiological aspects in esophageal atresia. *Proceedings of Symposium on Oesophageal Atresia*, World Congress of International Society for Disease of the Esophagus (Munich).

Pilcher, R. S. (1951) Cited by McIntosh and Wright (1986).

Romsdahl, M. M., Hunter, J. A. and Grove, W. J. (1966) Tracheo-oesophageal fistula and esophageal atresia: surgical management and results at a university hospital. *J. Thorac. Cardiovasc. Surg.*, **52**, 571–8.

Schimke, R. N., Leape, L. L. and Holder, T. M. (1972) Familial occurrence of esophageal atresia: a preliminary report. *Birth Defects: Original Article Series*, Vol. VIII, no. 2, pp. 22–23.

Sloan, H. and Haight, C. (1956) Congenital atresia of the esophagus in brothers. *J. Thorac. Surg.*, **32**, 209–15.

Stevenson, R. E. (1972) Extra vertebrae associated with esophageal atresias and tracheo-esophageal fistulas. *J. Pediatr.*, **81**, 1123–9.

Strodel, W. E., Coran, A. E., Kirsh, M. M. *et al.* (1979) Esophageal atresia: a 41-year experience. *Arch. Surg.*, **114**, 523–7.

Warkany, J., Roth, C. B. and Wilson, J. G. (1948) Multiple congenital malformations. A consideration of etiologic factors. *Pediatrics*, **1**, 462–71.

Warren, J., Evans, K. and Carter, C. O. (1979) Offspring of patients with tracheo-oesophageal fistula. *J. Med. Genet.*, **16**, 338–40.

Wayson, E. E., Garnjobst, W., Chandler, J. J. *et al.* (1965) Esophageal atresia with tracheo-esophageal fistula: lessons of a quarter century's experience. *Am. J. Surg.*, **110**, 162–7.

Woolley, M. D., Chinnock, R. F. and Paul, R. H. (1961) Premature twins with esophageal atresia and tracheo-esophageal fistula. *Acta Paediatr.*, **50**, 423–30.

3 Embryology

S. W. BEASLEY

3.1 Normal development of the oesophagus and trachea

The primitive foregut distal to the pharynx and proximal to the stomach remains tubular, and elongates to form the oesophagus. During the fourth week a depression develops on the ventral wall of the foregut which is called the laryngotracheal groove. Classical descriptions (Gray, 1972; Gray and Skandalakis, 1972) suggest that the groove deepens and its lips fuse from its caudal end to form a septum which converts the groove into a tube, the laryngotracheal tube (Figure 3.1). The tissue between the separating laryngotracheal tube and primitive oesophagus is known as the tracheo-oesophageal septum. The tube remains open at its cephalic end, where it connects with the pharynx. Two lateral outgrowths arise from its caudal end to form the stem bronchi and the right and left lung buds. This concept of the tracheo-oesophageal septum separating the ventral trachea from the dorsal oesophagus has been widely accepted since 1887 (His, 1887).

3.2 When does oesophageal atresia occur?

The primordium of the tracheopulmonary anlage is detectable on the anterior wall of the primitive foregut 21 days after fertilization. By the time the embryo is 8 mm (32 days) development of the tracheo-oesophageal septum and separation of the trachea and oesophagus is complete. This would suggest that the insult which causes oesophageal atresia is likely to have occurred before 32 days of gestation. The absence of striated muscle in the oesophagus beyond the tracheo-oesophageal fistula in oesophageal atresia has been taken as further evidence that oesophageal atresia occurs during the early period of separation of the trachea from the oesophagus (Pringle, 1983) because normally one would expect to find striated muscle in the middle third of the oesopha-

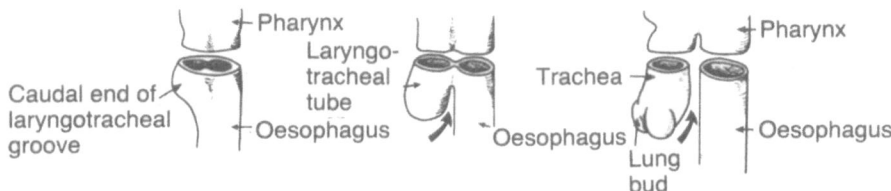

Figure 3.1   The classical concept of closure of the laryngotracheal groove and its separation from the oesophagus by the tracheo-oesophageal septum.

gus. In addition, there have been two reports of fully developed oesophageal atresia and tracheo-oesophageal fistula in embryos between 32 and 34 days of age (Ysander, 1925; Gruenwald, 1940).

These observations have led Tondury (1975) to propose that hereditary and environmental factors which affect the embryo before 23 days would produce severe lesions such as complete absence of the trachea or oesophagus, whereas later in the fourth week – as sensitivity regresses and the respiratory system has developed further – less-pronounced defects can be expected, such as the typical oesophageal atresia with distal tracheo-oesophageal fistula. After 32 days this type of foregut malformation cannot be expected at all.

3.3   Theories of embryogenesis of oesophageal atresia

While the morphology of the early development of the normal foregut in the human is well documented in general terms (Gray and Skandalakis, 1972) the disturbances which result in oesophageal atresia and tracheo-oesophageal fistula are poorly understood. Morphological descriptions often reflect the author's own impression of the mechanism of deformity (Smith, 1957; Kluth *et al.*, 1987) and there may be several interpretations of the same observation.

It should be acknowledged that interpretation of morphological features in the early embryo can be extremely difficult, as is evident by the controversy surrounding the significance of the tracheo-oesophageal septum. Although it is possible that the processes causing each anatomical variant of oesophageal atresia may be completely different, it is more likely that the same process produces a spectrum of abnormalities of which isolated tracheo-oesophageal fistula represents one end, and complete laryngo-oesophageal cleft, tracheal agenesis, or long-gap oesophageal atresia without fistula the other end.

Theories of the embryological development of tracheo-oesophageal abnormalities fall into four major groups:

1. Intraembryonic pressure
2. Epithelial occlusion
3. Differential growth
4. Vascular accident

3.3.1 INTRAEMBRYONIC PRESSURE

Pressure from an enlarged embryonic heart

The combination of embryonic cardiomegaly and marked dorsal curvature of the cervical region has been suggested as a mechanism which could compress the oesophagus and trachea against the vertebral column, producing oesophageal atresia (Schmitz, 1923). This theory does not take into account the fact that oesophageal atresia develops during a stage when the spine as such does not yet exist, and at most all a large heart could do would be to displace the oesophagus within the jelly-like consistency of the embryo. In addition, observations of oesophageal atresia in acardiac and microcardiac fetuses makes this an unlikely explanation (Smith, 1957).

Pressure from abnormal vessels

The association of oesophageal atresia with a right retro-oesophageal subclavian artery has led to speculation that persistence of the caudal portion of the right dorsal aorta may press on the developing oesophagus from behind (Fluss and Poppen, 1951). This hypothesis is not consistent with dissections of embryos with oesophageal atresia, in which the vessel is too insignificant to exert excessive pressure on the oesophagus. It would seem unlikely that the vascular anatomy is causally related to the tracheo-oesophageal abnormalities.

Pressure by the pneumatoenteric recesses

Excessive accumulation of fluid in these recesses which connect with the pericardial cavity has been suggested as a mechanism which puts excessive pressure on the foregut (Broman, 1904). However, these recesses develop too late to affect the early development of the oesophagus (Smith, 1957). As Smith has pointed out, the extremely gelatinous nature of the embryo at this early stage would appear to permit considerable displacement of developing structures such that mechanical pressure *per se* would be an unlikely cause for malformations during the embryonic stage.

Embryonic hyperflexion

In this theory oesophageal atresia and tracheo-oesophageal fistula result from abnormal differential growth of the dorsal structures during embryogenesis, causing hyperflexion of the embryo (Piekarski and Stephens, 1976). This creates disturbances in the alignment, direction and extent of the laryngo-tracheal groove and lateral endodermal ridges. To test this hypothesis chick embryos have been hyperflexed to the limit of fatal cardiac compression during the critical period of foregut development (stages 21–28) and the effect on the trachea and oesophagus examined (Kleckner *et al.*, 1984). In total, 42 chickens were evaluated and in only one was there a tracheo-oesophageal fistula, the orientation of which was the reverse of that seen in humans where the tracheal end is cranial to the oesophageal end. Again, during the critical phase of development it is difficult to imagine that the embryo is rigid enough to exert excessive pressure on any one part.

3.3.2   EPITHELIAL OCCLUSION

Failure of recannalization after physiological occlusion of the lumen of the oesophagus has been suggested as a possible cause of atresia (Kreuter, 1905). Although epithelial proliferation leads to narrowing of the oesophagus in the region just caudal to the bifurcation of the trachea between 46 and 52 days complete occlusion of the lumen does not appear to occur. Established oesophageal atresia has been observed in embryos well before this period of narrowing, and total occlusion of the lumen has never been observed. In addition, luminal obliteration does not account for the development of tracheo-oesophageal fistulae.

3.3.3   DIFFERENTIAL GROWTH THEORIES

Yamasaki (1933) was the first to suggest that oesophageal atresia could be the result of dysfunction of active cellular proliferation. He based his theory on the observation that the primitive foregut had a thin layer of cells on the dorsal side whereas there was profuse epithelium on its ventral side. He postulated that rapid growth of the trachea and pulmonary primordium consumed so much of the growth potential (the concept of 'tissue availability') that the posterior parts of the primitive foregut gained insufficient cellular material to complete oesophageal development.

Gruenwald (1940) thought that if the trachea rapidly elongated it could carry the developing oesophagus downwards so rapidly that it lost the ability to differentiate adequately as a separate structure (Figure

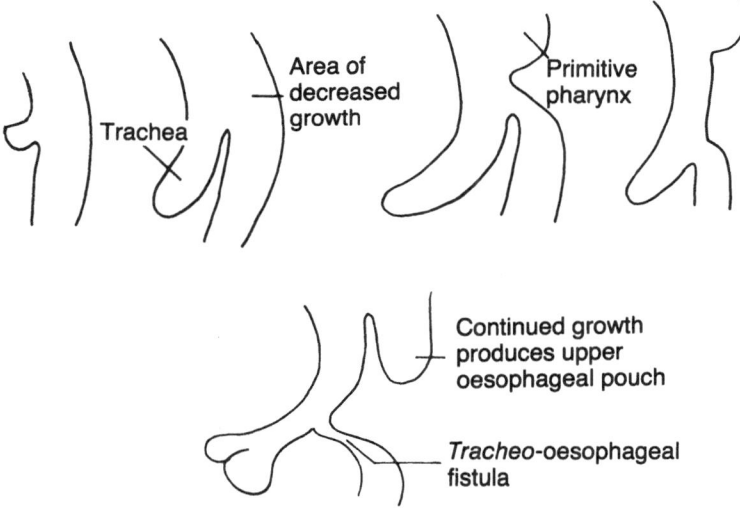

Figure 3.2   The rapid elongation of the trachea causes a 'thinning out' of the segment of oesophagus along the dorsal wall, leaving a tracheo-oesophageal communication. Continued elongation of the proximal trachea results in the fistula occupying a position near the bifurcation. The proximal oesophagus continues to grow producing an upper oesophageal pouch.

3.2). Once tracheal growth was complete the cranial segment of the oesophagus could continue to differentiate and may even make up some of the deficit and overlap the lower segment. Presence of oesophageal tissue on the dorsal wall of the trachea and of muscular bands passing between the upper segment of the oesophagus to the trachea have been cited as evidence that oesophageal tissue has been stretched thin by rapid elongation of the trachea.

Another explanation which has been proposed is that there is faulty union of the epithelial ridges which divide the foregut internally (Rosenthal, 1931). Disturbance in the direction of the separation of the trachea from the oesophagus may occur if there is excessive growth dorsally. This may divide the foregut in such a way as to produce oesophageal atresia. The epithelial ridges in the region of the lateral oesophageal grooves (Forssner, 1907; Lewis, 1912) may also play a role, although this possibility was not mentioned by Rosenthal. The grooves run in a caudal and dorsal direction immediately behind the tracheo-oesophageal ridges to the dorsal wall of the oesophagus. Their overgrowth could well result in oesophageal atresia and distal tracheo-oesophageal fistula (Figure 3.3). The importance of the epithelium of the foregut as the crucial site of

INTERNAL RIDGE OF LATERAL OESOPHAGEAL FOLD

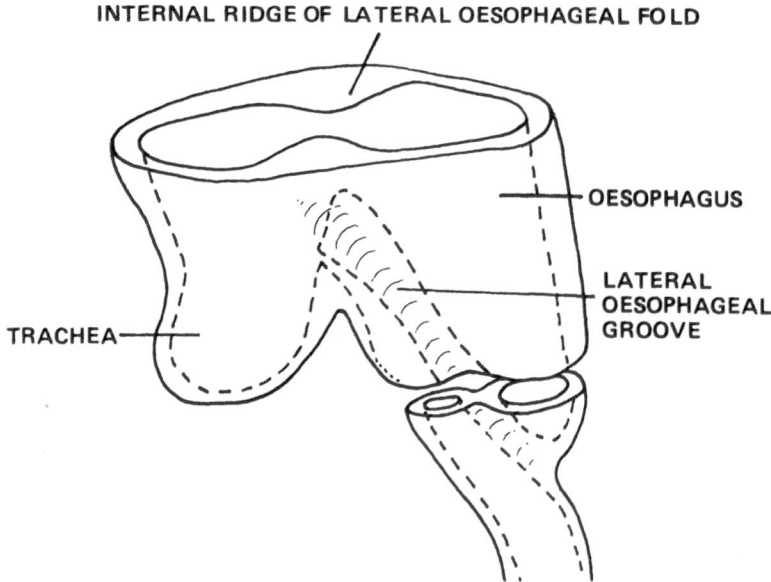

OESOPHAGUS

LATERAL
OESOPHAGEAL
GROOVE

TRACHEA

Figure 3.3 The foregut of a 4 mm human embryo. Over-development of the internal ridges of the lateral oesophageal groove would occlude the oesophagus along the line of the groove. Maintenance of a communication between the trachea and lower oesophagus (as shown by the broken line) would produce oesophageal atresia and distal tracheo-oesophageal fistula.

the primary organizational defect which determines how the trachea separates from the oesophagus seems widely accepted and has been highlighted by Smith (1957). The concept of a disturbance in the differentiation and growth pattern of the epithelial lining emanates from the apparent independence in timing of elongation of the trachea and oesophagus, bronchial branching and tracheo-oesophageal separation.

Although there is acceptance of the broad concept that oesophageal atresia may result from a disruption of the normal growth pattern of the cells surrounding the tracheo-oesophageal space, there is still no agreement as to the sequence of morphological changes which occurs. Some of the interpretatiosn proffered are described below.

Faulty development of the tracheo-oesophageal septum

In this model, the ventral trachea differentiates from the primitive foregut by a process of septation (His, 1887; Rosenthal, 1931; Gray and Skandalakis, 1972). Upward growth of the tracheo-oesophageal septum and progression of the lateral oesophageal groove separate the trachea from the oesophagus. If this growth is maldirected or deficient, tracheo-oesophageal septation will be abnormal and a variety of oesophageal and tracheal anomalies may ensue.

The tracheo-oesophageal septum has been the focus of much controversy in relation to its role in the separation of the trachea from the oesophagus. Some workers have considered it to be the key to the understanding of how oesophageal atresia develops (Rosenthal, 1931) whereas other workers have doubted that it even exists (Zwa Tun, 1982; Kluth and Habenicht, 1987). Zwa Tun could find no evidence to verify its importance, and proposed that respiratory tract development occurred by continued growth of the primitive lung bud in a caudal direction, with the implication that the so-called tracheo-oesophageal septum was the result of this development, rather than an essential prerequisite of it.

Overgrowth of lateral oesophageal ridges

Over-development of the internal ridges related to the lateral oesophageal grooves may occlude the tracheo-oesophageal space and oesophagus along the line of the grooves as they run caudally and posteriorly. If this over-development occurs excessively obliquely, the lateral oesophageal thickening may allow persistence of a communication between the trachea and lower oesophagus, producing a distal tracheo-oesophageal fistula (Figure 3.3).

Ventral displacement of the dorsal fold of foregut

This model is based on observations of the foregut in chick embryos using scanning electron microscopy (Kluth and Habenicht, 1987). Reduction in the size of the tracheo-oesophageal space has been observed but formation of a tracheo-oesophageal septum, with caudo-cranial extension, has not been demonstrated. Rather than considering the thickening of the lateral tracheo-oesophageal wall as the cranial limit of the advancing tracheo-oesophageal septum, this theory considers that the lateral oesophageal fold is just one of a number of folds which can be identified around the tracheo-oesophageal space: below the space is the tracheo-oesophageal fold (Figure 3.4), above it is the cranial fold, the primordium of the larynx, and posteriorly is the dorsal fold of the oesophagus (Figure 3.5). According to Kluth *et al.* (1987), if the dorsal fold of the foregut bends too far ventrally descent of the larynx is impaired. The tracheo-oesophageal space thus remains partially undivided and lies in a ventral position; and the ventral position causes it to differentiate into trachea (Figure 3.6). Kluth and Habenicht (1987) have used their concept to explain a variety of foregut malformations (Figure 3.7).

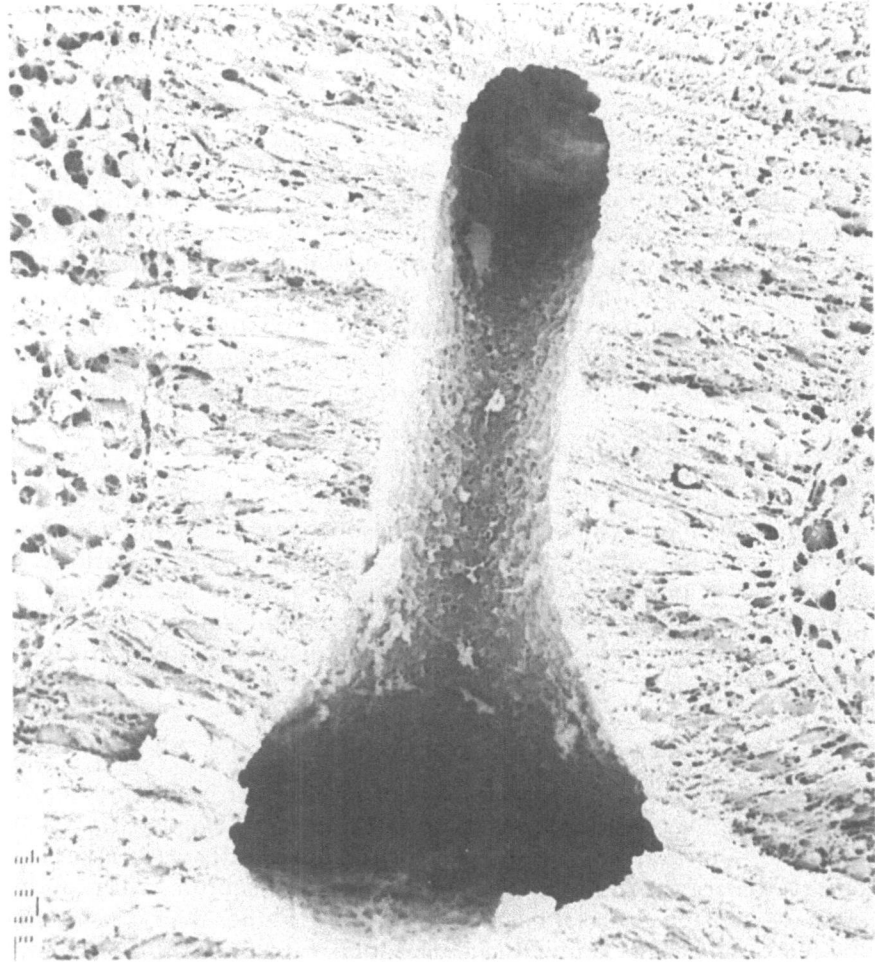

Figure 3.4 Scanning electron microscopy of the foregut of a chick embryo (approximately 84 h incubation). Transverse section through foregut showing the oesophagus (top), trachea and mainstem bronchi (bottom) separated by the tracheo-oesophageal fold. There is no sign of fusion of the lateral wall components. (Reproduced with permission from Kluth and Habenicht (1987).)

Disturbance of the mesenchymal control of differentiation

In this model, oesophageal atresia results from imbalance in longitudinal growth and septum formation (Tondury, 1975). This development is dependent on a mesenchymal factor which controls the differentiation of the tracheal mucosa anteriorly and the oesophagus posteriorly. Dis-

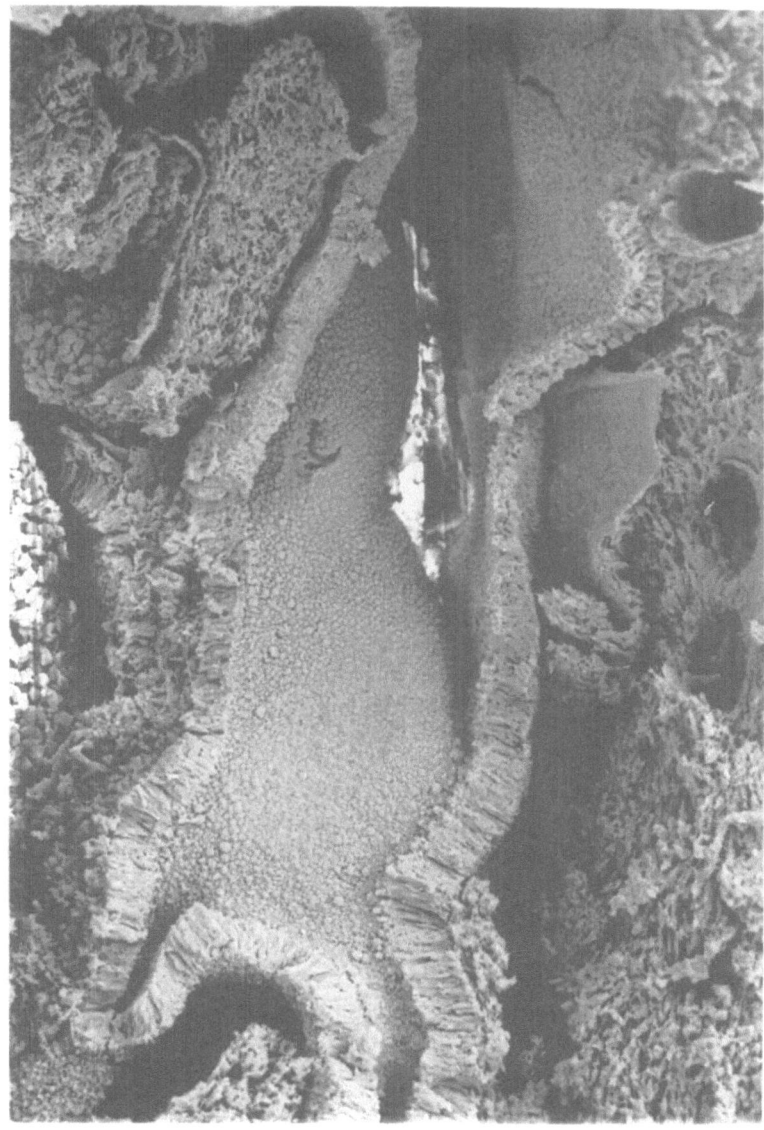

Figure 3.5 Scanning electron microscopy of a sagittal section through the foregut of a chick embryo (approximately 96 h incubation). The ventral aspect of the embryo is to the left of the photograph. The folds of the foregut approach each other reducing the size of the tracheo-oesophageal space. A dorsal fold develops and can be seen indenting the tracheo-oesophageal space from the right in the lower part of the photograph. (Reproduced with permission from Kluth and Habenicht (1987).)

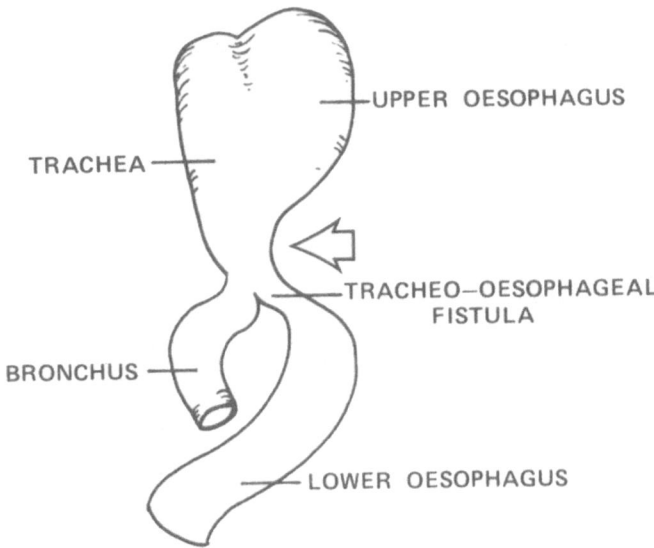

Figure 3.6 A system of folds developing in the primitive foregut reduces the size of the tracheo-oesophageal space. Kluth and Habenicht (1987) believe that excessive ventral displacement of the dorsal fold of the foregut (arrow) may cause the tracheo-oesophageal space to remain partly undivided and ventral resulting in differentiation into trachea.

turbance iñ the balance usually favours the trachea. Oesophageal atresia ensues if a disproportionately large part of the endodermal epithelium of the foregut is integrated into the trachea, and too little is reserved for the oesophagus. The similarities with the original concept proposed by Yamasaki (1933) are obvious. An isolated tracheo-oesophageal fistula may result if this disturbance is limited to a small part of the septum. The concept of disturbance of mesenchymal control of differentiation has also been used to account for regional defects in oesophageal atresia (Dickens and Myers, 1987).

The three models described above may represent different interpretations of the same process, and are not necessarily mutually exclusive. The exact mechanism of the deformity remains controversial.

3.3.4 DISTURBED BLOOD SUPPLY

Segmental bowel atresias are widely believed to be due to local disorders of microcirculation *in utero*. Interruption of the arterial circulation has been shown to cause intestinal atresia in dog fetuses (Barnard,

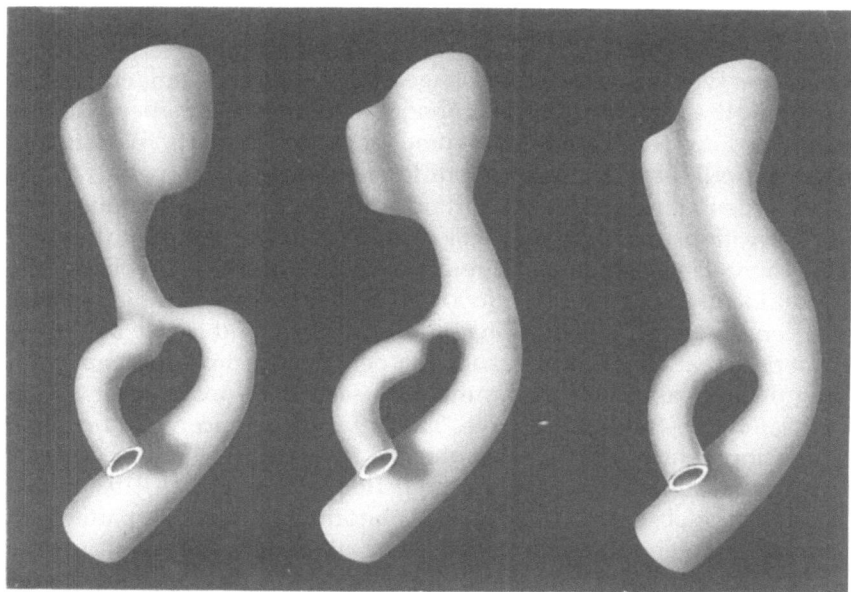

Figure 3.7   Presumed pathogenesis of foregut malformations. Left: in oesophageal atresia and distal tracheo-oesophageal fistula the dorsal fold bends too far ventrally, impeding descent of the larynx. The ventral position of the tracheo-oesophageal space causes it to differentiate into trachea. Middle: in tracheal atresia the foregut is deformed on the ventral side. Abnormal dorsal displacement of the tracheo-oesophageal space causes it to differentiate into oesophagus. Right: in laryngotracheo-oesophageal cleft there is inadequate development of the foregut folds leading to persistence of the primitive tracheo-oesophageal space. (Reproduced with permission from Kluth and Habenicht (1987).)

1956; Louw, 1966). Likewise, isolated rectal atresia can be induced in rabbit fetuses by partial or complete interruption of the blood supply (Stone and Wilkinson, 1983). Extrapolation of the results of these experiments to oesophageal atresia has encouraged the suggestion that interruption of part of the segmental arterial supply to the upper part of the thoracic oesophagus might result in isolated oesophageal atresia. However, in bowel atresias these disturbances in the vascular supply occur relatively late, whereas oesophageal atresia occurs at a much earlier stage, before the vascular structure is fully established, and at a time when the embryo is so small it is difficult to see how areas of hypoxia could occur. How this mechanism might also produce a tracheo-oesophageal fistula is not clear.

3.4   Unifying model of the development of oesophageal atresia

The factors which produce oesophageal atresia and its variants remain unknown. It seems unlikely that abnormal vessels and hyperflexion of the embryo are responsible, but some factor which alters the rate and timing of cell proliferation and differentiation in the region of the oesophagus and developing lung bud could well explain the microscopic observations made by embryologists. At the beginning of the third week there is enormous proliferative cellular activity involving the ventral side of the foregut. It is followed immediately by a rapid increase in the length of both the oesophagus and trachea, and it may be during this period that, for some reason, the oesophagus fails to keep pace, giving the appearance of a prominent dorsal fold or posterior deviation of the lateral oesophageal groove. The latter occurrence would explain the development of tracheo-oesophageal fistula as well as the appearance of tracheal remnants within the fistula (Hokama *et al.*, 1986).

Study of the observed chromosomal abnormalities and the patterns of associated congenital malformations may ultimately shed light on the basic cause and nature of the process which results in oesophageal atresia. The genetic basis for oesophageal atresia is yet to be established.

References

Barnard, C. N. (1956) The genesis of intestinal atresia. *Surg. Forum*, 7, 393–396.

Broman, I. (1904) Die Entwickelungsgeschichte der Buisa omentalis und ahnlicher Rozessbildungen bei den Wirbeltieren. Wiesbaden, 611 pp.

Dickens, D. R. V. and Myers, N. A. (1987) Oesophageal atresia and vertebral anomalies. *Pediatr. Surg. Int.*, 2, 178–281.

Fluss, S. and Poppen, K. J. (1951) Embryogenesis of tracheo-esophageal fistula and esophageal atresia. *Arch. Pathol.*, 52, 168–81.

Forssner, H. (1907) Die angeborenen Darm – und Osophagus-atresien. *Anat. Hefte*, 34, 1–163.

Gray, H. (1972) *Gray's Anatomy: Descriptive and Applied*, 34th edn. (eds D. V. Davies and R. E. Coupland), Longmans, London, p. 236.

Gray, S. W. and Skandalakis, J. E. (1972) *Embryology for Surgeons*, W. H. Saunders, Philadelphia, pp. 63–100.

Gruenwald, P. (1940) A case of atresia of the esophagus combined with tracheoesophageal fistula in a 9 mm human embryo, and its embryological explanation. *Anat. Rec.*, 78, 293–302.

His, W. (1887) Zur Bildungsgeschichte der Lungen beim menschlichen Embryo. *Arch. Anat.*, 89–106.

Hokama, A., Myers, N. A., Kent, M. *et al.* (1986) Esophageal atresia with tracheo-oesophageal fistula: a histopathological study. *Pediatr. Surg. Int.*, 1, 117–21.

Kleckner, S. C., Pringle, K. C. and Clark, E. B. (1984) The effect of chick embryo hyperflexion on tracheoesophageal development. *J. Pediatr. Surg.,* 19, 340–4.

Kluth, D. (1976) Atlas of esophageal atresia. *J. Pediatr. Surg.,* 11, 901–19.

Kluth, D. and Habenicht, R. (1987) The embryology of usual and unusual types of esophageal atresia. *Pediatr. Surg. Int.,* 2, 223–7.

Kluth, D., Steding, G. and Seidl, W. (1987) The embryology of foregut malformations. *J. Pediatr. Surg.,* 22, 389–93.

Kreuter, E. (1905) Die angeborenen Verschliessungen und Verengungen des Darmkanals im Lichte der Entwicklungsgeschichte. *Dtsch. Z. Chir.,* 79, 1–89.

Lewis, F. T. (1912) The development of the oesophagus. in *Manual of Human Embryology,* Vol. 2(17), (eds Keibel and Mall), Philadelphia, pp. 355–68.

Louw, J. H. (1966) Jejunal atresias and stenosis. *J. Pediatr. Surg.,* 1, 8–23.

Piekarski, D. H. and Stephens, F. D. (1976) The association and embryogenesis of tracheo-oesophageal and anorectal anomalies. in *Anorectal Malformations and Associated Diseases, Progress in Pediatric Surgery,* Vol. 9 (eds P. P. Rickham, W. C. Hecker and J. Prevot), Baltimore, University Park Press, pp. 63–76.

Pringle, K. C. (1983) Pathology of esophageal atresia with tracheo-esophageal fistula. Presented at 16th Annual Meeting of Pacific Association of Pediatric Surgeons, Fukuoka, Japan.

Rosenthal, A. H. (1931) Congenital atresia of the esophagus with tracheo-esophageal fistula: report of eight cases. *Arch. Pathol.,* 12, 756–72.

Schmitz, J. A. (1923) Ueber die formale Genese der Oesophagus-missbildungen. *Virchow's Arch. Pathol. Anat. Physiol.,* 247, 278–93.

Smith, E. I. (1957) The early development of the trachea and the esophagus in relation to atresia of the esophagus and tracheoesophageal fistula. *Contrib. Embryol. Carnegie Institution of Washington,* 36, 41–57.

Stone, H. H. and Wilkinson, A. W. (1983) Experimental production of rectal stenosis and atresia in the rabbit. *J. Pediatr. Surg.,* 18, 89–90.

Tondury, G. (1975) Zur Pathogenese der Oesophagus-tresie. *Z. Kinderchir.,* 16, 118–33.

Wailoo, M. P. and Emery, J. L. (1979) The trachea in children with tracheo-oesophageal fistula. *Histopathology,* 3, 329–38.

Yamasaki, M. (1933) Ein menschlicher Embryo von 8.5 mm Scheitel-Steisslange mit fehlerhaften und ungewohnlichen Bildungen. Arb. aus dem Anat. Inst. d. Kaiserlich-Japanischen Universitat 2. Sendai 15, 27–59.

Ysander, F. (1925) Human diplo-terata. Inaugural dissertation. Uppsala. Quoted by I. Smith.

Zwa Tun Ha (1982) The tracheo-esophageal septum – fact or fantasy? *Acta Anat.,* 114, 1–21.

4 Anatomy

S. W. BEASLEY

4.1 The oesophagus

The oesophagus is a muscular tube which commences at the lower end of the pharynx at the level of the cricoid cartilage and traverses the mediastinum before entering the stomach at the cardia. The cervical portion lies in front of the prevertebral fascia immediately behind the trachea. In the superior mediastinum it remains in contact with the posterior aspect of the trachea. At a lower level, it is situated slightly to the left of the midline behind the left bronchus, which is occasionally seen to indent it on a barium swallow. The oesophagus inclines forward as it descends, losing its contact with the vertebral column to pass in front of the descending aorta. It pierces the diaphragm opposite the tenth thoracic vertebra to enter the abdomen where its anterior surface becomes invested with peritoneum.

4.1.1 STRUCTURE

The empty oesophagus has a stellate appearance in cross-section with the transverse diameter greater than the anteroposterior diameter (Figure 4.1). The deep longitudinal folds of the mucosa (which give the lumen a stellate appearance) and the laxity of the subjacent submucosa enable the lumen to distend dramatically when accepting a bolus of food. The thick mucosal layer is of the stratified squamous type and contains superficial oesophageal glands. The highly vascular submucosa which lies external to the lamina propria and muscularis mucosae contains deep mucous glands, the inner nerve plexus and multiple lymph follicles. The mucosa is loosely bound and is surrounded by two layers of muscle: the inner circular layer which is continuous with the inferior constrictor muscle of the pharynx at its upper end, and with the oblique fibres of the stomach at its lower end; and the outer longitudinal layer. The longitudinal fibres arise as a short tendon from the dorsal

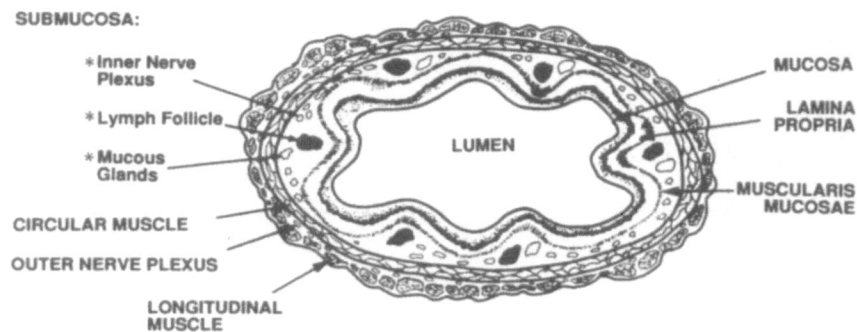

SUBMUCOSA:

* Inner Nerve Plexus

* Lymph Follicle

* Mucous Glands

CIRCULAR MUSCLE

OUTER NERVE PLEXUS

LONGITUDINAL MUSCLE

LUMEN

MUCOSA

LAMINA PROPRIA

MUSCULARIS MUCOSAE

Figure 4.1 Cross-section through the oesophagus showing its stellate lumen. When empty, the lumen is broadest in the coronal plane. Note that there is no serosal layer external to the longitudinal muscle layer.

aspect of the cricoid cartilage. As they diverge to invest the oesophagus they leave a small V-shaped deficiency posteriorly, exposing the inner circular muscle fibres. The upper third of the oesophageal muscle is striated whereas the lower two-thirds is smooth. External to the longitudinal muscle is a relatively thin and loose layer of adventitia which contains no mesothelial covering. The surgical significance of this is that there is no layer which can effectively seal off the oesophagus following perforation (Amoury, 1986).

4.1.2 RELATIONS OF THE OESOPHAGUS

The cervical oesophagus

The cervical oesophagus lies in front of the prevertebral fascia, and behind the trachea. In the lower part of the neck the oesophagus deviates slightly to the left, making it slightly more accessible from the left when a surgical approach to this region is required. On the other hand, the thoracic duct is vulnerable during a left cervical approach. The recurrent laryngeal nerves run in the groove between the trachea and oesophagus and are closely related to both structures. The lateral lobes of the thyroid are anterolateral to the upper oesophagus and lateral to these are the carotid sheaths containing the carotid arteries, internal jugular veins and vagus nerves (Figure 4.2).

The thoracic portion

During its descent through the thorax the oesophagus lies in the posterior mediastinum where it has the trachea and heart in front and the thoracic vertebrae behind. During inspiration the oesophagus may

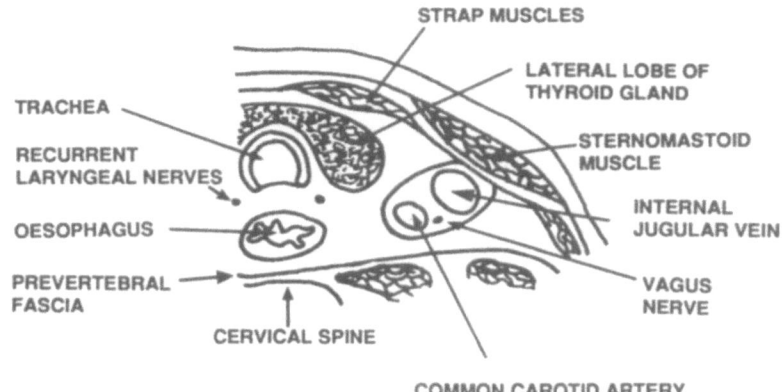

Figure 4.2 Cross-section through the lower neck to show the anatomical relationships of the cervical oesophagus.

move forward in its lower part allowing the pleura and medial portions of the lung to extend between it and the vertebral column.

In the left hemithorax the arch of the aorta passes dorsally to the left of the oesophagus and may indent the oesophagus. The descending aorta lies behind and to the left of the thoracic oesophagus. The left main bronchus, as it crosses the front of the oesophagus, may also indent it slightly.

On the right side the azygos vein crosses the oesophagus. During a right thoracic approach in oesophageal atresia this vein will usually be divided. For much of its length, the thoracic oesophagus is in contact with the pleura, but nowhere is it actually attached to the pleura (Last, 1978). During extrapleural dissection of the pleura the sympathetic chain and splanchnic nerves are clearly evident (Figure 4.3).

The vagus nerves can be seen coursing downwards and posteriorly from the groove between the trachea and upper oesophagus to run over the surface of the lower oesophageal segment before dividing into a plexus. At the lower end of the oesophagus the fibres of the plexus reunite to form the right vagus which runs behind the oesophagus and the left vagus which runs in front of it.

The abdominal portion

The part of the oesophagus which lies below the diaphragm is known as the abdominal portion. It pierces the diaphragm at the oesophageal hiatus opposite the tenth thoracic vertebra. The hiatus is formed mainly by the decussating fibres of the right crus although fibres of the left crus may also contribute. The crural fibres arise from the second, third and

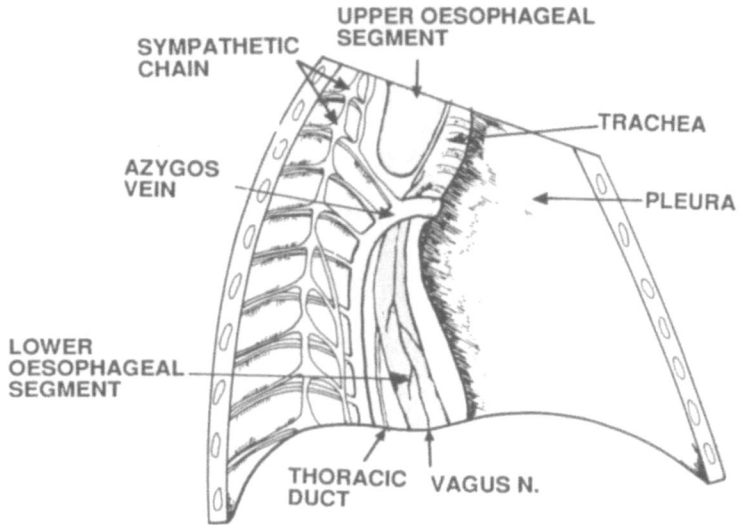

SYMPATHETIC CHAIN

UPPER OESOPHAGEAL SEGMENT

TRACHEA

AZYGOS VEIN

PLEURA

LOWER OESOPHAGEAL SEGMENT

THORACIC DUCT   VAGUS N.

Figure 4.3 The right hemithorax: the view of the posterior mediastinum as seen during an extrapleural approach to the oesophagus in oesophageal atresia (Modified from Amoury (1986)).

fourth lumbar vertebral bodies and insert in the central tendon of the diaphragm. Connective tissue which supports the oesophagus within the hiatus (the phreno-oesophageal ligament) is confined by the parietal pleura above and the peritoneum below. The abdominal oesophagus is short, but may be important in preventing gastro-oesophageal reflux.

4.1.3 INNERVATION OF THE OESOPHAGUS

The oesophagus is innervated by the autonomic nervous system. Its sympathetic supply arises from preganglionic neurons in the thoracic and upper lumbar spinal cord; the postganglionic fibres enter the oesophageal plexus by visceral branches of the sympathetic trunks and by branches of the greater splanchnic nerves (Gardner *et al.*, 1975). There is no information on whether the sympathetic supply of the oesophagus in oesophageal atresia is significantly different from that of the normal oesophagus.

The parasympathetic neurons are located in the nuclei of the vagus, with preganglionic fibres passing with the vagus nerves. In the oesophageal wall they synapse with short postganglionic neurons situated in the intramural myenteric and submucosal plexuses. These innervate the smooth muscle and secretory cells. There is some indirect evidence that the parasympathetic supply is abnormal in oesophageal atresia, result-

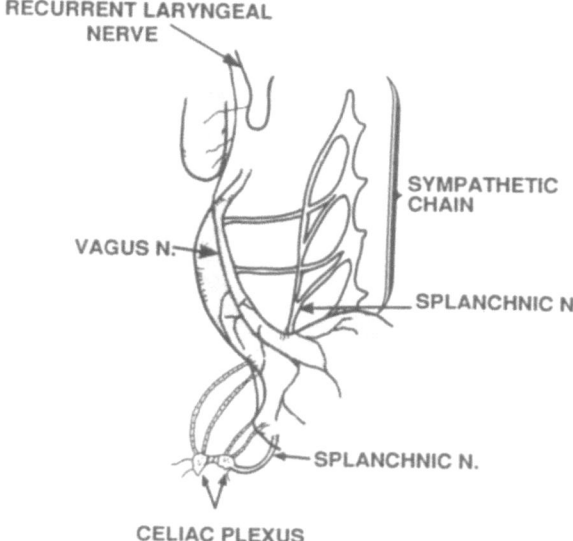

RECURRENT LARYNGEAL
NERVE

SYMPATHETIC
CHAIN

VAGUS N.

SPLANCHNIC N.

SPLANCHNIC N.

CELIAC PLEXUS

Figure 4.4 The autonomic supply of the oesophagus, as it is presumed to exist in oesophageal atresia (Modified from Amoury (1986)).

ing in dysmotility of the lower oesophageal segment (Chapter 5). In addition to this, the vagal fibres are vulnerable during dissection and mobilization of the oesophagus at the time of surgical repair. This may contribute further to abnormalities of oesophageal function in repaired oesophageal atresia. Figure 4.4 illustrates the presumed arrangement of the autonomic supply to the oesophagus in oesophageal atresia.

4.1.4 VASCULAR SUPPLY OF THE OESOPHAGUS

The cervical portion of the oesophagus is supplied by the inferior thyroid artery, a branch of the thyrocervical trunk (Last, 1978). The inferior thyroid artery gives off oesophageal and tracheal branches which run vertically downwards on their respective structures as far as the arch of the aorta in the superior mediastinum where they may anastomose with oesophageal branches from the aorta and bronchial arteries (Figure 4.5). It is these vessels which supply the upper oesophageal segment in oesophageal atresia.

The remainder of the thoracic portion of the oesophagus (i.e. from below the tracheal bifurcation) is normally supplied entirely by segmental oesophageal branches from the aorta, which are of relatively small calibre. These form a rich anastomosis with adjacent vessels as well as

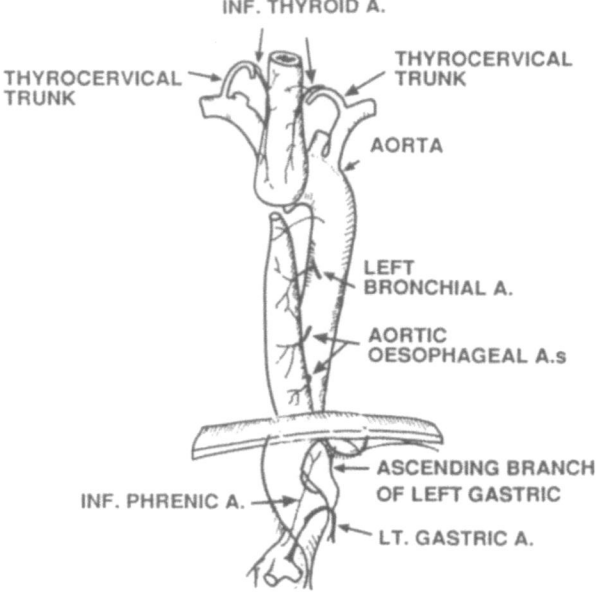

INF. THYROID A.

THYROCERVICAL TRUNK

THYROCERVICAL TRUNK

AORTA

LEFT BRONCHIAL A.

AORTIC OESOPHAGEAL A.s

ASCENDING BRANCH OF LEFT GASTRIC

INF. PHRENIC A.

LT. GASTRIC A.

Figure 4.5   The arterial supply of the oesphagus in oesophageal atresia (Modified from Amoury (1986)).

with branches from intercostal and bronchial arteries. In oesophageal atresia without fistula this part of the oesophagus is often missing and the vessels do not exist. In oesophageal atresia with a distal fistula these vessels supply the upper part of the distal oesophagus. The lower part of the distal oesophagus is supplied by the ascending branch of the left gastric artery with some support from the inferior phrenic artery (Figure 4.5). In oesophageal atresia this supply is no different from that of the normal oesophagus (Lister, 1964).

Surgical implications

The surgical significance of the vascular anatomy in oesophageal atresia is that the cervical and abdominal portions of the oesophagus are supplied richly by vessels which run along the oesophagus, whereas the thoracic portion is supplied segmentally, and has the most tenuous blood supply (Lister, 1964). Excessive mobilization of the thoracic oesophagus, therefore, may render it ischaemic. In many patients with oesophageal atresia it is possible to avoid oesophageal mobilization completely. In others (for example, oesophageal atresia without a tracheo-oesophageal fistula) an oesophageal anastomosis may only be achievable after extensive mobilization of both oesophageal segments.

Knowledge of the vascular anatomy of the oesophagus enables the surgeon to be confident in dealing with mobilization of the upper pouch: this mobilization can be extensive and continued well up into the neck with little risk of devascularization because the arterial supply from the inferior thyroid artery remains intact (Beasley, 1991). On the other hand, excessive mobilization of the lower oesophagus, by disrupting its segmental supply, may devascularize it and therefore should be limited. In short, where the gap between the oesophageal ends necessitates oesophageal mobilization, full mobilization of the upper segment should be performed first, and the lower segment mobilized only as much as is required to achieve an end-to-end anastomosis. Circular and spiral myotomies may further compromise the blood supply to the upper segment.

4.2 The oesophagus in oesophageal atresia

4.2.1 UPPER OESOPHAGEAL SEGMENT

In the fetus, swallowing begins at about 14 weeks' gestation, and by the end of pregnancy, several hundred millilitres of amniotic fluid are swallowed each day. In oesophageal atresia the fluid cannot be swallowed, and the upper pouch becomes dilated and relatively thick-walled. This hypertrophy is obvious at operation.

The length of the upper pouch is variable. In most infants with oesophageal atresia it extends to about the level of the arch of the azygos vein. Its length can be estimated preoperatively by the length of tube that can be introduced through the mouth into the oesophagus (taking into account the size of the infant) and is often evident on plain X-ray. At operation the lower limit of the upper pouch is readily identified when the anaesthetist introduces a stiff catheter into the oesophagus.

4.2.2 LOWER OESOPHAGEAL SEGMENT

In the usual type of oesophageal atresia, the lower oesophageal segment arises from the posterior wall of the trachea. Tracheal elements may persist for a variable length (Hokama *et al.*, 1986) but these are not evident at operation. The lower oesophageal segment has a smaller calibre than the blind upper pouch, and may be seen to expand with air during assisted ventilation. Recognition of vagal fibres coursing over its surface assist in its identification at operation.

4.3   The trachea

The trachea commences below the cricoid cartilage at the level of the lower border of the sixth cervical vertebra (Last, 1978). The exact anatomical level of its bifurcation into the two main bronchi is dependent on the phase of respiration, but is at or below the lower border of the manubrium (T4). The wall of the trachea is a fibro-elastic membrane supported by C-shaped rings of hyaline cartilage. The defect posteriorly is reinforced by unstriated trachealis muscle, contraction of which reduces the cross-sectional area of the lumen. The trachea is lined with ciliated respiratory epithelium.

4.3.1   TRACHEOMALACIA

In oesophageal atresia the trachea is rarely normal. There is almost always some degree of tracheomalacia, with deficiency in the amount of cartilage and an increase in the length of the transverse muscle of the posterior tracheal wall (Wailoo and Emery, 1979). The cartilage is shorter than normal and fails to give adequate support to the tracheal wall which has a perimeter greater than normal. A more comprehensive description of tracheomalacia is given in Chapter 22.

4.3.2   TRACHEO-OESOPHAGEAL FISTULAE

In most patients with oesophageal atresia, there is a fistulous connection between the posterior wall of the trachea and the distal oesophageal segment. In others there may be a connection with the upper oesophagus (Chapter 11), or rarely multiple fistulae. In isolated tracheo-oesophageal fistula ('H' fistula) the communication runs obliquely, arising from the trachea at a higher level than its entry into the oesophagus (Chapter 13).

4.4   Unusual types of congenital tracheo-oesophageal abnormality

Although over 80% of patients have oesophageal atresia and distal tracheo-oesophageal fistula, there is an enormous range of anatomical variations in congenital tracheo-oesophageal abnormalities. These have been described in detail by Kluth (1976) in his atlas of oesophageal atresia. Although he described 96 variants, there may be subtle differences within each subgroup and some cases do not fall readily into any subgroup (Burren and Beasley, 1990). Some knowledge of the range of abnormalities which may occur may assist the surgeon in the recognition of unusual variations when they are encountered at the time of thoracotomy.

4.4.1 VOGT CLASSIFICATION

The observation that the type of oesophageal atresia and tracheo-oesophageal fistula influenced management encouraged the development of classification systems to enable easy identification of each anatomical variant. A widely used classification has been that proposed by Vogt (1929) (Figure 4.6), but confusion with other classifications using letters or numbers or both, and difficulties in its application to unusual variants, have gradually led to its abandonment in favour of descriptive terms. For example, the Vogt type 2 anomaly is now described as oesophageal atresia without a tracheo-oesophageal fistula.

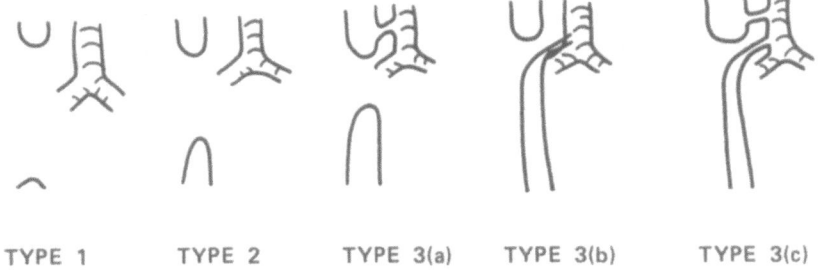

TYPE 1   TYPE 2   TYPE 3(a)   TYPE 3(b)   TYPE 3(c)

Figure 4.6   The Vogt classification of oesophageal atresia.

4.4.2 GROSS CLASSIFICATION

Gross (1953), likewise, classified oesophageal atresia into its main types (Figure 4.7). Again, inability to fit rare variations into the classification has limited its usefulness, although many surgeons still refer to it.

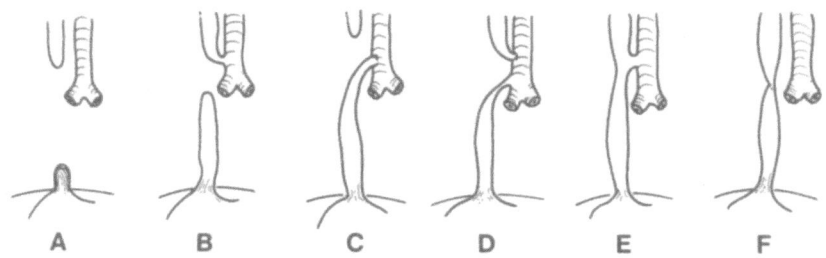

A   B   C   D   E   F

Figure 4.7   The Gross classification of oesophageal atresia.

4.4.3 KLUTH CLASSIFICATION

In 1976 Kluth attempted to document and classify every type of oesophageal atresia reported. His classification has been summarized here into the 10 major types he recognized. It should be noted that the classification encompasses all tracheo-oesophageal abnormalities, including isolated tracheal abnormalities. The classification is useful in highlighting the enormous variations which may occur, but its complexity will limit its acceptance. It has been included to facilitate description of the less common varieties of oesophageal atresia.

Type I. Oesophageal atresia in which a distal oesophagus cannot be demonstrated as a hollow viscus above the diaphragm (7 subtypes) (Figure 4.8).

Type II. All cases of oesophageal atresia in which there are proximal and distal segments without a fistula (5 subtypes) (Figure 4.9).

Type IIIa. Atresia of the oesophagus with tracheo-oesophageal fistula(e) of the proximal segment only (3 subtypes) (Figure 4.10).

Type IIIb. Oesophageal atresia with tracheo-oesophageal fistula(e) of the distal segment only (20 subtypes) (Figure 4.11).

Type IIIc. Atresia of the oesophagus with tracheo-oesophageal fistulae from the proximal and distal segments (5 subtypes) (Figure 4.12).

Type IV. The oesophagus demonstrates external continuity but its lumen is divided into a proximal and a distal segment by a transverse or oblique membrane (membranous atresia) (7 subtypes). There may or may not be an associated tracheo-oesophageal fistula (Figure 4.13).

Type V. Complete and partial duplication of the oesophagus, or atresia with intramural duplication. In addition to the patent oesophagus, there is a second one of variable length in communication with the main oesophageal lumen or the stomach. Atresia with intramural duplication is morphologically similar to atresia by membrane, but the dividing wall between the segments also contains a layer of muscularis (7 subtypes).

Type VI. Oesophagobronchial communications (12 subtypes). A fistula from the oesophagus reaches a main bronchus or a secondary bronchus. It may also communicate with an intra- or extralobar pulmonary seques-

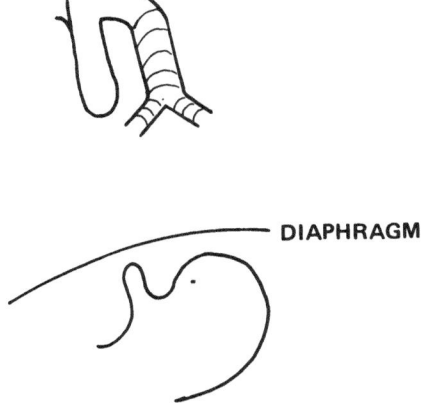

DIAPHRAGM

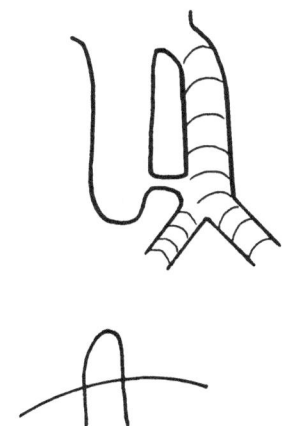

Figure 4.8   Type I anomalies.

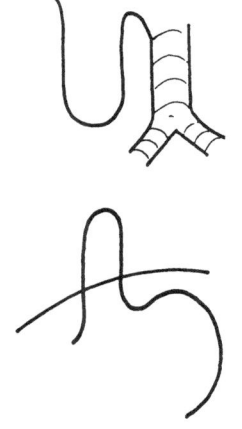

Figure 4.9   Type II anomalies.

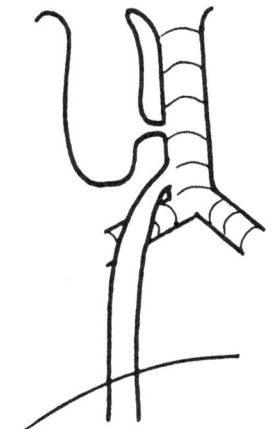

Figure 4.10   Type IIIa anomalies.

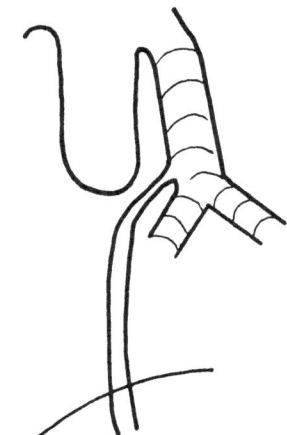

Figure 4.11   Type IIIb anomalies.

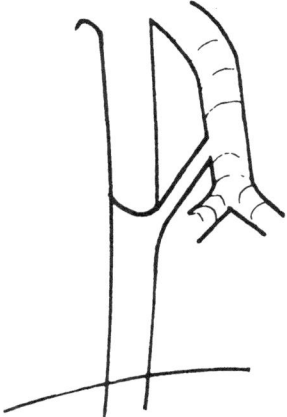

Figure 4.12   Type IIIc anomalies.

Figure 4.13   Type IV anomalies :
oesophageal membrane.

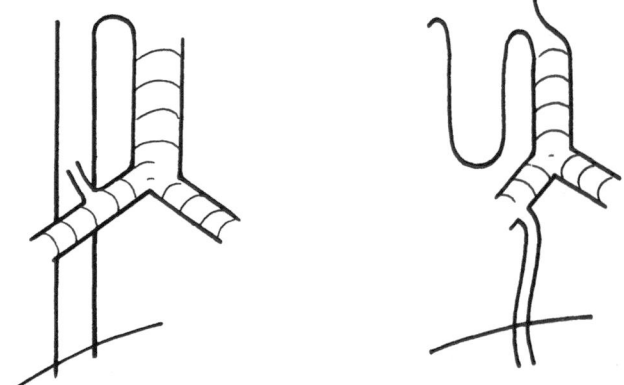

Figure 4.14   Type VI anomalies : oesophagobronchial communications.

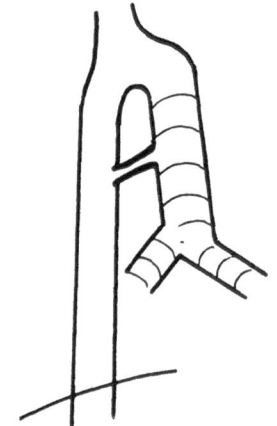

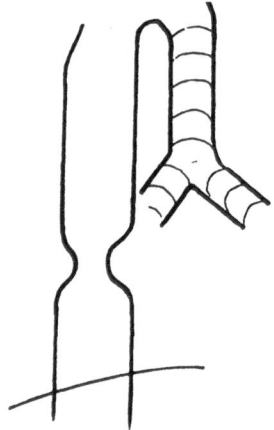

Figure 4.15   Type VII anomalies:
the 'H' fistulae.

Figure 4.16   Type VIII anomalies:
oesophageal stenoses.

tration. It may even replace a main bronchus. Alternatively, the distal oesophagus commences from the bronchus (Figure 4.14).

Type VII. 'H' fistula. A fistula runs between the oesophagus and trachea in the absence of oesophageal atresia (7 subtypes) (Figure 4.15).

Type VIII. Oesophageal stenoses. Congenital narrowing of the oesophageal lumen (7 subtypes) (Figure 4.16).

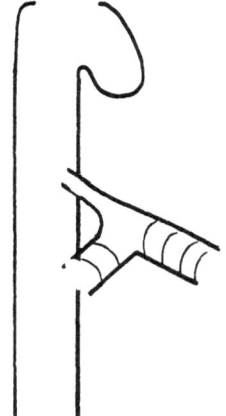
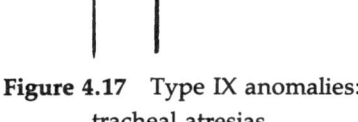
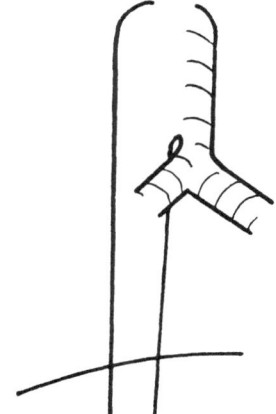

Figure 4.17 Type IX anomalies: **Figure 4.18** Type X anomalies:
tracheal atresias. ·fissure formation.

Type IX. Tracheal atresias. Agenesis or atresia of the trachea combined with tracheo-oesophageal fistula (4 subtypes) (Figure 4.17).

Type X. Fissure formation. Laryngeal fissure, sometimes in association with oesophageal atresia or lower tracheo-oesophageal fistulae (12 subtypes) (Figure 4.18).

There is little doubt that as further unusual cases are reported, the number of subgroups will expand. It behoves the surgeon to be cognizant of the possibility of variations in anatomy during thoracotomy for repair of oesophageal atresia.

References

Amoury, R. A. (1986) Structure and function of the esophagus in infancy and early childhood. in *Paediatric Esophageal Surgery* (ed. K. W. Ashcraft and T. M. Holder), Grune & Stratton, Orlando, pp. 1–29.

Beasley, S. W. (1991) Influence of anatomy and physiology on the management of oesophageal atresia. *Prog. Pediatr. Surg.*, **27** (in press).

Burren, C. P. and Beasley, S. W. (1990) Oesophageal septum and intramural distal tracheo-oesophageal fistula. *Pediatr. Surg. Int.*, **5**, 198–9.

Gardner, E., Gray, D. J. and O'Rahilly, R. (1975) *Anatomy*, 4th edn, W. B. Saunders, Philadelphia, pp. 280–1.

Gross, R. E. (1953) *Surgery of Infancy and Childhood*, W. B. Saunders, Philadelphia, p. 76.

Hokama, R., Myers, N. A., Kent, M. *et al.* (1986) Esophageal atresia with tracheo-esophageal fistula: a histopathological study. *Pediatr. Surg. Int.*, **1**, 117–21.

Kluth, D. (1976) Atlas of esophageal atresia. *J. Pediatr. Surg.*, **11**, 901–19.

Last, R. J. (1978) *Anatomy: Regional and Applied*, 6th edn, Churchill Livingstone, Edinburgh, pp. 224–8, 238–40.

Lister, J. (1964) The blood supply to the oesophagus in relation to oesophageal atresia. *Arch. Dis. Child.*, **39**, 131–7.

Vogt, E. C. (1929) Congenital esophageal atresia. *Am. J. Roentgenol.*, **22**, 463–5.

Wailoo, M. P. and Emery, J. L. (1979) The trachea in children with tracheo-oesophageal fistula. *Histopathology*, **3**, 329–38.

5 Pathophysiology

K. B. STOKES

Following repair of oesophageal atresia, function of the oesophagus rarely attains complete normality. The suboptimal function is in part because of inherent abnormalities of the oesophagus, its sphincters and its motility, and in part results from the surgery required to correct the atresia.

5.1 Normal physiology of the oesophagus

Organized oesophageal function begins *in utero* with fetal ingestion of amniotic fluid during the fourth month of gestation. Later, approximately 450 ml (about half the total volume of amniotic fluid) is swallowed each 24 hours (Pritchard, 1965).

Following birth, sucking with reflex swallowing is required and this is a well-developed function in the term infant. However, in the premature child, sucking and swallowing may be less well co-ordinated: there may be delay in opening of the cricoid sphincter, and oesophageal peristalsis may not be well organized (Gryboski, 1965, 1969).

Discussion of the normal physiology of the oesophagus involves consideration of the function of the two sphincters, one at each end of the oesophagus, together with the motility of the oesophagus itself.

5.1.1 PHARYNGO-OESOPHAGEAL SPHINCTER

The exact anatomical basis of this sphincter remains uncertain, although the cricopharyngeus appears to constitute its main element. The sphincter is identifiable on manometry as a zone of elevated pressure extending for a distance of 2.5–4.5 cm in the adult. The maximal resting pressure is 15–45 mmHg (Carre, 1987).

Once a bolus of food is swallowed, it is propelled by a high pressure wave created by the pharyngeal constrictor muscles. Before this wave reaches the pharyngo-oesophageal sphincter, it relaxes and pressure within the sphincteric zone drops abruptly, allowing unimpeded passage of the bolus. With the arrival of the pharyngeal pressure wave, the sphincter then closes and the pressure within it rises to 45–90 mmHg (twice the normal resting pressure). This high pressure prevents regurgitation of oesophageal contents into the pharynx and airway.

Following passage of the bolus well into the oesophagus, the pharyngo-oesophageal sphincter pressure returns to resting levels.

5.1.2 OESOPHAGEAL PERISTALSIS

At rest, the oesophagus is collapsed. Its intraluminal pressure is similar to the intrapleural pressure, ranging between 3 and 8 mmHg below atmospheric pressure.

Primary peristaltic wave

The food bolus is propelled along the oesophagus by a primary peristaltic wave which is the continuation of the propulsive pharyngeal wave. The primary peristaltic wave creates a pressure of 30–100 mmHg, moving at a speed of 2–4 cm/s. This wave corresponds to a 4–8 cm length of contracted oesophagus. The typical pattern of an oesophageal swallowing complex showing the primary peristaltic wave is illustrated in Figure 5.1 (Carre, 1987).

The primary wave occurs in response to efferent vagal impulses which are conveyed sequentially to progressively more distal areas of oesophageal wall. Provided the vagus nerves are intact, transverse section of the oesophagus does not impede the progress of the peristaltic wave across the gap into the distal oesophagus (Carveth *et al.*, 1962; Haller *et al.*, 1966). Primary waves are abolished by high bilateral vagotomy (Carveth *et al.*, 1962).

Secondary propulsive waves

Secondary propulsive waves reinforce the primary waves and are of similar speed and amplitude. These waves originate in the oesophagus below the pharyngo-oesophageal sphincter and are reflexly initiated by oesophageal distension caused by the food bolus. The neural mechanism of primary and secondary waves is identical.

Tertiary waves

Tertiary waves are also recorded but these are nonpropulsive.

Function during the first month of life

Pressure tracings of the pharynx and pharyngo-oesophageal sphincter, and from the body of the oesophagus in infants over the age of one

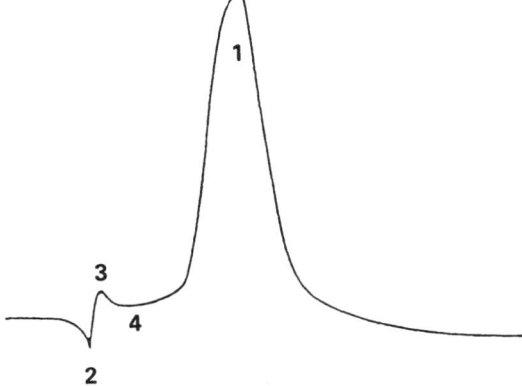

Figure 5.1 A typical oesophageal swallowing complex showing the primary peristaltic wave (1) preceded by a negative (2) and two positive deflections (3, 4). (Modified from Carre, 1987.)

month, are identical in pattern and magnitude to those recorded in adults (Colley and Creamer, 1958). Hollwarth (1979) reported poorer propulsive peristalsis in the oesophagus during the first month of life. For the first ten days of life, only approximately 60% of induced swallows are followed by normal propulsive contractions. During the first month of life the rate increases to 80%, which is within the normal range. Disordered motor co-ordination of oesophageal and sphincteric function may be encountered in the healthy newborn infant and have spontaneously resolved by one month of age.

In addition, inco-ordinate peristaltic activity has been recorded in newborn premature infants and this corresponds to the period when an immature suck–swallow pattern is also recognized.

5.1.3 THE GASTRO-OESOPHAGEAL SPHINCTER

Literature on this sphincter is vast and controversial, and there is on-going debate as to which factors contribute to the prevention of reflux of gastric contents into the lower oesophagus. The anatomy of the gastro-oesophageal region in relation to radiological and manometric observations is shown in Figure 5.2.

Forces predisposing to gastro-oesophageal reflux

The effective force predisposing to gastro-oesophageal reflux is represented by the excess of intragastric pressure over intra-oesophageal pressure. These forces, as studied by Marchand (1957) and Botha (1962), are summarized in Table 5.1.

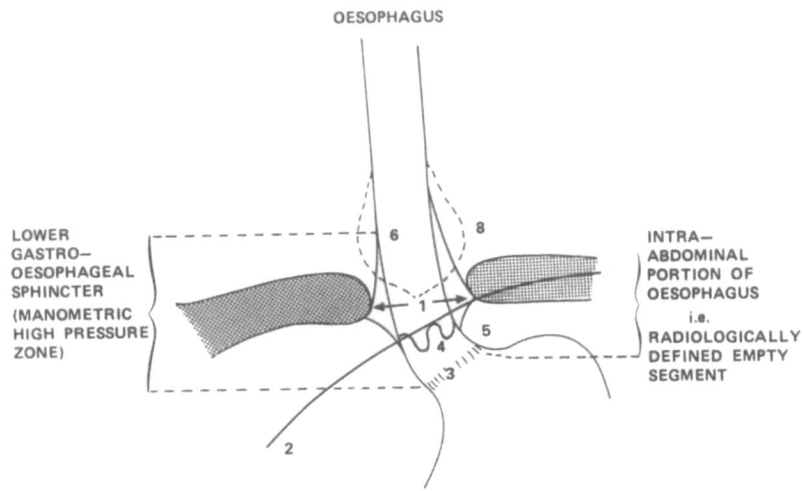

OESOPHAGUS

LOWER
GASTRO—
OESOPHAGEAL
SPHINCTER
(MANOMETRIC
HIGH PRESSURE
ZONE)

INTRA—
ABDOMINAL
PORTION OF
OESOPHAGUS
i.e.
RADIOLOGICALLY
DEFINED EMPTY
SEGMENT

Figure 5.2 Diagrammatic representation of gastro-oesophageal region. (1) Hiatus formed by diaphragmatic crura. (2) Position of diaphragm as portrayed by conventional radiography. (3) Site of gastro-oesophageal junction. (4) Irregular interdigitating junction of squamous and junctional columnar epithelium (Z line). (5) Cardia incisura. (6) Upper limit of attachment of phreno-oesophageal membrane. (7) Epiphrenic ampulla. (Modified from Carre, 1987.)

Table 5.1 Forces predisposing to gastro-oesophageal reflux during quiet respiration

	End of Expiration (mmHg)	End of Inspiration (mmHg)
Supin position		
Intra-oesophageal pressure	− 3	− 8
Intragastric pressure	+ 2	+ 7
Gradient across diaphragm	5	15
Upright position		
Intra-oesophageal pressure	− 3	− 8
Intragastric pressure	− 2	+ 2
Gradient across diaphragm	1	10

Straining, coughing and sneezing produces considerable elevation in intra-abdominal pressure causing the intragastric pressure to rise to + 40− + 60 mmHg. During the Valsalva manoeuvre, intragastric pressure may reach +85 mmHg. However, there is a concomitant elevation in intrathoracic pressure to between +30 and +60 mmHg, with the resultant gastro-oesophageal differential not exceeding 25 mmHg. The greatest transdiaphragmatic pressure differential is created by deep inspiration during which intrathoracic pressure becomes increasingly negative and intra-abdominal pressure becomes increasingly positive. During deep inspiration the pressure gradient may exceed 75 mmHg.

There are three principal mechanisms which have been invoked to explain competence at the gastro-oesophageal junction:

1. Compression of the lower oesophagus by the diaphragmatic crura
2. Valvular mechanisms
   (a) Mucosal valve
   (b) Flap valve
3. Intrinsic gastro-oesophageal sphincter

Compression by the diaphragmatic crura

The lower oesophagus is angulated forward and to the left as it passes through the slit-like opening in the diaphragm opening formed by the fibres of the right crus. It has been postulated that the margins of the crus at the oesophageal hiatus act as a diaphragmatic pinchcock to prevent reflux (Winans and Harris, 1967; Habibulla, 1972; Lobello *et al.*, 1978). Although the presence of the high pressure zone at the lower end of the oesophagus seems independent of diaphragmatic action, the squeezing action of the diaphragm is probably of considerable importance in maintaining a barrier against reflux (Habibulla, 1972; Edwards, 1982).

Valvular mechanisms

Various valvular mechanisms at the gastro-oesophageal junction have been described and include mucosal and flap valves. Mucosal folds at the gastro-oesophageal junction are gathered together in close apposition in the form of a rosette, which some believe may have an important antireflux action (Botha, 1958a).

Hill (1989) describes the existence of an anatomical one-way flap valve which closes so effectively against the lesser curve that it may be difficult to find. The valve offers no resistance to aboral flow of oesophageal contents into the stomach, but considerable resistance to retrograde flow. Hill postulates that the gastro-oesophageal sphincter consists of

Table 5.2 Factors affecting tone of lower oesophageal sphincter

	Increased tone	Decreased tone
Hormone	Gastrin/pentagastrin Motilin Bombesin substance P Cerulein Prostaglandin F_2	Secretin Cholecystokinin Gastric inhibiting polypeptide Vasoactive intestinal polypeptide Glucagon Prostaglandins E_1, E_2, A_2
Drugs	Metoclopramide Domperidine Indomethacin	Theophylline Diazepam Morphine Alcohol Smoking
Neurotransmitter drugs	Cholinergic (bethanecol) Anticholinesterase Alpha adrenergic agonist (norepinephrine) Alcohol Smoking	Anticholinergic drugs (e.g. atropine) Dopamine Beta-adrenergic agonist Alpha-adrenergic antagonist
pH of Stomach	Gastric alkalinization	Gastric acidification
Food	Protein meal Coffee	Fat Chocolate Peppermint
Miscellaneous	Histamine 5-Hydroxytryptamine	Inflammation

the lower oesophageal (physiological) sphincter, the gastro-oesophageal valve and the collar sling musculature anchored posteriorly.

Gastro-oesophageal sphincter

The existence of a physiological sphincter at the gastro-oesophageal junction has been well established. Manometric studies have identified a high pressure zone at the lower end of the oesophagus, extending 1–3 cm above and below the hiatus. Resting pressures in this zone exceed intragastric pressures by 15–30 mmHg. Following deglutition, a decrease of pressure within the high pressure zone occurs within 1.5–2 s due to relaxation of the sphincter. This ensures that the sphincter relaxation occurs ahead of arrival of the food bolus or fluid. A number of factors have been shown to affect the tone of the lower oesophageal sphincter (Table 5.2). Although the various factors recorded in Table 5.2 are known to influence sphincter tone, their physiological significance remains uncertain. For example, gastrin is thought to cause a significant increase in lower oesophageal sphincter tone only when given in pharmacological doses. Prostaglandin E, released by inflammation, is probably responsible for the additional decrease of lower oesophageal sphincter pressure seen in oesophagitis (Hollwarth and Uray, 1985).

The neural control of the gastro-oesophageal sphincter is independent of oesophageal continuity and normal peristaltic activity. When challenged by an increase in intragastric pressure such as that caused by abdominal compression, the sphincter contracts actively, with the incremental increase in sphincter pressure exceeding the increase in intragastric pressure by 50% or more. This response of the sphincter to increased intragastric pressure is impaired by truncal vagotomy, even though the resting tone of the sphincter is not influenced by this procedure. This suggests that efferent vagal activity remains intact, while the afferent limb of the reflex arc responsible for the normal sphincter response to abdominal compression must have been interrupted by vagotomy (Crispin *et al.*, 1967).

Carre and Astley (1958) first demonstrated the presence of a high-pressure sphincteric zone in the terminal oesophagus in children similar to that noted in adults. Sphincteric pressures in early infancy have been shown to be of equal magnitude to those of older children (Hollwarth, 1979). The high pressure zone measures 0.5–1 cm length at birth and gradually increases in length to 2.5 cm by 3 months of age. At birth, very little of the high pressure zone lies within the abdomen and it is not until 3 months of age that the length of the abdominal portion of the sphincter equals that of the thoracic part. These manometric findings accord well with anatomical studies in which it has been noted that there is almost complete absence of any abdominal portion of the oesophagus at birth (Botha, 1958b).

Maturation of an effective antireflux barrier is not achieved until 3 months of age (Boix-Ochoa and Canals, 1976). These authors found the decisive factor in the general development of an effective antireflux barrier was the increase in length of the intra-abdominal portion of the oesophagus rather than any enhancement of the sphincteric zone.

5.1.4 MOTOR DISORDERS OF THE OESOPHAGUS IN GASTRO-OESOPHAGEAL REFLUX

There is increasing evidence to indicate that in gastro-oesophageal reflux oesophagitis is not due primarily to abnormally high acid secretion, but rather to failure of the lower oesophageal sphincter to prevent excessive reflux and failure of oesophageal peristalsis to clear the refluxed acid (Castell, 1988). There is no question that patients with more severe reflux disease have lower oesophageal contraction pressures and a greater likelihood of peristaltic dysfunction. Considerably less certain, however, is whether the abnormal oesophageal motility is a cause or result of the chronic reflux.

Mahony *et al.* (1988) studied the mechanisms of gastro-oesophageal reflux in children with oesophageal manometry and pH monitoring. The pathophysiology of gastro-oesophageal reflux involves the interplay of oesophageal motility, lower oesophageal sphincter activity and gastric emptying. Disturbance of the mechanisms of clearance of gastric contents refluxed into the oesophagus may thus result from disturbance of the oesophageal motor apparatus. Data from their study provide evidence of the nature of disordered motor activity in patients with gastro-oesophageal reflux:

1. Oesophageal motor function was more disturbed in those children with both gastro-oesophageal reflux and reflux oesophagitis than in those with gastro-oesophageal reflux alone. The amplitude of contractions and lower oesophageal sphincter pressures were significantly lower than in controls and were often bizarre in nature.
2. Infants with trivial symptoms had reflux occurring synchronously with swallowing, whereas reflux occurred asynchronously with swallowing in those with serious symptoms (including reflux oesophagitis).
3. Acid clearance was slower in patients in whom reflux occurred asynchronously with swallowing, and slowest in those with oesophagitis and where secondary peristalsis was ineffective.

These events may result solely from the inflammatory response to prolonged acid exposure. It is possible that prolonged exposure of the oesophagus to acid which results in inflammation may lead to a vicious circle being established with further deterioration of oesophageal motor activity and even worse acid clearance.

5.2 Function of the oesophagus in oesophageal atresia

Information concerning oesophageal function in oesophageal atresia is based largely on studies performed following surgical repair of the anomaly. However, there is one study which describes oesophageal function prior to surgical intervention (Romeo *et al.*, 1987) and there are several studies of the function of the oesophagus in patients born with tracheo-oesophageal fistula without associated oesophageal atresia (Kirkpatrick *et al.*, 1961; Johnston and Hastings, 1966).

5.2.1 STUDIES OF OESOPHAGEAL FUNCTION PRIOR TO SURGICAL INTERVENTION

Romeo *et al.* (1987) studied 20 newborn infants with oesophageal atresia by recording intraluminal pressures of 16 proximal and 12 distal oesophageal segments. They found that the upper oesophageal sphincter function in response to swallowing was mostly normal. There was incomplete relaxation of the upper oesophageal sphincter in less than 50% of swallows in two infants only. The significance of this is uncertain as upper oesophageal sphincter function may be similarly affected in the normal newborn infant during the first week of life.

The oesophageal body of both proximal and distal segments showed a positive basal tone with total motor inco-ordination in all cases. Relaxation of the lower oesophageal sphincter was complete in 9/10 patients assessed. Normal lower oesophageal sphincter pressures were found with a good gastro-oesophageal gradient in all but two patients.

Pre-operative manometric studies on patients with H-type tracheo-oesophageal fistula reveal unco-ordinated peristalsis and gastro-oesophageal reflux (Kirkpatrick *et al.*, 1961; Johnston and Hastings, 1966).

5.2.2 STUDIES OF OESOPHAGEAL FUNCTION FOLLOWING REPAIR OF OESOPHAGEAL ATRESIA

Cinefluorographic studies

The upper oesophageal sphincter is normal in oesophageal atresia. Cinefluorographic studies of the function of the body of the oesophagus

(Haight, 1957; Kirkpatrick *et al.*, 1961; Desjardins *et al.*, 1964; Shepard *et al.*, 1967) show that the primary peristaltic wave becomes dissipated above the line of the oesophageal anastomosis and that below this line, secondary contractions occur which result in both antegrade and retrograde flow, the so-called 'yo-yo' phenomenon.

In more severe cases, the retrograde flow may be sufficient to enter the pharynx and spill over into the airway (Kirkpatrick *et al.*, 1961). 'Spastic' contractions may involve the distal segment of the oesophagus: these are in contrast to the propulsive and progressive contractions seen in normal patients. An aperistaltic segment extends both proximal and distal to the level of the anastomosis (Burgess *et al.*, 1968).

Manometric studies

Shepard *et al.* (1967) have demonstrated a paucity of peristaltic activity at and immediately below the oesophageal anastomosis. The area of dysmotility extends for a variable distance (4–13 cm) below the anastomosis, involving between 10 and 60% of the length of the oesophagus. Below this area and above the lower oesophageal sphincter, some abnormal motor activity can be observed. This activity includes spasm with simultaneously elevated pressure, biphasic, tertiary and retrograde waves. Other workers (Haller *et al.*, 1966; Burgess *et al.*, 1968; Laks *et al.*, 1972), have confirmed that almost the whole length of the oesophagus has abnormal function.

Following deglutition the primary peristaltic wave is lost a short distance below the upper oesophageal sphincter and an aperistaltic segment extends both proximal and distal to the level of the anastomosis. These features continue into the teenage years (Burgess *et al.*, 1968) but cause surprisingly few adverse symptoms in adult life (Chapter 25).

5.2.3   LOWER OESOPHAGEAL SPHINCTER FUNCTION

The function of the lower oesophageal sphincter in oesophageal atresia has been the source of considerable controversy and studies have been contradictory in their findings.

Burgess *et al.* (1968) demonstrated normal resting sphincteric pressures and a normal sphincteric response to swallowing. Likewise, Shepard *et al.* (1967) found normal sphincteric relaxation to allow oesophageal emtpying. On the other hand, Lind *et al.* (1966) demonstrated failure of lower oesophageal sphincter relaxation and postulated dysfunction similar to achalasia of the oesophagus.

Orringer *et al.* (1977) who performed both manometric and intra-oesophageal pH studies on 22 patients between 6 and 32 years after repair of the oesophageal atresia made three important observations:

1. *Abnormal lower oesophageal sphincter function.* In five patients there was complete loss of tone in the lower oesophageal sphincter with no identifiable high pressure zone (HPZ). The average mean and peak HPZ pressures in the remaining 17 patients tended to be approximately half the comparable values for healthy young adult controls. In all patients with an identifiable HPZ, however, normal reflex relaxation occurred with deglutition.
2. *High incidence of gastro-oesophageal reflux.* Moderate to severe acid reflux was documented in 13 patients, including the five in whom no distal oesophageal HPZ was found. An increased incidence of gastro-oesophageal reflux occurred in patients requiring mobilization of more than 3 cm of distal oesophagus to achieve the oesophageal anastomosis.
3. *Abnormal acid clearance from the oesophagus.* Abnormal acid clearing ability was seen in 21 of 22 patients studied, reflecting disturbance of lower oesophageal motor function.

The clinical implication of gastro-oesophageal reflux and impaired acid clearing ability combined is an increased incidence of complications secondary to reflux, such as oesophagitis and pulmonary infection secondary to aspiration.

Jolley *et al.* (1980), in a study of patterns of gastro-oesophageal reflux following repair of oesophageal atresia using pH monitoring and gastro-oesophageal scintigraphy, found that two-thirds of the 25 patients had significant gastro-oesophageal reflux. Slow gastric emptying, which was observed in association with gastro-oesophageal reflux, may have the same neurological basis as the oesophageal dysfunction.

5.3 Aetiology of oesophageal motor dysfunction associated with oesophageal atresia

Is the underlying basis of oesophageal dysfunction in oesophageal atresia congenital, acquired, or a combination of both? Both preoperative and postoperative studies suggest a basic underlying congenital aetiology, although acquired factors may affect the ultimate functional result. Studies in puppies (Carveth *et al.*, 1962; Haller *et al.*, 1966) show no disruption of oesophageal motility following transection and resuture of the oesophagus, even after mobilization of the oesophagus. However, injury to oesophageal branches of the vagus nerve produce an aperistaltic segment, similar to that found in the clinical setting following repair of oesophageal atresia (Carveth *et al.*, 1962). Damage to vagal nerves during mobilization of the oesophageal segment might cause disordered oesophageal motility, even when the vagal trunks remain intact, as demonstrated by normal Hollander tests (Burgess *et al.*, 1968).

Post-operative manometric studies following repair of oesophageal atresia show that almost the entire length of the oesophagus has abnormal motility, regardless of the extent of dissection or tension at the anastomosis, suggesting a possible congenital aetiology. Oesophageal function studies on patients who have undergone end-to-side oesophageal anastomosis revealed the same motility disturbance. Patients with H-type tracheo-oesophageal fistula also show oesophageal dysmotility (Kirkpatrick *et al.*, 1961; Johnston and Hastings, 1966). The most compelling evidence for an inherent congenital disorder remains that of Romeo *et al.* (1987) in their studies showing motility disorders in both proximal and distal oesophageal segments prior to surgical repair.

5.4   Conclusion

Although there remains controversy as to the underlying aetiology of oesophageal dysfunction associated with oesophageal atresia, the weight of evidence supports the likelihood of an inherent congenital motor dysfunction. The most convincing evidence is afforded by preoperative manometric studies performed on patients with oesophageal atresia as well as those with H-type tracheo-oesophageal fistulae. These studies have demonstrated definite motility disorders prior to surgical intervention.

Acquired factors related to the surgical procedure are important in contributing further to the functional disturbance. The finding of normal lower oesophageal sphincter pressures prior to surgery contrast with the abnormal postoperative studies reported by Orringer *et al.* (1977) and Jolley *et al.* (1980). An iatrogenic basis for lower oesophageal dysfunction is strongly suggested by these contrasting preoperative and postoperative findings.

The most troublesome problems recorded after repair of oesophageal atresia are dysphagia and recurrent respiratory symptoms. Although in some instances these problems may be due to an anastomotic stricture, recurrent tracheo-oesophageal fistula or tracheal instability, they are much more commonly due to disordered oesophageal motility, including lower oesophageal sphincter disturbance and gastro-oesophageal reflux. The consequences of reflux are often augmented in oesophageal atresia by delay in oesophageal clearance of gastric acid due to poor oesophageal motility. This predisposes these patients to oesophagitis, anastomotic stricture and aspiration pneumonia.

References

Atkinson, M., Edwards, D. A. W., Honour, A. J. and Rowlands, E. N. (1957) Comparison of cardiac and pyloric sphincters; a manometric study. *Lancet*, ii, 918–1008.

Boix-Ochoa, J. and Canals, J. (1976) Maturation of the lower oesophagus. *J. Pediatr. Surg.*, 11, 749–56.

Botha, G. S. M. (1958a) Mucosal folds at the cardia as a component of the gastro-oesophageal closing mechanism. *Br. J. Surg.*, 45, 569–80.

Botha, G. S. M. (1958b) The gastro-oesophageal region in infants. *Arch. Dis. Child.*, 33, 78–94.

Botha, G. S. M. (1962) *The Gastro-Oesophageal Junction*, J. & A. Churchill, London, p. 369.

Burgess, J. N., Carlson, H. C. and Ellis, F. J. Jr (1968) Esophageal function after successful repair of esophageal atresia and tracheo-esophageal fistula – a manometric and cine-fluorographic study. *J. Thorac. Cardiovasc. Surg.*, 56, 667–73.

Carre, I. J. (1987) Some physiological mechanisms of the upper gastrointestinal tract. in *Paediatric Gastroenterology* 2nd edn (eds C. M. Anderson, V. Burke and M. Gracey), Blackwell Scientific Publications, Oxford, pp. 1–31.

Carre, I. J. (1987) Disorders of the oropharynx and oesophagus. in *Paediatric Gastroenterology* 2nd edn (eds C. M. Anderson, V. Burke and M. Gracey), Blackwell Scientific Publications, Oxford, pp. 32–77.

Carre, I. J. and Astley, R. (1958) The gastro-oesophageal junction in infancy. *Thorax*, 13, 159–64.

Carveth, S. W., Schlegel, J., Code, F. F. and Ellis, F. H. Jr (1962) Esophageal motility after vagotomy, phenicotomy, myotomy and myomectomy in dogs. *Surg. Gynecol. Obstet.*, 114, 31–42.

Castell, D. O. (1988) Esophagitis, a motility disorder. *Motility, Clin. Perspect. Gastroenterol.*, 2, 4–6.

Code, C. F., Creamer, B., Schlegel, J. F., Olsen, A. M., Donoghue, F. E. and Anderson, H. A. (1958) *An Atlas of Esophageal Motility in Health in Disease*, C. C. Thomas, Springfield, Illinois, p. 134.

Colley, J. R. T. and Creamer, B. (1958) Sucking and swallowing in infants. *Br. Med. J.*, ii, 422–3.

Crispin, J. S., McIver, D. K. and Lind, J. F. (1967) Manometric study of the effect of vagotomy on the gastro-oesophageal sphincter. *Can. J. Surg.*, 10, 299–303.

Desjardins, J. G., Stephens, C. A., Moes, C. A. F. (1964) Results of surgical treatment of congenital tracheo-esophageal fistula with a note on cinefluorographic findings. *Ann. Surg.*, 160, 141–5.

Dodds, W. J., Hogan, W. J., Helm, J. M. and Dent, J. (1981) Pathogenesis of reflux esophagitis. *Gastroenterology*, 81, 376–94.

Edwards, D. A. W. (1982) The anti-reflux mechanism, its disorders and their consequences. *Clin. Gastroenterol.*, 11, 479–96.

Erbelding, K. P., Siemens, F. and Angerpointner, T. A. (1985) Progress in the diagnosis of gastroesophageal reflux in childhood; 24 hour pH monitoring. *Progress in Pediatric Surgery*, vol. 18, Springer-Verlag, Berlin, pp. 32–7.

Fotter, R., Hollwarth, M. and Uray, E. (1985) Correlation between manometric and roentgenologic findings of diseases of the esophagus in infants and children. *Progress in Pediatric Surgery*, vol. 18, Springer-Verlag, Berlin, pp. 14–21.

Fyke, F. E. Jr and Code, C. F. (1955) Resting and deglutition pressures in the pharyngo-esophageal region. *Gastroenterology*, 29, 24–34.

Fyke, F. E. Jr, Code, C. F. and Schlegel, J. F. (1956) The gastroesophageal sphincter in healthy human beings. *Gastroenterologia (Basel)*, 86, 135–50.

Golubuva, E. L., Shuleikina, K. V. and Vainshtein, I. I. (1959) The development of reflex and spontaneous activity of the human fetus in the process of embryogenesis. *Obstet. Gynecol. (USSR)*, 3, 59–62.

Gryboski, J. D. (1965) The swallowing mechanism of the neonate. 1. Esophageal and gastric motility. *Pediatrics*, 35, 445–52.

Gryboski, J. D. (1969) Suck and swallow in the premature infant. *Pediatrics*, 43, 96–102.

Gryboski, J. D., Thayer, W. R. Jr and Spiro, H. M. (1963) Esophageal motility in infants and children. *Pediatrics*, 31, 382–95.

Habibulla, K. S. (1972) The diaphragm as an antireflux barrier. A manometric, oesophagoscopic and transmucosal potential study. *Thorax*, 27, 692–702.

Haight, C. (1957) Some observations in esophageal atresia and tracheo-esophageal fistulas of congenital origin. *J. Thorac. Surg.*, 34, 141–72.

Haller, J. A., Broker, A. F. and Talbert, J. L. (1966) Esophageal function following resection. Studies in newborn puppies. *Ann. Thorac. Surg.*, 2, 180–7.

Hill, L. D. (1989) Myths of the esophagus. *J. Thorac. Cardiovasc. Surg.*, 98, 1–11.

Hollwarth, M. (1979) Die entwicklung der speiserohrenfunktion bei neugeborenen – eine manometrische studie 2. *Kinderchir*, 27, 201–15.

Hollwarth, M. and Uray, E. (1985) Physiology and pathophysiology of the esophagus in childhood. *Progress in Pediatric Surgery*, vol. 18, Springer-Verlag, Berlin, pp. 1–13.

Johnston, P. W. and Hastings, N. (1966) Congenital tracheoesophageal fistula without esophageal atresia. *Am. J. Surg.*, 112, 233.

Jolley, S. G., Herbst, J. J., Johnson, D. G. *et al.* (1979) Patterns of postcibal gastro-esophageal reflux in symptomatic infants. *Am. J. Surg.*, 138, 946–50.

Jolley, S. G., Johnson, D. G., Roberts, C. C. and Herbst, J. J. (1980) Patterns of gastro-esophageal reflux in children following repair of esophageal atresia and distal tracheo-esophageal fistula. *J. Pediatr. Surg.*, 15, 857–62.

Jolley, S. G., Johnson, D. G., Herbst, J. J., Pena, A. *et al.* (1978) An assessment of gastro-esophageal reflux in children by extended pH monitoring of the distal esophagus. *Surgery*, 84, 16–24.

Kirkpatrick, J. A., Cresson, S. L. and Pilling, G. P. IV (1961) The motor activity of the esophagus in association with esophageal atresia and tracheo-esophageal fistula. *Am. J. Roentgenol. Radium Ther.*, 86, 884–7.

Koch, A., Gass, R. and Bettex, M. (1985) Significance of esophageal manometry and long-term pH monitoring for the evaluation of gastroesophageal reflux in infancy and childhood. *Progress in Pediatric Surgery*, vol. 18, Springer-Verlag, Berlin, pp. 22–31.

Laks, H., Wilkinson, R. H. and Schuster, S. R. (1972) Long-term results following correction of esophageal atresia with tracheoesophageal fistula. A clinical and cine-fluorographic study. *J. Pediatr. Surg.*, 7, 591–7.

Lind, J. F., Blanchard, R. J. and Guhda, H. (1966) Esophageal motility in tracheo-esophageal fistula and esophageal atresia. *Surg. Gynecol. Obstet.*, **123**, 557–64.

Lobello, R., Edwards, D. A. W., Gummer, J. W. P. and Stekelmman, M. (1978) The anti-reflux mechanism after cardiomyotomy. *Thorax*, **33**, 569–73.

Mahony, M. J., Migliavacca, M., Spitz, L. and Milla, P. J. (1988) Motor disorders of the esophagus in gastro-esophageal reflux. *Arch. Dis. Child.*, **63**, 1333–8.

Marchand, P. (1957) A study of the forces productive of gastro-oesophageal regurgitation and herniation through the diaphragmatic hiatus. *Thorax*, **12**, 189–202.

Moroz, S. P., Espinoza, J., Cumming, W. A. and Diamant, N. E. (1976) Lower oesophageal sphincter function in children with and without gastro-oesophageal reflux. *Gastroenterology*, **71**, 236–41.

Myers, W. F., Roberts, C. C., Johnson, D. G. and Herbst, J. J. (1985) Value of tests for evaluation of gastro-esophageal reflux in children. *J. Pediatr. Surg.*, **20**, 515–20.

Orringer, M. B., Kirsh, M. M. and Sloan, H. (1977) Long-term esophageal function following repair of esophageal atresia. *Ann. Surg.*, **186**, 436–43.

Pritchard, J. A. (1965) Deglutition by normal and anencephalic fetuses. *Obstet. Gynecol.*, **25**, 289–97.

Romeo, G., Zuccarello, B., Proietto, F. *et al.* (1987) Disorders of esophageal motor activity in atresia of the esophagus. *J. Pediatr. Surg.*, **22**, 120–4.

Shepard, R., Fenn, S. and Sieber, W. K. (1967) Evaluation of esophageal function in post-operative esophageal atresia and tracheo-esophageal fistula. *Surgery*, **59**, 608–18.

Shermeta, D. W., Whittington, P. F., Seto, D. S. *et al.* (1977) Lower esophageal sphincter dysfunction in esophageal atresia. Nocturnal regurgitation and aspiration pneumonia. *J. Pediatr. Surg.*, **12**, 871–6.

Winans, C. S. and Harris, L. D. (1967) Quantitation of lower esophageal sphincter competence. *Gastroenterology*, **52**, 773–8.

PART THREE
Diagnosis and Perioperative Care

6 Diagnosis

N. A. MYERS and S. W. BEASLEY

Occasionally, the diagnosis of oesophageal atresia may be suspected before birth, but in the vast majority the diagnosis cannot be made with certainty until after birth. In patients with oesophageal atresia it is necessary first to demonstrate complete oesophageal obstruction. Once this has been done the type of anomaly and the presence of other major anomalies must be determined. Associated congenital anomalies are found in approximately 50% of babies with oesophageal atresia and their recognition is important in deciding treatment priorities (Chapter 14).

The presence, size and anatomical location of a tracheo-oesophageal fistula may modify the clinical picture in infants with oesophageal atresia, but symptomatology alone does not enable absolute confirmation of the type of anomaly. Additional evidence is obtained by passage of a catheter through the mouth (Figure 6.1) and by radiology or endoscopy. These investigations will almost always indicate the exact anatomical nature of the anomaly.

The clinical features of a baby with a tracheo-oesophageal fistula without atresia (the 'H' fistula) differ significantly from those of the baby with oesophageal atresia (Chapter 13). Babies with an isolated tracheo-oesophageal fistula can swallow but tend to 'choke on feeds' and have cyanotic episodes. There may be considerable delay in diagnosis.

6.1 Antenatal diagnosis

6.1.1 POLYHYDRAMNIOS

Polyhydramnios is an associated finding in 95% of cases with oesophageal atresia without fistula, in 90% of those with a proximal fistula, but in only 35% of those with a distal fistula. In all pregnancies complicated by polyhydramnios the diagnosis of oesophageal atresia

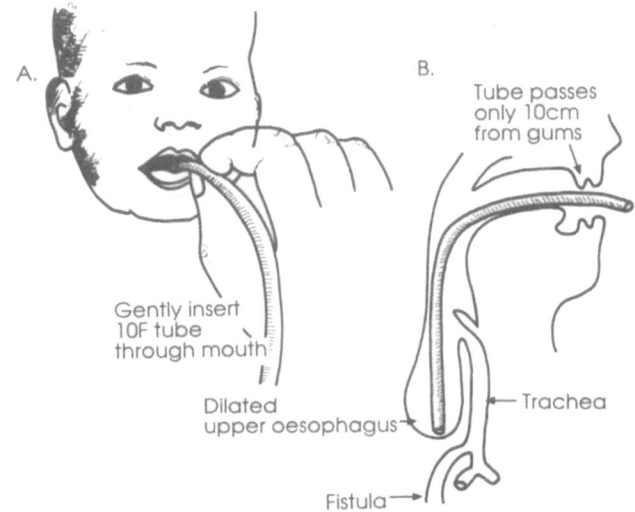

Figure 6.1 Technique of passage of a no. 10 tube into the oesophagus in infants suspected of having oesophageal atresia. When oesophageal atresia is present the catheter becomes arrested at about 10 cm from the gums. (Reproduced with permission from Hutson and Beasley, 1988.)

should be suspected and the baby should be appropriately examined and investigated at birth (Beasley *et al.*, 1989b). This includes attempted passage of a tube through the mouth into the stomach.

Now that there is increasing expertise in the antenatal ultrasound diagnosis of oesophageal atresia all pregnancies, particularly those complicated by polyhydramnios, should have careful ultrasonographic examination of the fetal oesophagus and stomach. It must be remembered that polyhydramnios is also present in many other congenital conditions and may even occur with a normal baby.

6.1.2 FETAL ULTRASONOGRAPHY

The technology available and the expertise of ultrasonographers performing fetal ultrasound has improved to such a degree in recent years that the diagnosis *in utero* of oesophageal atresia is becoming practical, with or without polyhydramnios to increase the suspicion. Evidence which should be sought and which may indicate oesophageal atresia includes direct visualization of the blind upper oesophageal pouch which may be seen filling and emptying, (Eyheremendy and Pfister, 1983), smallness of or inability to detect the stomach (Jassani *et al.*, 1982) and a paucity of fluid in the intestine. The last two features are particularly suggestive of atresia without fistula (Farrant, 1980). In the absence of these findings the ultrasonographer may observe abnormal swallowing movements with regurgitation (Bowie and Clair, 1982; Cooper *et al.*, 1985) and an abdominal diameter smaller than the biparietal diameter (Pretorius *et al.*, 1983). Apparent fetal vomiting may further substantiate the diagnosis (Bowie and Clair, 1982).

6.1.3 AMNIOGRAPHY

This technique has been performed in the past by injecting radioopaque material into the liquor as a means of radiological imaging of the gastrointestinal tract, but has not gained widespread acceptance and has been largely replaced by ultrasonography. Passage of a contrast medium into the fetal intestine in oesophageal atresia is known to occur and may give rise to a false negative diagnosis (Holzgreve and Golbus, 1983).

6.1.4 AMNIOCENTESIS

If oesophageal atresia is suspected prenatally the question of an abnormal karyotype must be addressed. Amniocentesis can be used to determine the karyotype and to plan the further management of the pregnancy. It can also be used to obtain amniotic fluid to estimate the level of acetylcholinesterase, which has been reported to be elevated in some cases of oesophageal atresia (Holzgreve *et al.*, 1983), but not consistently so (Holzgreve and Golbus, 1983).

6.2 Postnatal diagnosis

The diagnosis of oesophageal atresia could be established at birth if all Obstetric Units followed the practice of routine passage (or attempted passage) of a tube into the stomach at birth in all babies (Figure 6.1). However, this routine has the potential disadvantage to the baby of traumatically induced apnoea by inadvertent injury to the larynx. Therefore, the passage of a size 10 catheter is recommended in all babies where, because of polyhydramnios during the pregnancy, the diagnosis is suspected at birth; where abnormalities of swallowing have been shown on ultrasonography or where the diagnosis is suspected after birth because of symptoms and signs. Table 6.1 shows the main presenting features of 488 babies with oesophageal atresia and distal tracheo-oesophageal fistula. In 92 infants passage of a tube was attempted because of the presence of other major congenital abnormalities, during

Table 6.1 Main clinical presentation of babies with oesophageal atresia and distal tracheo-oesophageal fistula

Presentation		No. of cases
Obstruction to passage of tube		92
Other abnormalities, including multiple and chromosomal	44	
During routine resuscitation	29	
Polyhydramnios	19	
Symptomatic		384
Mucousy baby (excessive drooling)	209	
Respiratory distress	44	
Cyanotic attacks with feeding	39	
Cyanotic attack without feeding	35	
Feeding problems: 'vomiting' or regurgitation or unable to feed satisfactorily	31	
Unable to swallow	14	
Failure of attempted gavage feeds	8	
Other	4	
Not clearly recorded		12
Total		488

routine resuscitation or because of polyhydramnios. In the remaining infants, the diagnosis of oesophageal atresia was suspected from other symptoms, of which the most common was excessive drooling (Figure 6.2).

Any baby drooling excessive saliva should be assumed to have oesophageal atresia, until successful passage of an oro-oesophageal

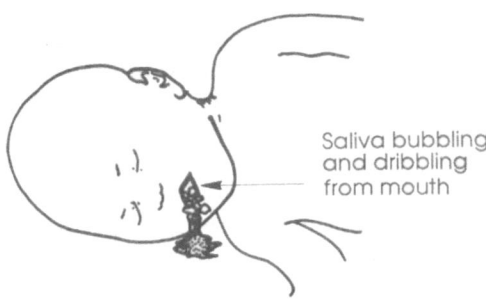

Saliva bubbling and dribbling from mouth

Figure 6.2 The infant with oesophageal atresia appears to be 'mucousy' and drools excessively. This occurs because the saliva accumulates in the upper oesophageal pouch as it cannot be swallowed. (Reproduced with permission from Hutson and Beasley, 1988.)

tube. However, the clinician should be aware that some premature infants may not appear to secrete much saliva. If for some reason the diagnosis is not recognized at birth and feeding is commenced, explosive rejection of the first feed will occur, usually with cyanosis, choking and respiratory distress; and this should immediately alert the clinician to the correct diagnosis.

6.2.1 DELAY IN DIAGNOSIS

In past years, many babies were offered milk before the diagnosis was suspected. Milk entering an obstructed oesophagus has a high chance of being aspirated into the lungs and causing aspiration pneumonia (Figure 6.3). Our aim over a long period of time has been to educate obstetricians and paediatricians to suspect oesophageal atresia when:

1. The baby is mucousy
2. There are cyanotic episodes (due to aspiration of saliva which has accumulated in a blind upper pouch)
3. There has been polyhydramnios
4. There are other anomalies, e.g. imperforate anus, radial dysplasia

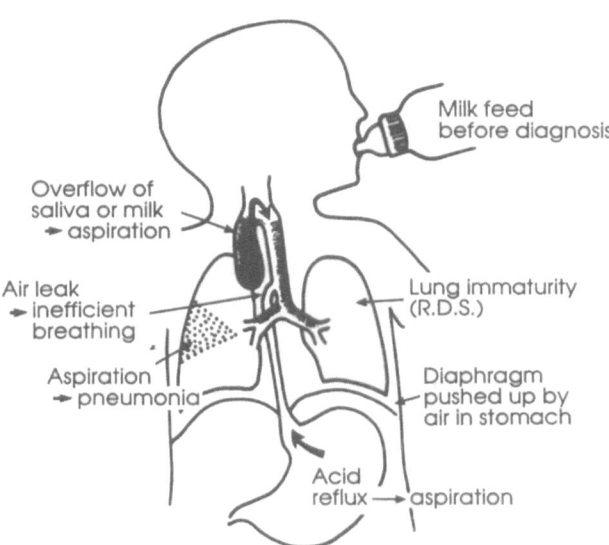

Figure 6.3 Factors contributing to respiratory problems in oesophageal atresia. Tracheomalacia, which is common in oesophageal atresia, may add to the respiratory difficulties (Reproduced with permission from Hutson and Beasley, 1988.)

6.2.2   CONFIRMATION OF DIAGNOSIS

If the diagnosis is suspected we recommend passage of a relatively
stiff 10 English gauge nasogastric tube through the mouth. If the tube
cannot be introduced beyond 8–11 cm the diagnosis of oesophageal
atresia is established and the baby should be transfered to a tertiary
centre. No further delineation of the anatomy is required before transfer. Contrast studies, if any, should be performed after transfer to the
tertiary institution. A smaller calibre tube is not used because it may curl
up in the upper pouch and give a misleading impression of oesophageal
continuity (Figure 6.4).

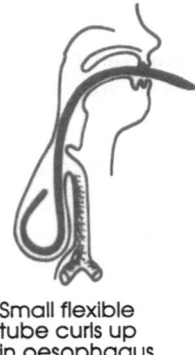

Small flexible
tube curls up
in oesophagus

Figure 6.4   A stiff 10 English gauge catheter is used because smaller tubes may
curl up in the upper pouch giving a false impression of oesophageal continuity.
Introduction of the tube through the nose should not be attempted because it
may injure the nasal passages. (Reproduced with permission from Hutson and
Beasley, 1988.)

6.2.3   DIAGNOSIS OF THE ANATOMICAL TYPE

Knowledge of the anatomical variant is necessary before definitive
treatment can be instituted. The presence or absence of a fistula between
the trachea and the blind upper oesophagus or lower segment of the
oesophagus must be established. In addition, it is useful to have some
indication of the distance between the oesophageal segments.

Plain X-rays are taken of the chest and abdomen (Figure 6.5). Often
the plain film will show the blind upper pouch in the upper mediastinum in both the AP and lateral views (Figures 6.5 and 6.6). Occasionally the lateral view will also demonstrate an open fistula and air in
the lower oesophagus. Tam *et al.* (1987) have used direct sagittal CT
scanning to demonstrate both oesophageal segments and to measure
the intervening gap.

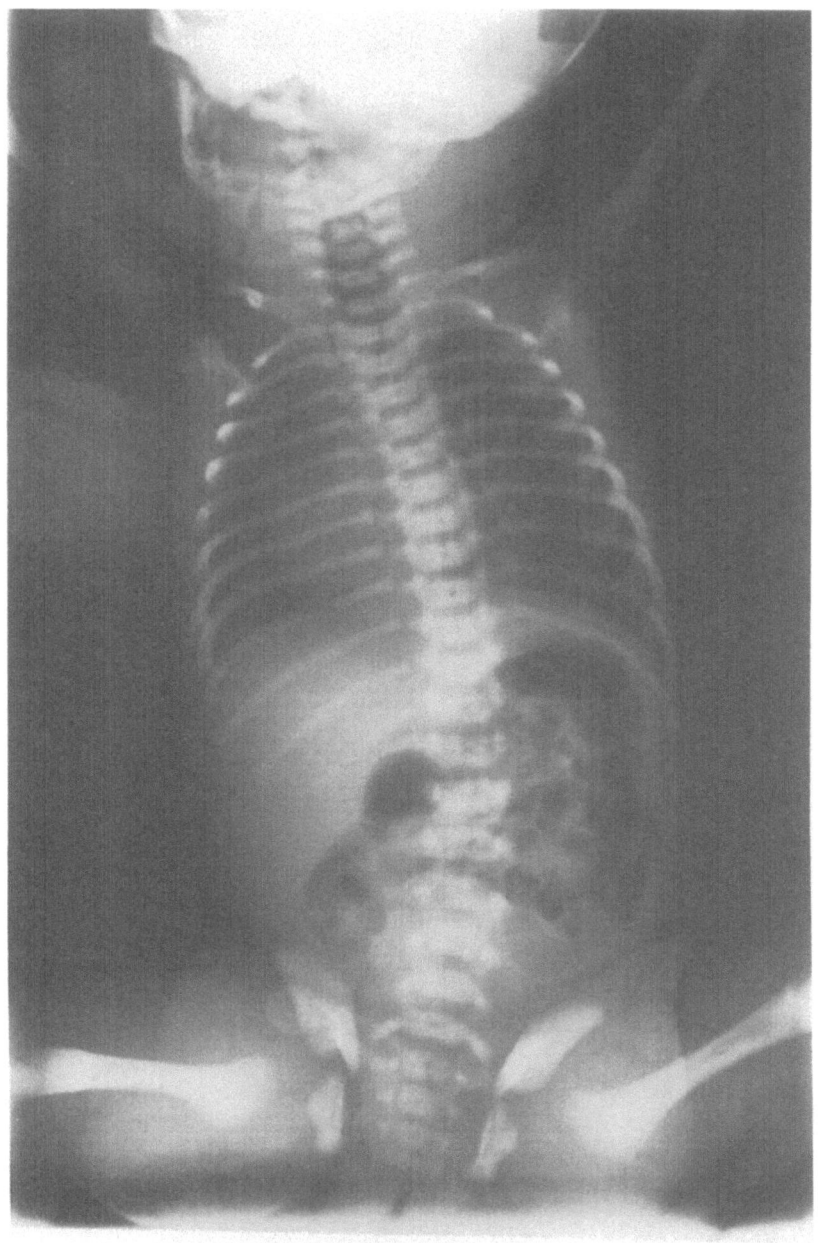

Figure 6.5 Plain radiology of the chest should also include the abdomen so that the presence or absence of gas below the diaphragm can be observed.

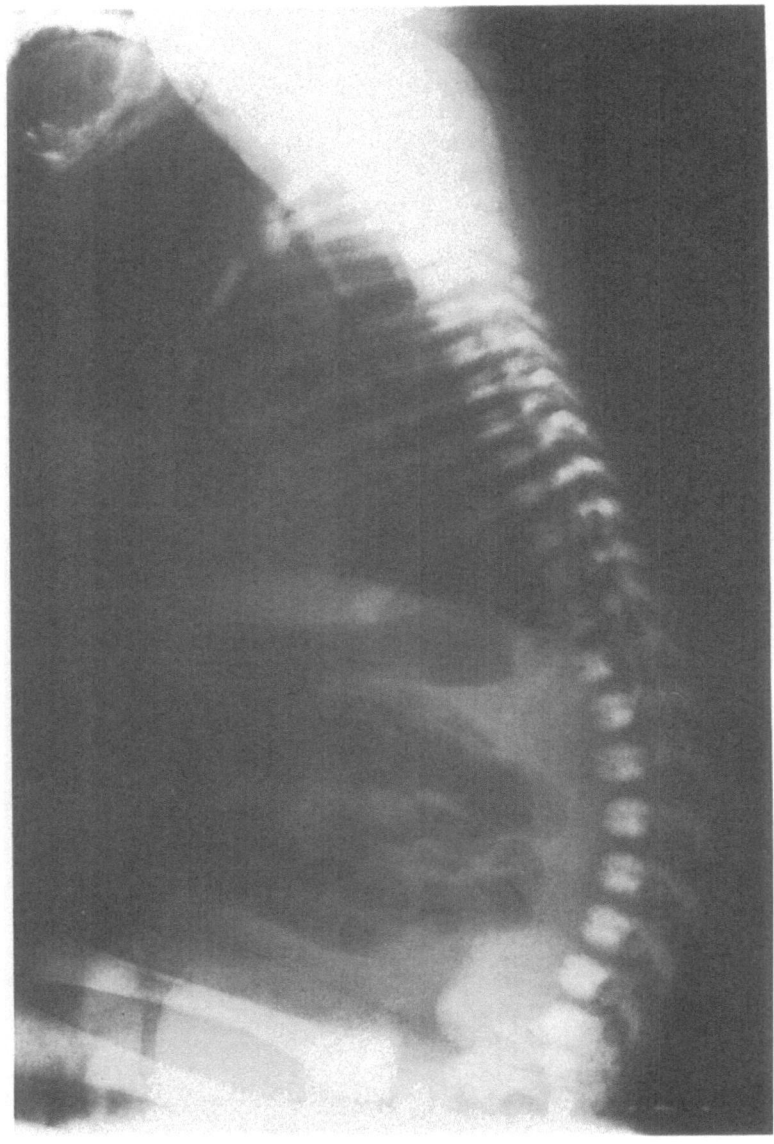

Figure 6.6 A lateral view of the chest showing the upper oesophageal segment. Air below the diaphragm confirms the presence of a distal tracheo-oesophageal fistula.

The gasless abdomen

If there is no gas in the abdomen for longer than a few minutes after birth the patient has either atresia without a fistula or atresia with a proximal fistula (Figures 6.7 and 6.8). The rare situation of a distal unopened fistula has been described (Waterston *et al.*, 1963) but has not been encountered in our experience. In the infant who has a gasless abdomen it is appropriate to perform a careful upper pouch contrast study to look for an upper pouch fistula (Beasley *et al.*, 1989a). If a fistula is found management should proceed along the lines described in Chapter 10. If an upper pouch fistula is not found, oesophageal atresia without fistula is assumed, and gastrostomy is performed as soon as the patient is fit enough to undergo the procedure. At the time of gastrostromy the length of the lower oesophagus can be demonstrated by passing a metal bougie up into the lower oesophagus. Subsequent management is described in Chapter 11.

Distal tracheo-oesophageal fistula

If the plain radiographs show gas in the abdomen the most likely anatomical arrangement is a blind upper pouch in association with a distal tracheo-oesophageal fistula (Figure 6.5). In our series only two out of 584 patients have had a double fistula and with care these can be identified at thoracotomy undertaken for repair of the anomaly. It has not been our recent practice to perform a routine upper pouch contrast study or to perform endoscopy. However, endoscopy has been recommended by some authors (Gans, 1983; Filston *et al.*, 1984; Kosloske *et al.*, 1988) and is performed routinely to define the position and number of fistulae.

Diagnosis of 'H' fistula

Patients with isolated tracheo-oesophageal fistulae present differently because they have an intact oesophagus. The infants are able to swallow but suffer choking and coughing with feeds, abdominal distension from air escaping through the fistula into the stomach, and recurrent chest infections (Chapter 13). Radiology is used to confirm the diagnosis (Beasley and Myers, 1988) but endoscopy also has its advocates (Gans and Berci, 1973; Gans and Johnson, 1977). This is discussed more fully in Chapter 13.

6.2.4 DIFFERENTIAL DIAGNOSIS

Any condition which causes respiratory stress, choking or cyanotic episodes, abdominal distension and excessive drooling of saliva should

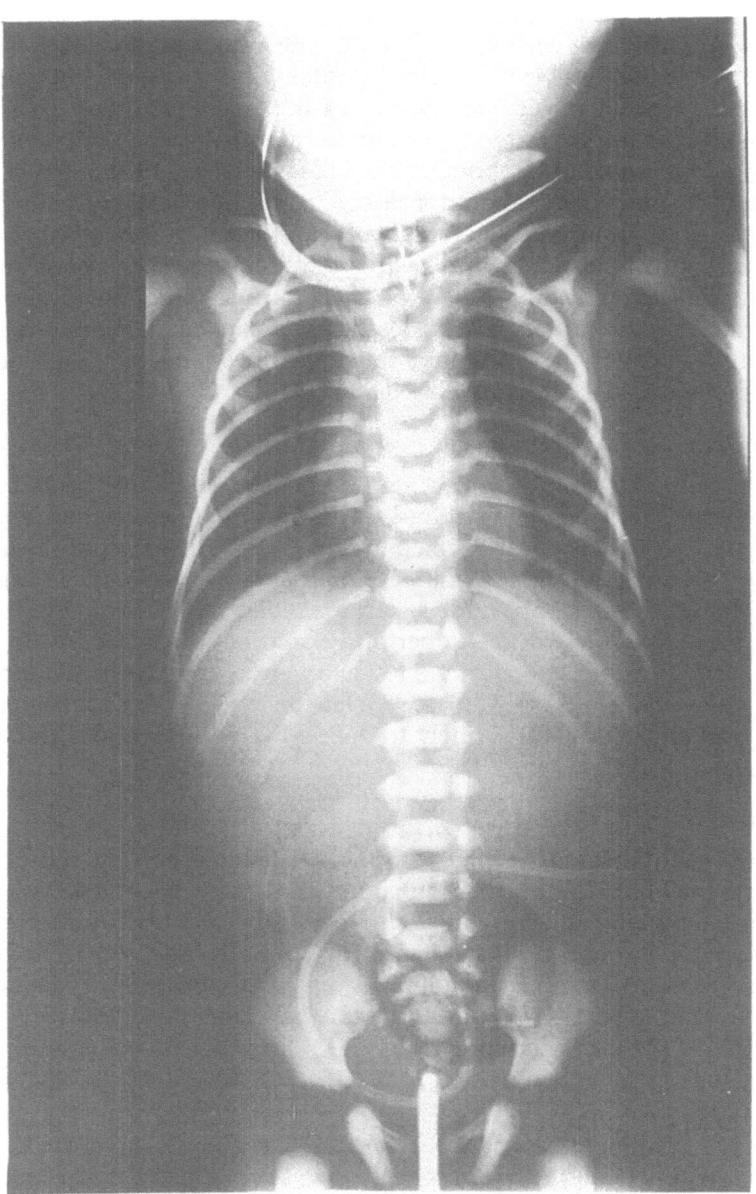

Figure 6.7 The gasless abdomen: the patient has either oesophageal atresia without a fistula (75%) or oesophageal atresia and a proximal fistula.

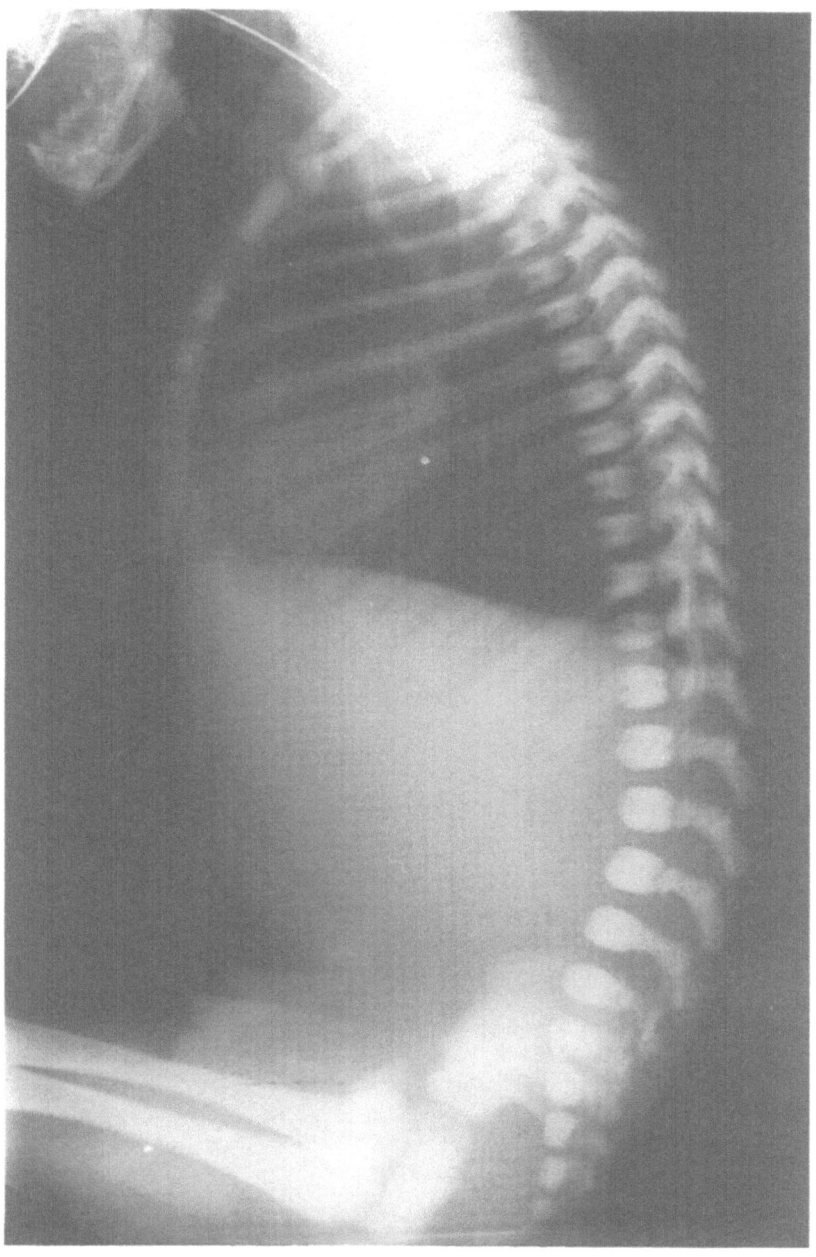

Figure 6.8 Lateral view of the gasless abdomen. There is no distal tracheo-oesophageal fistula.

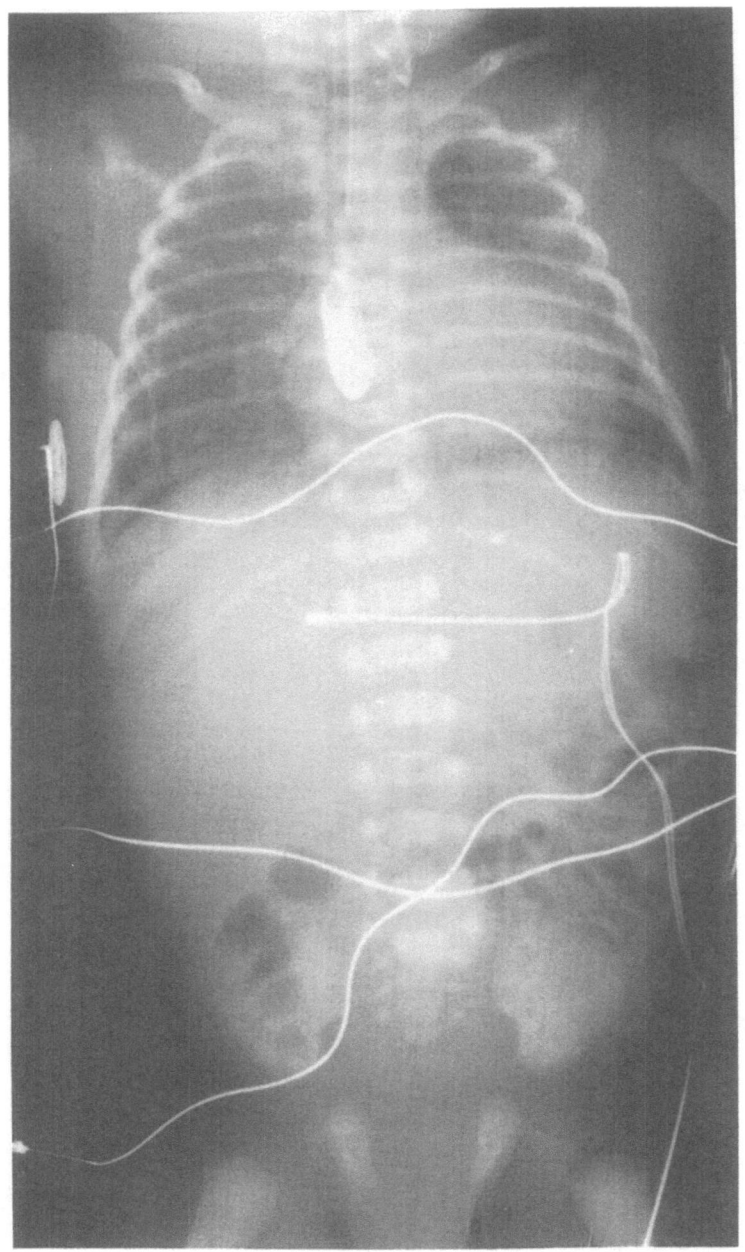

Figure 6.9 Barium in the oesophagus and a relatively small amount of gas in the abdomen (at 17 hours of age).

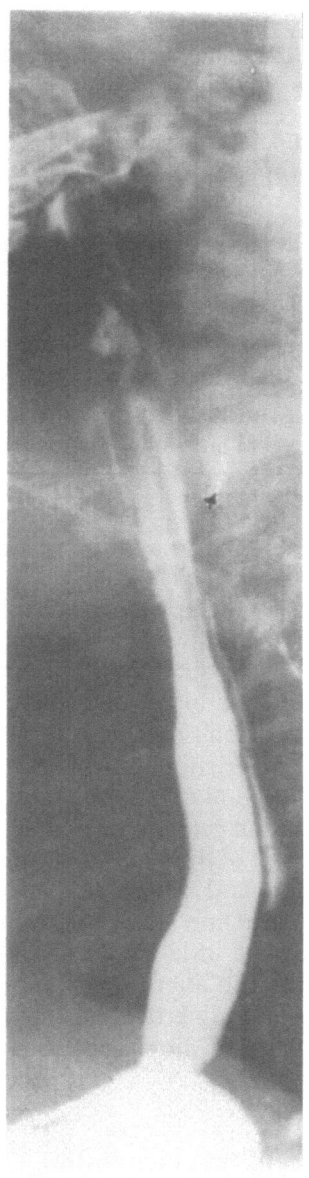

Figure 6.10 A lateral chest and abdominal radiograph demonstrating the 'normal' oesophageal lumen (nasogastric tube *in situ*) anteriorly and residual barium in the traumatic pseudodiverticulum posteriorly.

Table 6.2   Differential diagnosis of oesophageal atresia and tracheo-oesophageal fistula

1.	Conditions associated with aspiration Nasopharyngeal inco-ordination Gastro-oesophageal reflux
2.	Conditions producing oesophageal obstruction Oesophageal stenosis Vascular ring
3.	Traumatic oesophageal pseudodiverticulum
4.	Miscellaneous Prematurity Cerebral birth injury

be considered in the differential diagnosis of oesophageal atresia. The most important of these conditions are those which allow aspiration into the respiratory tract; those which produce oesophageal obstruction; and traumatic oesophageal pseudodiverticulum (Table 6.2). The traumatic pseudodiverticulum is a rare but important differential diagnosis for oesophageal atresia (Cohen and Myers, 1987). Copious drooling of saliva is associated with inability to pass a nasogastric tube into the stomach and is seen characteristically in premature babies who require intensive neonatal resuscitation. The pseudodiverticulum results from traumatic passage of a suction catheter or endotracheal tube through the mucosa of the posterior wall of the pharynx (Edison and Holinger, 1973; Wells *et al.*, 1974; Cohen and Myers, 1987). If a contrast study is performed the level of obstruction is low in the chest and radiography of the abdomen usually reveals little gas in the alimentary tract (Figure 6.9). A lateral chest radiograph after introduction of contrast may show residual barium in the pseudodiverticulum (Figure 6.10). The diagnosis is confirmed by endoscopy and thoracotomy can be avoided.

6.3   Diagnosis of other congenital anomalies

Associated anomalies are present in over 50% of babies with oesophageal atresia and/or tracheo-oesophageal fistula. When a baby is diagnosed at birth as having oesophageal atresia it is necessary to examine the infant for one or more associated anomalies. Diagnosis of congenital anomalies, including chromosomal defects, affecting other systems is described in detail in Chapters 14 to 17.

References

Beasley, S. W. and Myers, N. A. (1988) The diagnosis of congenital tracheo-oesophageal fistula. *J. Pediatr. Surg.*, **23**, 415–17.

Beasley, S. W., Auldist, A. W. and Myers, N. A. (1989a) Current surgical management of oesophageal fistula and tracheo-oesophageal atresia. *Aust. N. Z. J. Surg.*, **59**, 707–12.

Beasley, S. W., Shann, F. A., Myers, N. A. and Auldist, A. W. (1989b) Developments in the management of oesophageal atresia and tracheo-oesophageal fistula. *Med. J. Aust.*, **150**, 501–3.

Bowie, J. D. and Clair, M. R. (1982) Fetal swallowing and regurgitation: observation of normal and abnormal activity. *Radiology*, **144**, 877–8.

Cohen, R. and Myers, N. A. (1987) Traumatic oesophageal pseudo-diverticulum. *Aust. Pediatr. J.*. **23**, 125–7.

Cooper, C., Mahony, B. S., Bowie, J. D., Albright, T. O. and Callen, P. W. (1985) Ultrasound evaluation of the normal fetal upper airway and esophagus. *J. Ultrasound. Med.*, **4**, 343–6.

Edison, B. and Holinger, P. H. (1973) Traumatic pharyngeal pseudodiverticulum in the newborn infant. *J. Pediatr.*, **82**, 483–5.

Eyheremendy, E. and Pfister, M. (1983) Antenatal real-time diagnosis of esophageal atresias. *J. Clin. Ultrasound*, **11**, 395–7.

Farrant, P. (1980) The antenatal diagnosis of oesophageal atresia by ultrasound. *Br. J. Radiol.*, **53**, 1202–3.

Filston, H. C., Rankin, J. S. and Grimm, J. K. (1984) Esophageal atresia: prognostic factors and contribution of pre-operative telescopic endoscopy. *Ann. Surg.*, **199**, 532–7.

Gans, S. L. (1983) Bronchoscopy. in *Pediatric Endoscopy* (ed. S. L. Gans), Grune & Stratton, Philadelphia, p. 39.

Gans, S. L. (1985) Editors note. *J. Pediatr. Surg.*, **20**, 242.

Gans, S. L. and Berci, G. (1973) Inside tracheo-esophageal fistula: new endoscopic approaches. *J. Pediatr. Surg.*, **8**, 205–11.

Gans, S. L. and Johnson, R. O. (1977) Diagnosis and management of 'H'-type tracheo-esophageal fistula in infants and children. *J. Pediatr. Surg.*, **12**, 233–6.

Holzgreve, W. and Golbus, M. S. (1983) Amniotic fluid acetylcholinesterase as a prenatal diagnostic marker for upper gastrointestinal atresias. *Am. J. Obstet. Gynecol.*, **147**, 837.

Holzgreve, W., Beller, F. K. and Pawlowitzki, I. H. (1983) Amniotic fluid acetylcholinesterase as a marker in prenatal diagnosis. *Am. J. Obstet. Gynecol.*, **145**, 641.

Hutson, J. M. and Beasley, S. W. (1988) *The Surgical Examination of Children*, Heinemann Medical, London, pp. 239–42.

Jassani, M. N., Gauderer, M. W. L., Faranoff, A. A. *et al.* (1982) A perinatal approach to the diagnosis and management of gastro-intestinal malformation. *Obstet. Gynecol.*, **59**, 33.

Kosloske, A. M., Jewell, P. F. and Cartwright, K. C. (1988) Crucial bronchoscopic findings in esophageal atresia and tracheo-esophageal fistula. *J. Pediatr. Surg.*, **23**, 466–70.

Mackellar, A. and Kennedy, J. C. (1972) Congenital diverticulum of the pharynx simulating esophageal atresia. *J. Pediatr. Surg.*, **7**, 408–11.

Pretorius, D. H., Meier, P. R. and Johnson, M. L. (1983) Diagnosis of esophageal atresia in utero. *J. Ultrasound Med.*, **2**, 475–6.

Tam, P. J. H., Chan, F. L. and Saing, H. (1987) Diagnosis and evaluation of esophageal atresia by direct saggital CT. *Pediatr. Radiol.*, **17**, 68–70.

Waterston, D. J., Bonham-Carter, R. E. and Aberdeen, E. (1963) Congenital tracheo-esophageal fistula in association with oesophageal atresia. *Lancet*, **i**, 55–7.

Wells, S. D., Leonidas, J. C., Conkle, D., Holder, T. M., Amoury, R. A. and Aschcraft, K. W. (1974) Traumatic prevertebral pharyngoesophageal pseudo-diverticulum in the newborn infant. *J. Pediatr. Surg.*, **9**, 217–22.

7 Transport of the neonate with oesophageal atresia

R. N. D. ROY

The over-riding principle of transport of the newborn is stabilization before transport, followed by supervision of transport by specialist nursing and medical personnel with appropriate equipment.

Ideally, in most regions this requires the tertiary hospital to provide a retrieval team that will travel out to the hospital of birth to perform the necessary stabilization of the infant, and to continue resuscitation during subsequent transport. For example, in the State of Victoria, the Newborn Emergency Transport Service (NETS) provides this facility (Roy and Kitchen, 1977) (Figure 7.1).

Transport of an infant with oesophageal atresia involves the same principles and practices applicable to all neonatal transport, as well as some specific management techniques. If these principles are followed, most babies with oesophageal atresia will arrive at the 'tertiary institution' in good condition.

7.1 Transport organization

7.1.1 COMMUNICATION

There must be ready access via telephone to the transport team 24 hours a day. In addition to arranging the transfer, the transport team can provide advice on the management of the infant until the retrieval team arrives.

7.1.2 STAFFING

Nursing

The nursing role in neonatal transport is vital to its success. If there is a high enough volume of transports (more than 500 per/year), it is prefer-

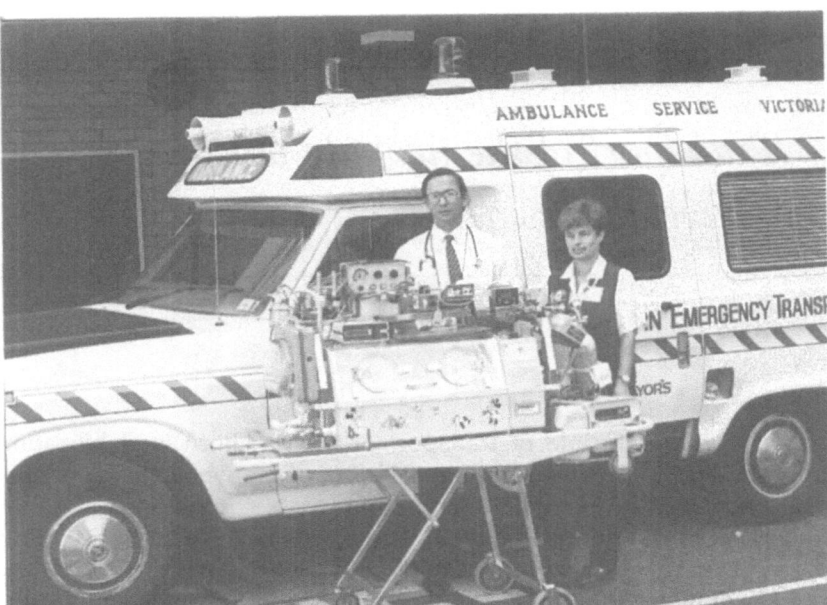

Figure 7.1 In Victoria, Australia, the Newborn Emergency Transport Service (NETS) is responsible for the initial stabilization and transport of infants with oesophageal atresia.

able to have staff fully dedicated to transport; alternatively, it is possible to train neonatal unit staff to act as transport nurses when required.

The nurse's role is multifaceted and includes organization of trips, nursing management of patients during stabilization and transport, documentation, provision of support and comfort to the parents and care of equipment. For patients with oesophageal atresia, the nurse may be able to conduct the transfer on his/her own if there are no associated complications and the distance is short. Where there are complications, the distance is great or air transport is required, a second person (in the NETS system, a doctor) should accompany the infant.

Medical

The retrieval team should be directed by a neonatal paediatrician. Medical personnel involved in transfers should be suitably experienced senior paediatric trainees or consultant neonatologists. For rapid response, there must be at least one doctor rostered for transport duties at all times.

7.1.3 EQUIPMENT

The following equipment is required:

1. A transport incubator capable of withstanding the expected environmental temperature changes and of running from a variety of power sources, including 240V AC, 12V and 24V DC. It should allow for adequate observation of the infant, access for procedures (e.g. aspiration of the upper oesophagus) and facility for securing the infant.
2. Oxygen and medical air in sufficient supply to last the length of the anticipated journey with reserve to accommodate unexpected delays.
3. Adequate suction apparatus.
4. Cardiac monitoring, preferably with a screen displaying the QRS complex.
5. Intravenous infusion apparatus: syringe pumps are preferred so that infusion volumes can be administered accurately.
6. Temperature monitor.
7. Oxygen concentration analyser.
8. Transcutaneous oxygen or oxygen saturation monitor.
9. Blood pressure measuring apparatus.
10. Equipment box containing drugs, disposable items and equipment for procedures such as endotracheal intubation, intravenous infusion and pneumothorax drainage.

7.1.4 CHOICE OF VEHICLE

The three usual vehicles for newborn transport are road, fixed wing and rotary wing aircraft (Figure 7.2). For transports of up to 160 km, road transport is preferred, unless the route is slow when rotary-wing aircraft may be preferred. Fixed wing aircraft are most useful beyond 160 km. A road vehicle should have adequate security and comfort for the staff, and allow adequate access to the patient and equipment. It may be a specially designed transport vehicle (as for NETS) which has additional gas supplies and power outlets, and a separate resuscitation area.

Travel by air has additional problems:

1. The pO_2 of ambient air decreases with increased altitude, and compensation for this necessitates increasing the inspired oxygen concentration, especially for infants with respiratory distress.
2. Confined gas expands with increasing altitude, e.g. an air-filled

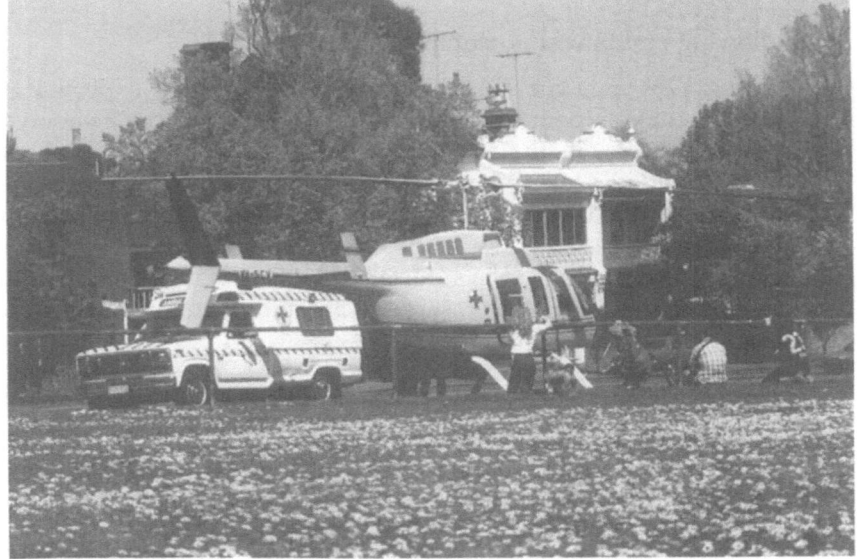

Figure 7.2   The type of newborn transport used depends on distance, available vehicles and facilities, and the urgency of transport. This NETS helicopter is landing adjacent to the Royal Children's Hospital, Melbourne.

   stomach associated with a tracheo-oesophageal fistula will expand by 50% at an altitude of 10 000 ft (3000 m).
3.   There is usually limited space in an aircraft for resuscitation and special procedures to be performed if the baby's condition deteriorates.
4.   Helicopters and small fixed wing aircraft may have payload limitations which restrict the number of personnel and equipment which may be carried.

7.2   Medical care before and during transport

7.2.1   GENERAL MEDICAL CARE

Gentle handling

Stabilization and transport is of necessity invasive (Roy, 1977; Roy and Brown, 1983). However, handling should be kept to a minimum because excessive disturbance increases the infant's oxygen consumption, exposes the infant to cold stress and may cause dramatic cardiovascular responses in an unstable infant. Specific reasons for gentle handling of the infant with oesophageal atresia are considered in section 7.2.2.

Temperature control

Cold stress increases oxygen requirement and may lead to acidosis. Care must be exercised to avoid excessive cooling in the delivery room and during subsequent stabilization and transport. The environmental temperature required in a standard incubator in the first six hours of life according to birthweight is shown in Table 7.1.

Table 7.1 Incubator temperature required

Weight (g)	Incubator temperature (°C)
< 1000	35–37
1000–1500	34–36
1500–2000	33–35
2000–2500	32–34
> 2500	30–31

Oxygen therapy

A number of infants with oesophageal atresia will have associated respiratory distress, either because of prematurity, other abnormalities, transient tachypnoea, and occasionally aspiration pneumonia or from diaphragmatic splinting caused by excessive escape of air through the fistula into the stomach.

Where blood gases can be measured by arterial blood sampling or transcutaneous monitoring, the pO_2 should be in the range of 50–80 mmHg, although it has been our experience that the pO_2 can be safely kept between 80–100 mmHg in infants over 34 weeks' gestation.

If no blood gas monitoring facilities are available, the infant must be kept pink at all times: a short period of hypoxia is more dangerous than several hours of hyperoxia.

Airway and posture

The specific aspects of airway and posture management of infants with oesophageal atresia are discussed in section 7.2.2. In general, the infant in transport should be nursed in the right lateral position to allow a spontaneously clear airway. Additional aspiration of the airway is required in the event of apnoea, with sudden changes in the pattern of breathing or with obvious accumulation of secretions.

Fluids and glucose

The need for institution of fluid therapy depends on the time it will take for the transport team to arrive and transport the infant to the tertiary hospital. There is no immediate need for fluids and glucose unless there are associated conditions such as hypoglycaemia or asphyxia; a routine intravenous infusion should be commenced by two to three hours of age. The initial intravenous maintenance fluid requirement is 10% glucose at 3 ml/kg/h.

7.2.2 CARE OF THE OESOPHAGEAL ATRESIA AND TRACHEO-OESOPHAGEAL FISTULA

Posture

The infant with oesophageal atresia should be nursed in the right lateral position, either flat or head up. The rationale for this is:

1. To provide a spontaneously clear airway should any fluid enter the pharynx;
2. To minimize regurgitation of gastric contents up the associated tracheo-oesophageal fistula; by being on the right side, gastric contents will move to the pylorus rather than the fundus near the cardia, and gastric emptying will be enhanced (Yu, 1975);
3. To decrease work of breathing and improve oxygenation (Hutchinson *et al.*, 1979). The neonate depends almost entirely on contraction of the diaphragm for effective ventilation which is more easily accomplished in this position.

Care of the upper pouch

The upper oesophagus should be 'suctioned' intermittently – every 10–15 min irrespective of whether there appear to be any excessive secretions, and more often if necessary. Saliva may accumulate 'silently' in large volumes in the upper pouch, regurgitate suddenly, and be aspirated into the lungs if not sucked out. It may occasionally compress the trachea from behind, particularly if tracheomalacia is marked.

The suction catheter should be firm but soft, such as 8 or 10 French (size 12 may be too traumatic). Y-Suction catheters are preferred, because they enable pressure adjustment to minimize mucosal damage.

Gentle handling

At all times, particular attention must be paid to the infant with a tracheo-oesophageal fistula to minimize crying, since crying tends to fill the stomach with air via the fistula; this in turn (a) increases the likelihood of regurgitation of gastric contents into the trachea; and (b) increases abdominal distension and impedes breathing.

7.2.3 CARE OF ASSOCIATED MEDICAL PROBLEMS

Prematurity

One-third of infants with oesophageal atresia are premature. They require attention to temperature control, oxygen therapy, earlier fluid and dextrose infusion, and observation for apnoea, respiratory distress and hypoglycaemia.

Intrauterine growth retardation

Infants with intrauterine growth retardation are at risk of hypogly-caemia, which must be avoided. Careful examination of such infants for associated anomalies should be made.

Respiratory distress

The majority of infants with oesophageal atresia and respiratory distress can be managed with increased ambient oxygen concentration (see section 7.2.1). However, 7% will require ventilation in transit. This presents additional problems if ventilation pressures are high since gastric distension (and rupture) may develop (Templeton *et al.*, 1985), making ventilation more difficult. This problem may be reduced by placing the tip of the endotracheal tube just proximal to the carina but distal to the fistula (Salem *et al.*, 1973).

7.3 Care of the family

Counselling the parents

The parents should be given an honest appraisal of the situation and, provided there are no associated severe anomalies, the prognosis for survival is good. This is the first and most important statement to be made to the parents, since often they will only hear the first statement made. An outline of the nature of oesophageal atresia should be given, with an explanation that further investigation may be necessary to determine the precise anatomical defect.

Description of further management

The transfer of their infant to an unfamiliar hospital, the complexity of equipment and procedures used, and the separation of the infant from the family and of the parents from their familiar and trusted supports, are fearful experiences (Chapter 19). The parents should be given a clear outline of the transport, of what to expect, and some details of the receiving unit, including names of the personnel who will be caring for their infant, if these are known. Contact telephone numbers and details of hospital visiting procedures must be provided to allow for continuing contact. This expedites the transfer of trust from their own chosen medical care team to the one they do not know, and have not chosen.

Parent–infant contact

The transfer of their infant can leave an enormous sense of loss in parents; it is thus of great importance for them to view, and if practicable, to touch, stroke and cuddle their infant (Chapter 19). A Polaroid photograph should be taken of the infant, and left with the parents to be a concrete reminder of their living infant.

Arrangements for the parents

Parents may require advice on their own travel and accommodation arrangements if they live far from the neonatal unit. Transfer and admission arrangements may be required for the mother.

The parents should be asked if they require their infant to be baptized, especially if the infant is very sick.

If the mother wishes to breast feed, this should still be possible, and arrangements need to be made for transport of her expressed breast milk.

Confirmation of safe transfer

Once transfer is completed, it should be automatic that the parents at the referring hospital are telephoned and informed of the safe arrival of their infant.

Documentation

Documents required to accompany the infant include:

1. History and examination sheet – NETS provides a standard referral sheet for all hospitals in the state
2. Permission for Transport and Treatment document signed by at least one parent
3. Progress notes (copies from the referring hospital)
4. Pathology reports and all X-rays
5. Transport team record sheet detailing observations and procedures performed during stabilization and transport.

Other items which should accompany the infant include the placenta; 10 ml of cord blood and 10 ml of maternal blood (clotted).

7.4   Experience with transport of 101 patients with oesophageal atresia

In the last eleven years, NETS has transported 132 infants with oesophageal atresia, with a range of 9–18 patients per year, for which detailed records are available for patients transported from 1980 onwards.

Details of the 101 patients transported since 1980 are shown in Tables 7.2 and 7.3. Prematurity was documented in 34%, and a low birthweight (< 2500 g) in 46%. The male : female ratio was 62% : 38%. A total of 33% had been born at one of the tertiary maternity hospitals, many being transferred there *in utero* because of maternal polyhydramnios. Oxygen was required during transport in 6%, and intubation and ventilation was required in 7%. Most patients arrived normothermic (Table 7.4).

Table 7.2   101 infants with oesophageal atresia transported 1980–7

Birthweight (g)	No.	Gestation (weeks)	No.
< 1000	0	< 28	1
1000–1499	8	29–30	4
1500–1999	20	31–32	8
2000–2499	20	33–34	11
> 2500	53	35–36	10
		> 37	67

Table 7.3   Procedures required in transit

Intravenous infusion	54
Oxygen administration	61
Assisted ventilation (intubation)	7

Table 7.4   Temperature on arrival at tertiary hospital

Hypothermic	< 36 °C	9
Normothermic	36–37.2 °C	84
Hyperthermic	> 37.2 °C	8

References

Hutchinson, A. A., Ross, K. R. and Russell, G. (1979) The effect of posture on ventilation and lung mechanics in preterm and light-for-date infants. *Pediatrics*, **64**, 429–32.

Roy, R. N. D. (1977) Neonatal transport. *Med. J. Aust.*, **2**, 862–6.

Roy, N. and Brown, M. (1983) *Stabilization and Transport of Newborn Infants*. NETS publication.

Roy, R. N. D. and Kitchen, W. H. (1977) NETS: A new system for neonatal transport. *Med. J. Aust.*, **2**, 855–8.

Salem, M. R., Wong, A. Y., Lin, Y. H., Firor, H. V. and Bennett, E. J. (1973) Prevention of gastric distension during anaesthesia for newborns with tracheoesophageal fistulas. *Anesthesiology*, **38**, 823–4.

Templeton, J. M. Jr, Templeton, J. J., Schnaufer, L., Bishop, H. C., Ziegler, M. M. and O'Neill, J. A. Jr (1985) Management of esophageal atresia and tracheoesophageal fistula in the neonate with severe respiratory distress syndrome. *J. Pediatr. Surg.*, **20**, 394–7.

Yu, V. Y. H. (1975) Effect of body position in gastric emptying in the neonate. *Arch. Dis. Child.*, **50**, 500–4.

8 Anaesthesia and perioperative care

T. C. K. BROWN, R. EYRES and N. A. MYERS

The overall results of correction of oesophageal atresia, with or without fistula, improved considerably with progress in neonatal anaesthesia and the evolution of paediatric intensive care in the 1960s, which in turn was associated with the advent of prolonged intubation and mechanical ventilation.

8.1 Preoperative care

8.1.1 ADMISSION

All infants with diagnosed oesophageal atresia should be admitted to the intensive care unit or special care neonatal unit. The transport team must ensure that adequate handover is given to the paediatric surgeon.

8.1.2 PREVENTION OF RESPIRATORY COMPLICATIONS

Diagnosis before commencement of feeds decreases the risk of aspiration, a problem which used to occur at the time of the first feed and led to respiratory complications, including aspiration pneumonia.

The infant should be nursed supine while intravenous lines are being inserted, blood is being taken for biochemistry and crossmatch and monitoring is established. The supine position enables ready access to the infant and allows frequent gentle suction of upper pouch to prevent aspiration of secretions (Figure 8.1).

8.1.3 TEMPERATURE HOMEOSTASIS

Neonatal transport has improved so that infants born in outlying hospitals arrive at the referral hospital in better general condition and hypothermia is rarely a problem (Table 7.4). On arrival in the intensive

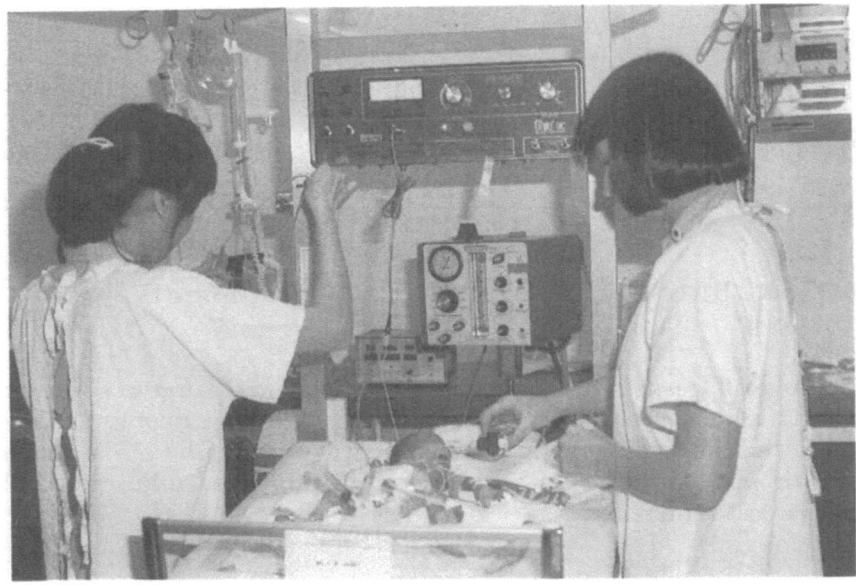

Figure 8.1 The supine position enables frequent gentle suction of the upper oesophageal pouch while intravenous lines are being inserted and monitoring is being established.

care or neonatal special care unit, these babies are nursed in a temperature-controlled environment, preferably under an overhead radiant heater which allows better access to the infant than does an incubator.

8.1.4 PREOPERATIVE INVESTIGATIONS

Preliminary investigations and management include:

1. *X-rays*: the X-ray should include the chest and abdomen to show the presence of gas in the abdomen and to enable assessment of the vertebral column. The AP chest radiograph gives information about the heart, the lung fields, and number of ribs. A lateral view of the chest may demonstrate the fistula and upper pouch.
2. *Investigation for associated anomalies*: preliminary assessment for associated cardiac, renal or other anomalies should be made. These include echocardiography and renal ultrasound. In the premature infant or following difficult delivery, the opportunity can be taken to perform cranial ultrasound as well.
3. *Biochemistry*: acid–base, electrolytes and pO_2 are measured and corrected as necessary.

4. *Blood crossmatch*: blood should be taken for haemoglobin, haematocrit and crossmatch preoperatively.

8.1.5 RESUSCITATION AND MONITORING

Intravenous access

An intravenous line is usually inserted to provide maintenance fluids and calories. 10% dextrose in 0.22% saline is commonly used. It is preferable to place the intravenous line in the right arm or hand as this will be uppermost and easily accessible during surgery. If a line is placed in the foot, an extension set will be needed. Abnormalities of fluids and acid–base are corrected.

Oxygenation

In the majority of babies, adequate oxygenation can be obtained by controlling the F_1O_2 in a head box, and endotracheal intubation is required rarely.

Early intubation may be necessary if there is:

1. Respiratory distress or respiratory failure, pneumonia, hyaline membrane disease or diaphragmatic splinting secondary to gastric distension
2. Airway instability due to severe tracheomalacia or airway obstruction from laryngeal anomalies
3. Recurrent or persistent soiling of the airway, either from spillover of secretions from the upper pouch or from gastric regurgitation through the fistula into the trachea, or
4. As an adjunct to the treatment of associated cardiac lesions.

Vitamin K

It should be ensured that the infant has received intramuscular Vitamin K_1 (phytomenadione).

Antibiotics

Antibiotics are given prior to surgery as prophylaxis. Unless there is pre-existing soiling of the lungs requiring continuation of a 'therapeutic' antibiotic regimen, a single dose of penicillin and gentamicin will suffice.

Monitoring

Continuous recording of pulse and ECG is established. Attachment of a urine bag allows the volume of urine passed to be recorded. If no urine is passed, preoperative renal ultrasound is mandatory (Chapter 16).

informed consent

Consent for operation should be obtained from the parents following discussion with them of the condition and its prognosis, and the significance of any known associated anomalies.

8.1.6   TIMING OF SURGERY

The baby should proceed to surgery as soon as convenient after preliminary assessment and management has been undertaken. Attitudes regarding the timing of operation, its urgency and whether primarily to divide the fistula or to create a gastrotomy before thoracotomy have varied. Current thinking is dominated by the view that early operation to divide the fistula (and anastomose the ends of the oesophagus) is desirable to limit lung soiling and the development of consequent respiratory complications.

8.1.7   TRANSPORT TO THEATRE

The specialist paediatric anaesthetist responsible for the infant during surgery is responsible for the transport of the infant from the intensive care unit to the operating suite. During transport, oxygen and suction equipment must be available, and the anaesthetist controls ventilation if required.

8.1.8   ON ARRIVAL IN THE OPERATING THEATRE

The overhead heater must be on and in place before the infant is transferred on to the operating table. All intravenous lines and monitoring devices are checked to ensure that they are in place and functioning normally before the anaesthetic is commenced (Figure 8.2). The diathermy plate is attached and rectal temperature probe inserted before induction, and checked at the time of positioning prior to skin preparation and draping. If there is an anorectal anomaly, a pharyngeal temperature probe is used. Where oximetry is available it must be used.

8.2   Anaesthesia

8.2.1   INDUCTION

Anaesthesia may be induced with thiopentone (about 1–2 mg/kg), or an opiate (morphine 10 μg/kg), fentanyl (1–2 μg/kg), with an inhala-

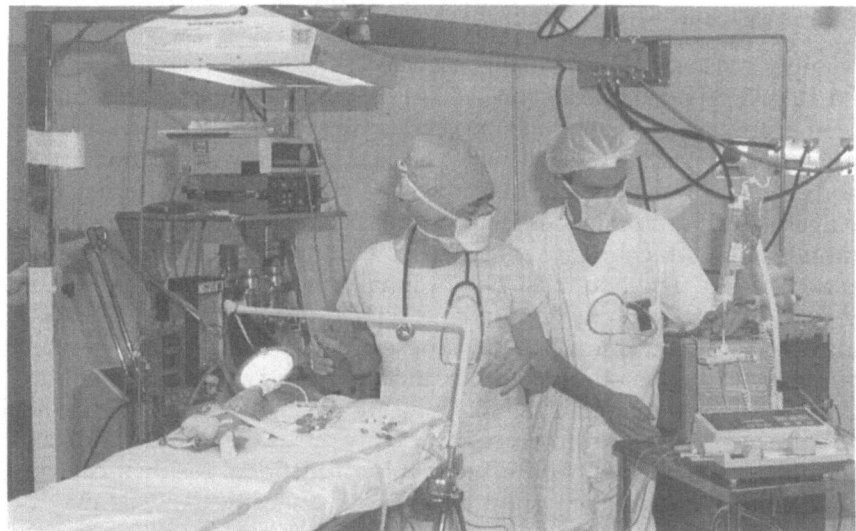

Figure 8.2 The overhead heater maintains normothernmia during attachment of monitoring devices, induction of anaesthesia and positioning prior to the commencement of surgery.

tion agent in oxygen or some combination of these. Atropine is usually given intravenously to reduce secretions. A muscle relaxant can be used safely, except in the occasional baby with an unusually large fistula and gastric distension. The baby is ventilated with oxygen and inhalation supplement and then intubated when appropriate. The tube should be inserted so that it is near the carina to splint the trachea against compression by retractors, but it must not be endobronchial and accidental intubation of the fistula must be avoided (Brown and Fisk, 1979).

8.2.2 INTUBATION

Intubation is accomplished with less stress and trauma if the infant is paralysed. On the rare occasions when the fistula is large and there is significant gastric distension, intubation without muscle relaxation may be employed to avoid Intermittent Positive Pressure Respiration (IPPR) until the chest is opened.

Alternatively, the brief period of paralysis and ventilation afforded by suxamethonium may be tolerable in these infants. Gastric distension and its detrimental effect on ventilation is thereby minimized.

8.2.3   ANALGESIA

It is now accepted that neonates are susceptible, and respond, to pain and therefore require adequate analgesia during surgery. This can be given as fentanyl or morphine. Neonates are sensitive to the respiratory depressive effects of narcotics which should be used with caution unless the baby is to be ventilated electively postoperatively. Alternatively, analgesia may be administered as an inhalation supplement, preferably with an agent which provides analgesia without too much cardiovascular depression. The two most potent inhalation analgesics are probably methoxyflurane and trichlorethylene which also provide analgesia in subanaesthetic concentrations, but these are now not available in many countries. The inhalation agent should be given with air and enough added oxygen to maintain full oxygen saturation. The use of air avoids the extra gastric distension caused by highly diffusible nitrous oxide and also decreases the reduction in ventilation functional residual capacity (RFC) of the lungs which often occurs with anaesthesia. This may be associated with alveolar collapse, decreased oxygenation, increased work of breathing, and an increased tendency to postoperative apnoeic spells (Brown and Fisk, 1979).

8.2.4   MAINTENANCE OF ANAESTHESIA

Anaesthesia is maintained with air, oxygen, and an inhalational agent with or without an opiate analgesic.

8.2.5   MONITORING

Monitoring should include observation of the patient, non-invasive pulse and blood pressure monitoring, pulse oximetry and temperature. A stethoscope may be attached to the left side of the chest for monitoring heart and breath sounds.

Attention to temperature homeostasis includes the use of a heating blanket, an overhead heater and a heated humidifier. Temperature is usually monitored by a rectal probe.

8.2.6   INTERCOSTAL BLOCKADE

Prior to closing the chest, the surgeon can inject local anaesthetic into the intercostal spaces above and below the thoracotomy, to provide postoperative analgesia. Up to 1 ml/kg 0.3% bupivacaine (3 mg/kg) can be used.

8.2.7 MANOEUVRES REQUIRED OF THE ANAESTHETIST DURING SURGERY

During thoracotomy

When the chest is being opened, extrapleural dissection is made easier if the anaesthetist reduces the ventilating pressure. This reduces the likelihood of injury to the pleura.

During lung retraction

During the intrathoracic part of the procedure, when the right lung is being retracted, the F_1O_2 should be increased. Manual ventilation allows the anaesthetist to keep slight positive pressure on the lungs which improves oxygenation. It will also allow early detection of tracheal compression by the assistant when retractors are not placed correctly. When this happens, the anaesthetist must inform the surgeon immediately, who likewise should be informed if there is any compression of the heart or great vessels. This will be detected by recognition of changes in blood pressure and pulse, and alteration in the intensity of the heart sounds.

Identification of upper pouch

The anaesthetist can be of assistance during the operation by passing a catheter (8 or 10 Fr gauge) into the upper pouch. This can help to push the upper pouch downwards to facilitate its identification from within the chest.

The distance from the gums to the anastomosis should be measured so that postoperatively the suction catheter is not inserted to the level of the anastomosis where it could cause damage. It must be ensured that the endotracheal tube is firmly fixed during this manoeuvre to avoid its accidental displacement.

Completion of anaesthesia

At the conclusion of the operation, the collapsed lung should be reinflated before the chest is closed. If a chest drain is inserted, residual air can be released through the tube.

The roll, placed under the left chest at the commencement of the procedure to improve exposure when the chest is opened, is removed to make rib apposition easier.

When it is not necessary to keep the baby paralysed and intubated postoperatively, neostigmine and atropine are given to reverse the muscle relaxation and allow early extubation. This can be achieved when the baby is in good condition, severe hyaline membrane disease is unlikely, respiration has not been depressed by opiates and the operative repair was accomplished easily. The endotracheal tube can be removed once the baby breathes adequately.

If the operation has been difficult, or depressant doses of opiates have been given, it may be preferable to continue an opiate infusion and ventilate the baby postoperatively for 24–48 hours. If no complications have occurred, the baby can then be weaned from the ventilator on to continuous positive airway pressure (CPAP) and then extubated when appropriate.

8.3 Special situations

8.3.1 RESPIRATORY DISTRESS SYNDROME

In the infant with severe respiratory distress syndrome, the aims should be to gain rapid cardiorespiratory stabilization, to use the minimum ventilatory pressures required to achieve adequate oxygenation and to divide the tracheo-oesophageal fistula early.

These infants do better if operated on early, before the hyaline membrane disease becomes fully established, and the complications of inadequate ventilation and ruptured stomach occur. The management of the infant with severe hyaline membrane disease is discussed more fully in Chapter 9.

8.3.2 THE 'H' FISTULA

In infants with an 'H' fistula (or a fistula between the upper oesophagus and trachea), there may be direct drainage of secretions into the lungs. The 'H' fistula is usually divided through a cervical incision above the thoracic inlet and requires the endotracheal tube to be taken over the forehead so that the anaesthetist is out of the surgeon's way, and to reduce the likelihood of accidental displacement.

8.3.3 OESOPHAGEAL REPLACEMENT

Oesophageal replacement is required in those patients in whom anastomosis is not possible (Chapter 12). These patients with a gastrostomy and cervical oesophagostomy return for replacement at about 12 months of age or 10 kg in weight. The principles of anaesthesia for thoracoabdominal surgery apply, and good intravenous access for blood transfusion is essential. A morphine infusion postoperatively (0.5 mg/kg in 500 ml at 20–40 ml/h) is recommended for at least 24 hours in these children (Beasley and Tibballs, 1987). This should be well tolerated in these children, as sensitivity to opiates decreases after the first few months.

8.4 Postoperative management

8.4.1 RETURN TO THE INTENSIVE CARE UNIT

The postoperative management is supervised by the surgeon who has performed the operative repair. The measures employed during transfer of the infant to the operating theatre apply equally to the transfer back to the intensive care unit postoperatively. The anaesthetic staff accompany the baby to the Intensive Care Unit before handing over to the staff of the unit.

The vital signs continue to be monitored, a chest X-ray obtained and the serum electrolytes and acid–base balance measured. Bacteriological cultures of secretions or drainage are obtained as required.

8.4.2 PHARYNGEAL SECRETIONS

During the early postoperative period the baby may have increased pharyngeal secretions and require continuing aspiration of the pharynx. Where there is an oesophageal anastomosis the suction tube must not be passed through it if injury to, or rupture of, the anastomosis is to be avoided. A marker indicating the maximum length of tube which can be passed safely through the mouth is placed on the side of the incubator (Figure 8.3). This serves as a reminder to the nursing attendants, and guards against inadvertent trauma to the anastomosis.

In the postoperative period, respiratory complications may be encountered and arise as a result of respiratory distress syndrome in the premature, aspiration, the effect of thoracotomy and tracheal instability (Chapter 22). Clinical evaluation of the respiratory status is complemented by X-ray studies and blood gas estimations. If an artificial airway is required, it should be supplemented by continuous positive airway pressure (CPAP) or intermittent positive pressure ventilation (IPPV).

In the vast majority of infants, extubation is possible at an early stage, and usually is carried out before the baby leaves the operating theatre.

8.4.3 ROLE OF SURGEON IN COMMUNICATION

The surgeon must communicate his operative findings, the procedure performed, and postoperative instructions to the unit staff, and is

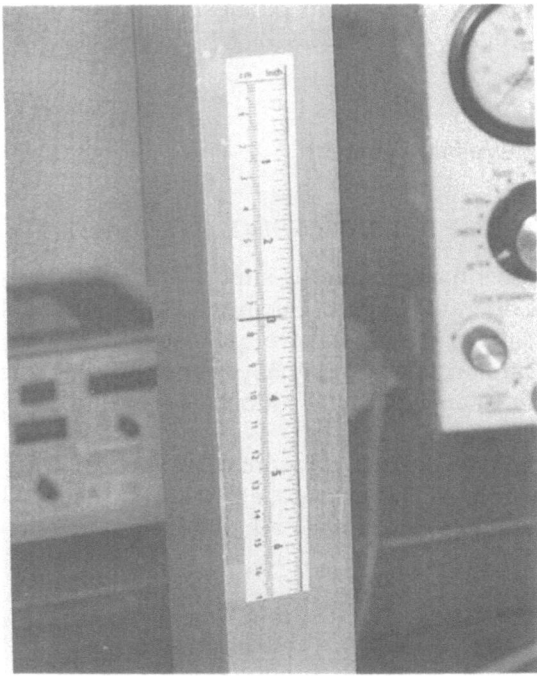

Figure 8.3 A marker attached to the infant's bed or incubator indicates the maximum length of tube which can be passed safely through the mouth for aspiration of pharyngeal secretion without causing injury to the oesophageal anastomosis.

responsible for informing the parents of the completion of the procedure.

Frequent discussion with the parents throughout the postoperative period continues to be of great importance, and the mother should be encouraged to visit and hold her baby at the first opportunity. Early involvement of the medical social worker provides great support to the family as a whole: this involvement may continue for many months (Chapter 19).

8.4.4 NUTRITION

The nutritional requirements of the baby must be respected and oral feeding should be commenced as soon as possible. Full-term babies should be able to feed orally from the third or fourth postoperative day, and in premature babies a transanastomotic tube can be passed at the time of operation, or when it is evident that the anastomosis has healed. This permits early gavage feeding.

If for any reason gastrostomy has been performed, alimentation is commenced via this route. In those with a gastrostomy because the gap between the oesophageal segments was too great to achieve an early primary anastomosis, relatively large feeds are offered to facilitate gastro-oesophageal reflux in the belief that this may enhance the growth of the lower oesophageal segment.

Where delay in the commencement of enteral feeding is anticipated, intravenous nutrition should be employed. In infants this can be administered through a peripheral intravenous line. The nutritional support given must take into account the rapidly changing requirements of the neonate according to his age and gestation.

8.4.5 CONTRAST STUDY OF OESOPHAGUS

A barium contrast study of the oesophagus should be performed to evaluate the calibre of the anastomosis, assess the degree of dysmotility of the distal oesophagus, and determine the presence and severity of gastro-oesophageal reflux. This should be done before the infant is discharged from hospital. It is reasonable to perform the barium study before commencing oral feeds, particularly if an anastomotic leak is suspected. It is usual to see some narrowing of the oesophagus at the anastomosis (Figure 8.4).

8.4.6 GENERAL OBSERVATIONS

During the postoperative period, close observation of the whole baby is required, bearing in mind that there may be other congenital anomalies not yet diagnosed. The vital signs, respiratory status and fluid balance (including urine output) are monitored. Where a chest drain has been used, its drainage should be checked. Normally, a small amount of serosanguinous fluid is drained during the first day, after which there is no drainage; the appearance of saliva in the tubing is diagnostic of anastomotic disruption.

Complications which must be recognized early are described in full in Chapter 21. In addition to respiratory and cardiovascular complications, complications associated with congenital anomalies and a number of problems specific to oesophageal atresia may also occur. These include anastomotic disruption, oesophageal stricture, recurrent tracheo-oesophageal fistula and severe tracheomalacia.

In close liaison with the nursing staff and social worker, the surgeon should ensure that he or she maintains good communication with the

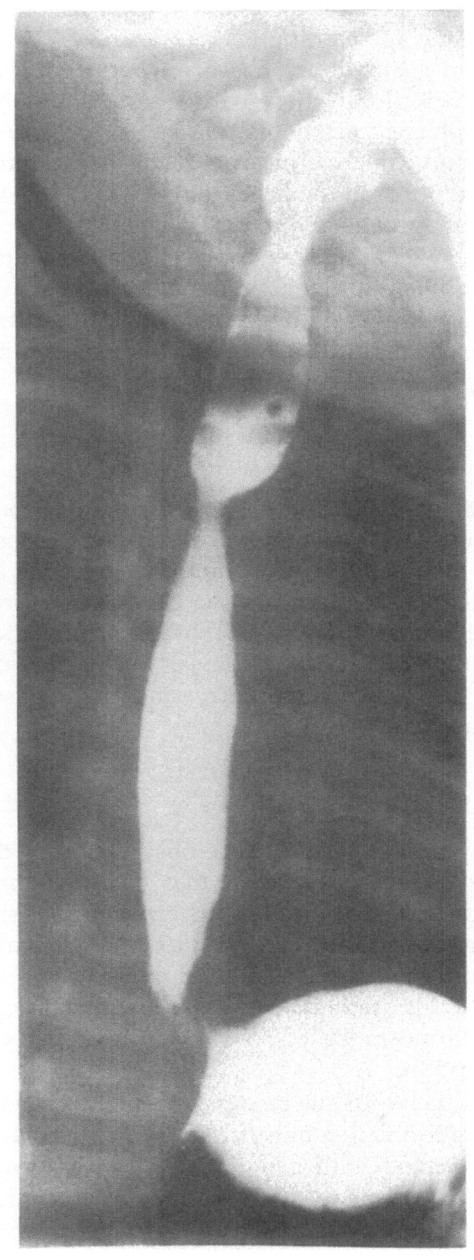

Figure 8.4 Early postoperative barium study of the oesophagus. Some narrowing of the oesophagus at the level of the anastomosis is common.

parents, and informs them of the infant's progress. The parents should receive at least a daily 'medical bulletin', indicating the baby's condition.

References

Beasley, S. W. and Tibballs, J. (1987) Efficacy and safety of continuous morphine infusion for postoperative analgesia in the paediatric surgical ward. *Aust. N. Z. J. Surg.*, **57**, 233–7.

Brown, T. C. K. and Fisk, G. S. (1979) *Anaesthesia for Children*, Blackwells Scientific Publishers, Oxford, pp. 154–8.

PART FOUR
Surgical Aspects

9 Oesophageal atresia with distal tracheo-oesophageal fistula

S. W. BEASLEY and A. W. AULDIST

In the most common variant of oesophageal atresia, the proximal oesophagus ends as a blind upper pouch and there is a distal tracheo-oesophageal fistula (Figure 9.1). The distal oesophagus joins the posterior aspect of the trachea, usually in the lower half of its intrathoracic part.

In oesophageal atresia with a distal tracheo-oesophageal fistula, the aim of treatment should be early total correction of the congenital abnormality with minimal complications and satisfactory long-term

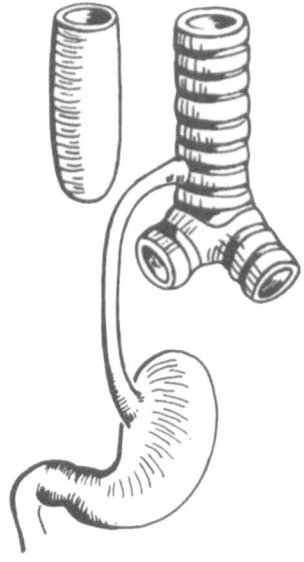

Figure 9.1 Oesophageal atresia with distal tracheo-oesophageal fistula.

function. In the early days of surgical experience with this condition it was appropriate to correct the anomaly in stages, particularly in premature or sick infants, but now that there is better supportive care available, the requirement for staged procedures is rare (Beasley *et al.*, 1989; Randolph *et al.*, 1989). Morbidity has been reduced to a minimum and mortality is essentially that of severe concomitant congenital anomalies.

9.1 Incidence

Oesophageal atresia with a distal tracheo-oesophageal fistula has occurred in 498 of our 584 patients. It is the commonest variant in all reported series (Table 9.1), ranging from 81 to 92%.

Table 9.1 Incidence of oesophageal atresia with distal tracheo-oesophageal fistula

Author	Year	Total number of cases	%
Spitz *et al.*	1987	148	85.0
Holder *et al.*	1964	1058	86.5
Bishop *et al.*	1985	295	92.0
German *et al.*	1976	102	81.4
Louhimo and Lindahl	1983	500	88.2
Waterston *et al.*	1962	218	87.0
Haight	1957	200	85.5
Strodel *et al.*	1979	365	85.9
RCH Melbourne	1988	584	85.0

9.2 Surgical anatomy

The surgeon should be aware of the range of anatomical variants. There may be wide separation of the ends with the upper oesophagus reaching just into the mediastinum, and occasionally the lower oesophagus enters the lower trachea at the carina. The upper oesophagus is comparatively thick-walled and has a diameter at least twice that of the distal oesophagus. This is because the upper oesophagus has been distended with swallowed amniotic fluid during intrauterine life, whereas the distal oesophagus has remained relatively empty. The lower oesophagus enters the posterior aspect of the trachea, and despite misleading illustrations in some publications which portray a narrow 'fistula' into the trachea, the oesophagus actually joins the trachea without any diminution in its calibre. The vagal nerves occupy their usual position in relation to the oesophagus and traverse the back of the trachea if there is separation of the ends. In some instances, the muscle of the upper oesophagus blends with that of the lower oesophagus obscuring the point of atresia; this necessitates careful definition of the anatomy, with a catheter in the upper oesophagus, before the fistula is divided and the upper oesophagus is opened.

9.3 Preoperative care

The patient is nursed in the Intensive Care Unit, in an open cot with an overhead heater and temperature control. The upper pouch is kept empty by suction at 10–15 minute intervals, or more frequently if necessary, while the patient is assessed for other anomalies and for complications such as aspiration. A peripheral line is inserted for intravenous access. The patient is given preoperative antibiotics (penicillin and gentamicin) in a single dose so there are adequate blood levels at the time of operation. Blood is crossmatched, although it is not usually required at operation (Chapter 8 provides further details of preoperative care).

9.3.1 VENTILATORY REQUIREMENTS

Endotracheal intubation is not usually necessary in the preoperative period but is used at the time of anaesthesia and care is taken not to over-inflate the stomach. In patients with severe lung disease, as in severe prematurity, the requirement for increased inspiratory pressure means that gastric distension is more likely to occur. Nevertheless, the provision of adequate oxygenation of the patient at all times is of paramount importance. The anaesthetic techniques are described fully in Chapter 8.

9.4 The operative procedure

9.4.1 POSITION

The infant is placed in the full lateral position with the right side uppermost, with a small towel folded underneath the body to give lateral flexion, and adhesive tape across the infant at the level of the iliac crest to secure the patient in position (Figure 9.2). The right arm is raised

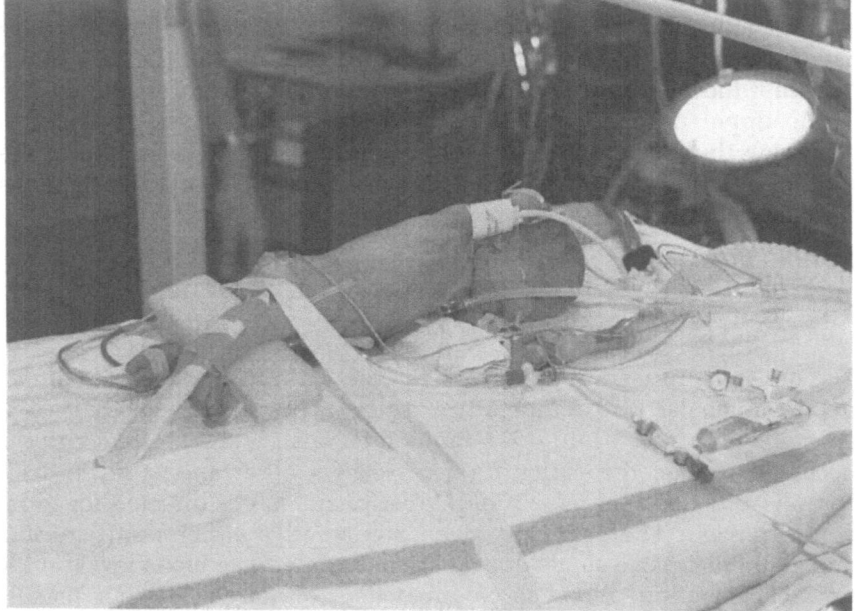

Figure 9.2   Position for thoracotomy: full lateral position with right side upper-most. Note the small towel folded underneath the body to give lateral flexion, and adhesive tape across the iliac crest for stability.

and allowed to lie on the head. This rotates the inferior angle of the scapula laterally to facilitate the thoracic approach. The anaesthetist must be assured of sufficient access so that a size 10 French tube can be inserted into the mouth to demonstrate the upper oesophagus during the operation without risk of displacement of the endotracheal tube.

9.4.2   INCISION AND APPROACH

A transverse incision is made just below the angle of the scapula (Figure 9.3) and after division of the latissimus dorsi muscle in the line of incision, the posterior fibres of the serratus anterior are divided as low as possible in the incision. To achieve this, the lower edge of the wound and divided latissimus dorsi are retracted inferiorly, and the serratus anterior separated from its origin on the chest wall with diathermy dissection. In this way the muscle remains fully innervated, as its supply from the long thoracic nerve courses from above and runs vertically downwards near its free posterior border. The chest is entered in the

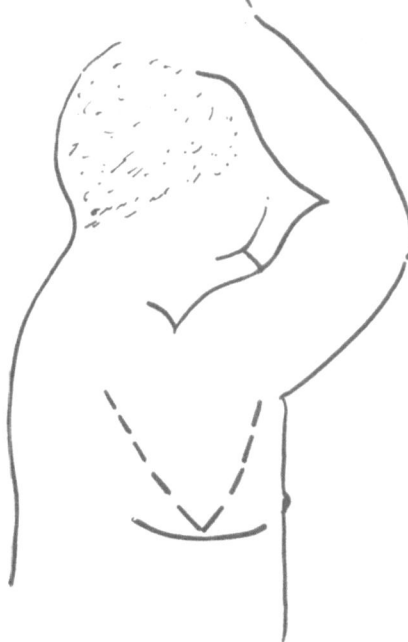

Figure 9.3 The incision, centred on the inferior angle of the scapula when the arm is placed over the right ear.

fourth or fifth intercostal space by dividing the intercostal muscles with diathermy. The dissection is stopped short of the pleura to allow mobilization in the extrapleural plane. The pleura is gently swept from the inner aspect of the chest wall. An intercostal retractor is inserted and extrapleural dissection continued until the posterior mediastinum is exposed. The azygos vein is readily identified: right-angled forceps passed beneath it (Figure 9.4) pick up 3/0 polyglycolic acid sutures between which the vein is then divided.

9.4.3 DIVISION OF THE FISTULA

The lower oesophagus can usually be identified in front of the aorta after incision with scissors of the fine endothoracic fascia of the posterior mediastinum. Identification is helped by seeing distension of the fistula during the inspiratory phase of anaesthesia. The first dissection around the lower oesophagus should be to identify the angle between the back of the trachea and the oesophagus (Figure 9.5), but on occasions this may not be readily identified, and a greater length of lower oesophagus

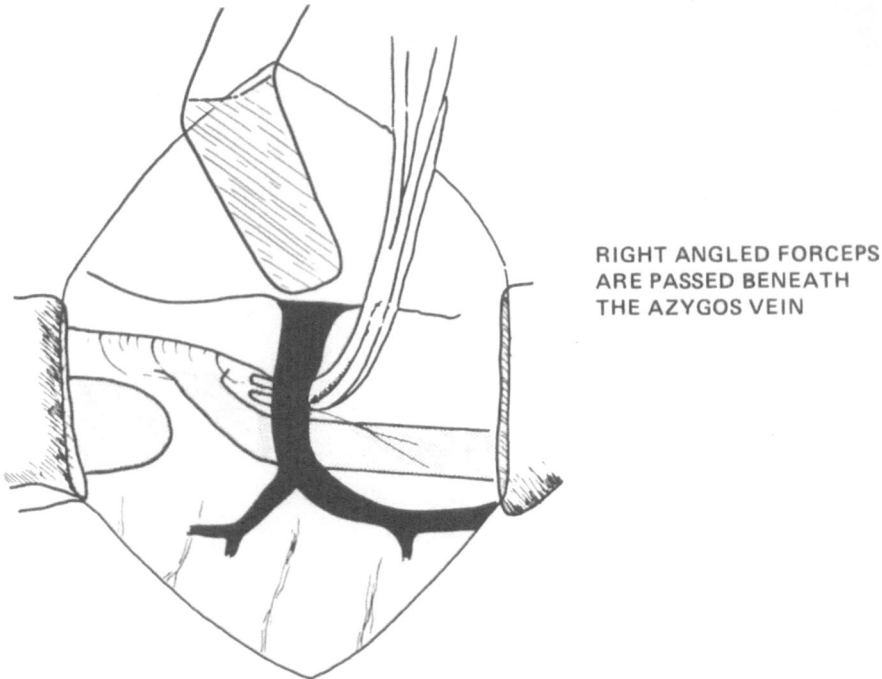

RIGHT ANGLED FORCEPS
ARE PASSED BENEATH
THE AZYGOS VEIN

Figure 9.4   Right-angled forceps passed beneath the azygos vein pick up 3/0 polyglycoglic acid sutures between which the vein is divided.

may need to be exposed. A vascular sling is passed around the upper part of the lower oesophagus after dissection has identified the angle between the lower oesophagus and the trachea (Figure 9.6). Care must be taken to avoid damage to the vagus nerve and the blood supply of the oesophagus. Once the sling has been positioned, gentle upward traction can be used to impede air escape from the trachea through the fistula, a

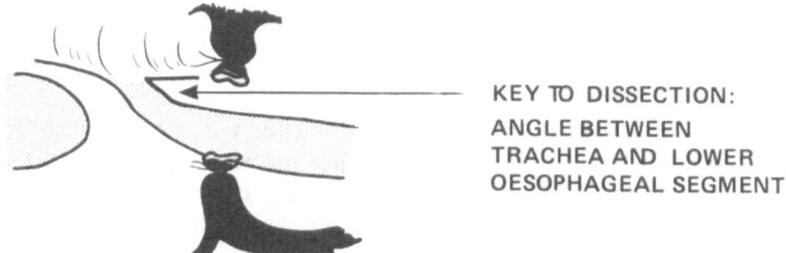

KEY TO DISSECTION:

ANGLE BETWEEN
TRACHEA AND LOWER
OESOPHAGEAL SEGMENT

Figure 9.5   The junction of trachea and distal oesophagus must be demonstrated.

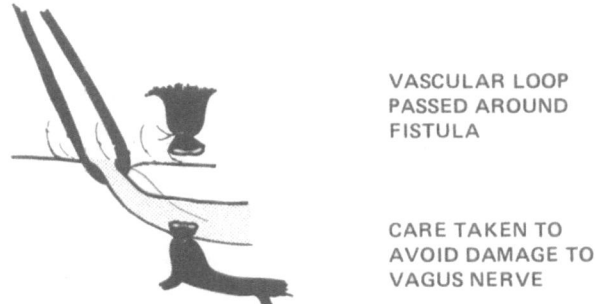

VASCULAR LOOP
PASSED AROUND
FISTULA

CARE TAKEN TO
AVOID DAMAGE TO
VAGUS NERVE

Figure 9.6 A vascular sling is passed around the tracheo-oesophageal fistula.

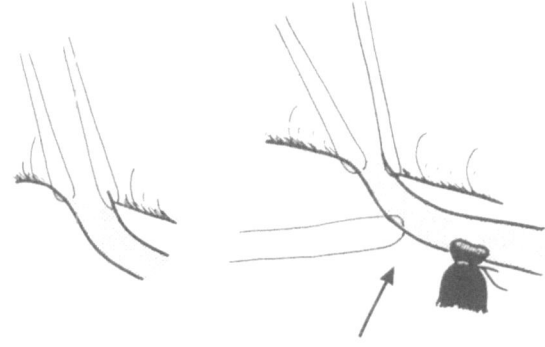

STAY SUTURE ON LOWER
SEGMENT (IF REQUIRED)

Figure 9.7 Two 4/0 polyglycolic acid sutures are placed on each side of the tracheo-oesophageal fistula prior to its division. These act as stay sutures and tend to reduce the air leak through the fistula.

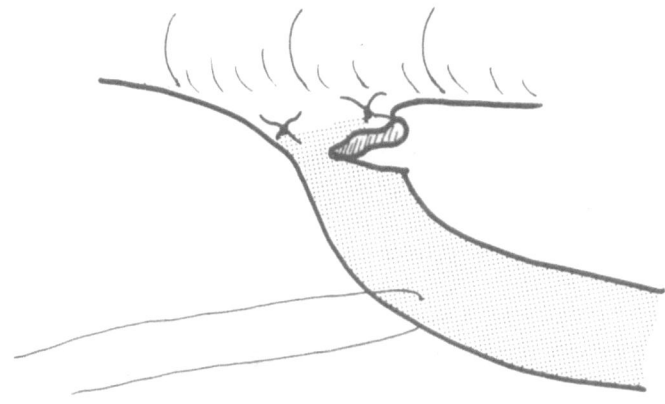

Figure 9.8 The two stay sutures are tied before the fistula is divided.

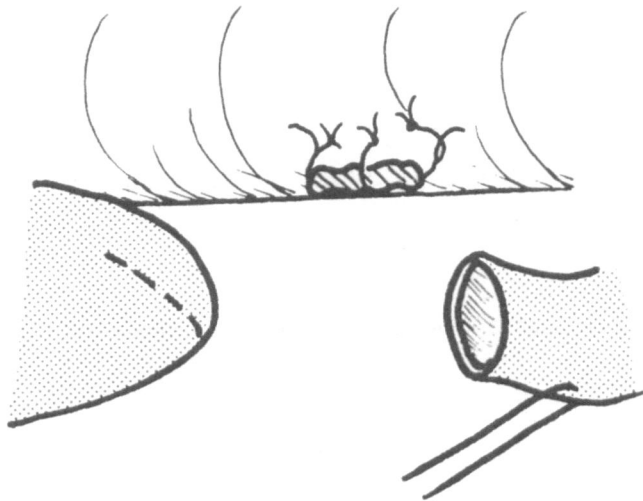

Figure 9.9 The fistula is closed with interrupted 4/0 polyglycolic acid sutures leaving about 3 mm of fistula at the tracheal end. The site of the upper pouch oesophagotomy is shown by the dotted line.

manoeuvre which may help ventilatory mechanics. Two 4/0 polyglycolic acid sutures are placed in the tracheal end of the lower oesophagus and tied to effect partial closure of the fistula before it is completely divided (Figures 9.7 and 9.8). The oesophagus is divided, leaving about 3 mm of fistula at the tracheal end. The fistula is then closed completely with interrupted 4/0 or 5/0 polyglycolic acid sutures; a stay suture inserted in the distal oesophagus is useful to limit further handling (Figure 9.9).

9.4.4 THE UPPER OESOPHAGUS

The upper oesophageal pouch is readily located when the anaesthetist passes a size 8 French nasogastric tube through the mouth into the oesophagus. As soon as the upper pouch is identified a stay suture is placed through its most distal part. This stay suture assists subsequent mobilization and avoids unnecessary handling of (and trauma to) the oesophagus.

The decision is now made as to whether further dissection of the upper oesophagus will be required, as this should be done only where there is a significant distance between the ends. Mobilization of the upper oesophagus commences with dissection of its posterior aspect: the most difficult dissection is between the upper oesophagus and the trachea. Continuity of the two structures by fibrous bands is often the cause of difficulty and is best addressed by sharp dissection, with care being taken not to enter the lumen of either the trachea or oesophagus. Mobilization of the upper oesophagus can be continued up into the neck as far as necessary, and apart from the posterior aspect, is readily achieved using pledgets.

9.4.5 THE ANASTOMOSIS

The oesophageal segments are united by an end-to-end interrupted anastomosis, in which the posterior medial portion of the anastomosis is completed first. A small disc of the upper oesophagus is excised at the site of the previously inserted stay suture at its apex (and sent for histological examination). Three interrupted 5/0 polyglycolic acid sutures are placed in the postero-medial aspect of the oesophagus (Figure 9.10). Each suture is accurately placed through all layers of each segment, taking moderately large 'bites' of tissue. Special care must be taken to ensure that the mucosal layer of the upper pouch of the oesophagus is included, as this tends to retract upwards out of view when the upper pouch is opened. When all three sutures have been placed, the two oesophageal ends are gently apposed and the sutures

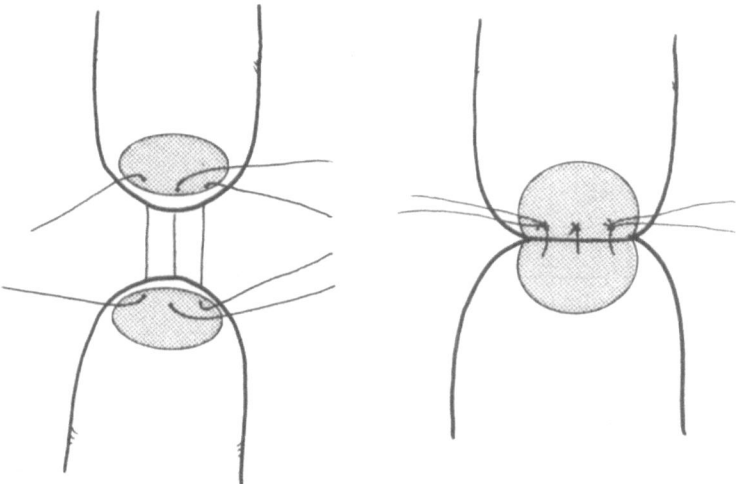

Figure 9.10 The end-to-end oesophageal anastomosis: the posteromedial layer is completed first. When all posteromedial sutures have been inserted, the two oesophageal ends are gently apposed and the sutures tied on the mucosal surface.

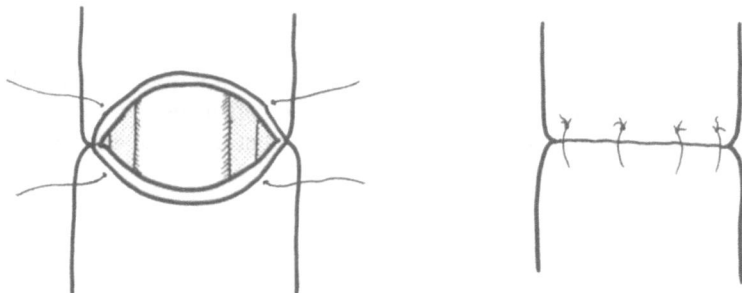

Figure 9.11   A nasogastric tube is passed through the partially completed anastomosis before the anterolateral sutures are inserted.

tied on the mucosal surface (Beasley *et al.*, 1989). The size 8 French nasogastric tube can now be passed beyond the upper pouch temporarily into the lower oesophagus before the anastomosis is completed. The anterior and lateral sutures, 4–6 in number and using 5/0 polyglycolic acid, are inserted, including all layers but with the knot tied on the outside (Figure 9.11).

Other methods of anastomosis, which involve an end-to-side anastomosis after ligation or transfixion of the fistula, have an unacceptable incidence of recurrent tracheo-oesophageal fistula and no demonstrable benefit (Chapter 21). Furthermore, they decrease the mobility of the oesophagus, limiting their application in long gap oesophageal atresia. We strongly recommend the simple end-to-end anastomosis as described.

9.4.6   CLOSURE

Before closure is commenced, the thoracic cavity is irrigated with warm antibiotic saline solution, which also enables confirmation that there is no air leakage from the closed fistula.

It has been customary to leave a small drain tube in the extrapleural plane in case of oesophageal anastomotic leak, but this is probably unnecessary where a good anastomosis without excessive tension has been accomplished. The intercostal space is closed with interrupted polyglycolic acid sutures placed around the fourth and fifth ribs. If no drain has been used, the anaesthetist fully expands the lung before the last intercostal suture is tied, so that extrapleural air can escape. The muscles are closed in layers, the serratus anterior being reattached at its origin. The skin is closed with a 5/0 subcuticular polyglycolic acid suture (Figure 9.12).

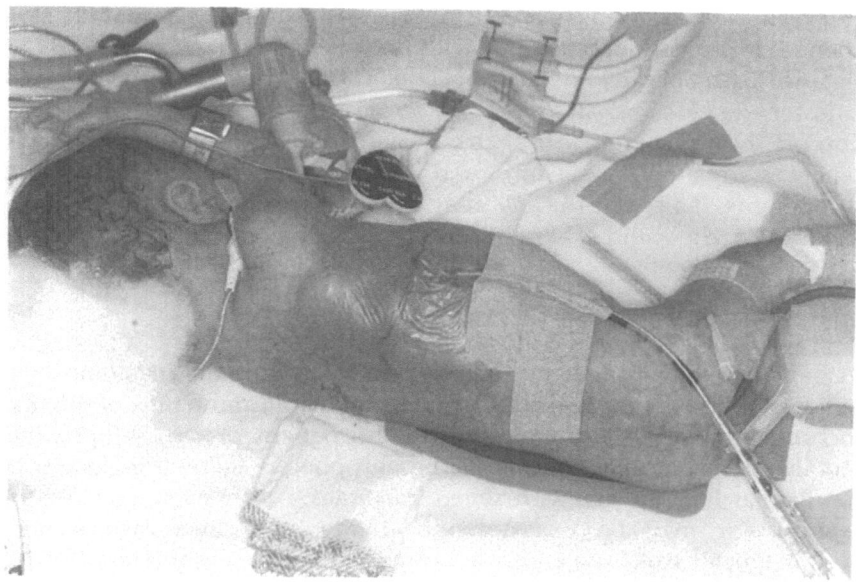

Figure 9.12 Completion of the operation. Where a good anastomosis has been accomplished an extrapleural chest drain is probably unnecessary.

9.5 Intraoperative difficulties

9.5.1 IDENTIFICATION OF LOWER OESOPHAGUS

The location of the lower oesophagus may not be immediately apparent and occasionally dissection down to the level of the carina may be necessary, or the oesophagus may be identified at a lower level in the chest and traced upwards. The vagus nerves act as a guide to the lower oesophagus. These nerves can be recognized as white fibres which leave the posterolateral aspect of the trachea to sweep downwards and encompass the lower oesophagus. It is important not to divide or apply traction to the fibres during dissection at the tracheo-oesophageal junction.

9.5.2 RIGHT AORTIC ARCH

A right aortic arch may be suspected on the plain film of the chest, or by preoperative echocardiography which is now carried out on most patients. If a right aortic arch is diagnosed with certainty preoperatively, it is recommended that operation is through a left thoracotomy, as a 'mirror image'. If the right arch is not recognized until the right chest is opened, it is possible to proceed with the anastomosis in the majority of instances. An operative decision will determine whether an anastomosis is best made medial to and below the aortic arch or lateral to (on the right side of) the right arch. An anastomosis to the right of a right arch is usually completely satisfactory, and does not cause compression of the oesophagus. It also has the advantage of being relatively easy to perform when the arch would otherwise obscure the level of the anastomosis.

9.5.3   THE LONG GAP

In our view it should always be possible to perform an anastomosis in patients with oesophageal atresia and distal fistula at the time of the first thoracotomy unless the condition of the patient precludes operative mobilization and anastomosis of the oesophagus following closure of the fistula. In a patient with severe respiratory distress syndrome, for example, it may be necessary to divide and close the tracheo-oesophageal fistula, and attach the closed lower oesophagus to the region of the paravertebral fascia. Anastomosis is then performed when the baby's condition will tolerate a second thoracotomy.

In other patients with a significant gap our recommendation is first to mobilize the upper oesophagus well up into the neck through the thoracotomy incision. As described previously, the most difficult part of this dissection is separation of the trachea from the upper oesophagus. If the upper oesophageal mobilization does not enable apposition of the oesophageal ends, the next step is gentle mobilization of the lower oesophagus leaving its blood supply intact as much as possible. It is rarely necessary to mobilize the lower oesophagus to a great extent, and even more rarely is a circular myotomy on the upper oesophagus required to obtain more length (Beasley *et al.*, 1989).

9.5.4   CONTINUOUS OESOPHAGUS

Apparent continuity of the upper and lower oesophagus at thoracotomy sometimes leads the surgeon to believe that his preoperative diagnosis was incorrect. Realization that the lumen of the oesophagus may be obstructed even though it appears intact externally, enables the correct diagnosis to be made. Obstruction to the advance of a catheter in the upper oesophagus helps to clarify the pathology. After the diagnosis has been established it is possible to perform an anastomosis with minimal dissection and minimal disruption of the nerve and vascular supply of the oesophagus.

9.5.5 DOUBLE FISTULA

At the time of dissection of the upper oesophagus the surgeon needs to be aware of the possibility of a second (upper pouch) fistula. This fistula may be transverse or oblique, extending upwards from the oesophagus to the trachea. Distension of the upper oesophagus during ventilatory inspiration may alert the surgeon to this possibility. It may also be encountered if mobilization of the upper pouch is required after division of the distal fistula. In our series the anomaly has been encountered infrequently (2 cases out of 584). In some centres where routine preoperative endoscopy is performed, a double fistula can be diagnosed during bronchoscopy; our experience of the rarity of the double fistula has led us to refrain from routine contrast radiography.

9.6 Extreme prematurity

The extremely premature infant is likely to develop severe hyaline membrane disease (HMD). This poses a particular problem if the infant has oesophageal atresia as well: should the distal tracheo-oesophageal fistula be divided before the HMD becomes fully established (at 24–48 h), or should the infant be ventilated until the HMD resolves before the fistula is controlled? The danger with the latter approach is that adequate ventilation of an infant with severe HMD may require high pressures over a prolonged period and is only effective if the airway resistance is lower than that of the fistula (Holmes *et al.*, 1987); if the fistula acts as a 'low-resistance vent' (Filston *et al.*, 1982), and there is major escape of air through it, ventilation becomes inadequate and the stomach distends with air (Figure 9.13) (Malone *et al.*, 1990). The consequences of this can be disastrous (Figure 9.14) with gastric perforation (Jones *et al.*, 1980), pneumoperitoneum, elevation of the diaphragm with splinting, hypoxia, cardiac arrest (Baraka and Slim, 1970) and death.

If a gastrostomy has been constructed, there may be preferential passage of air through the fistula, and satisfactory ventilation becomes impossible (Karl, 1985). To overcome this, other manoeuvres have been described. These include: distal positioning of the endotracheal tube with the bevel facing anteriorly to occlude the fistula (Salem *et al.*, 1973); retrograde placement of a balloon catheter in the lower oesophagus (Kadowaki *et al.*, 1982; Karl, 1985); bronchoscopic placement of a Fogarty balloon catheter in the fistula (Filston *et al.*, 1982); silastic banding of the oesophagus (Leininger, 1972) or gastric division (Randolph *et al.*, 1968). These manoeuvres are either unreliable in their effect or excessively

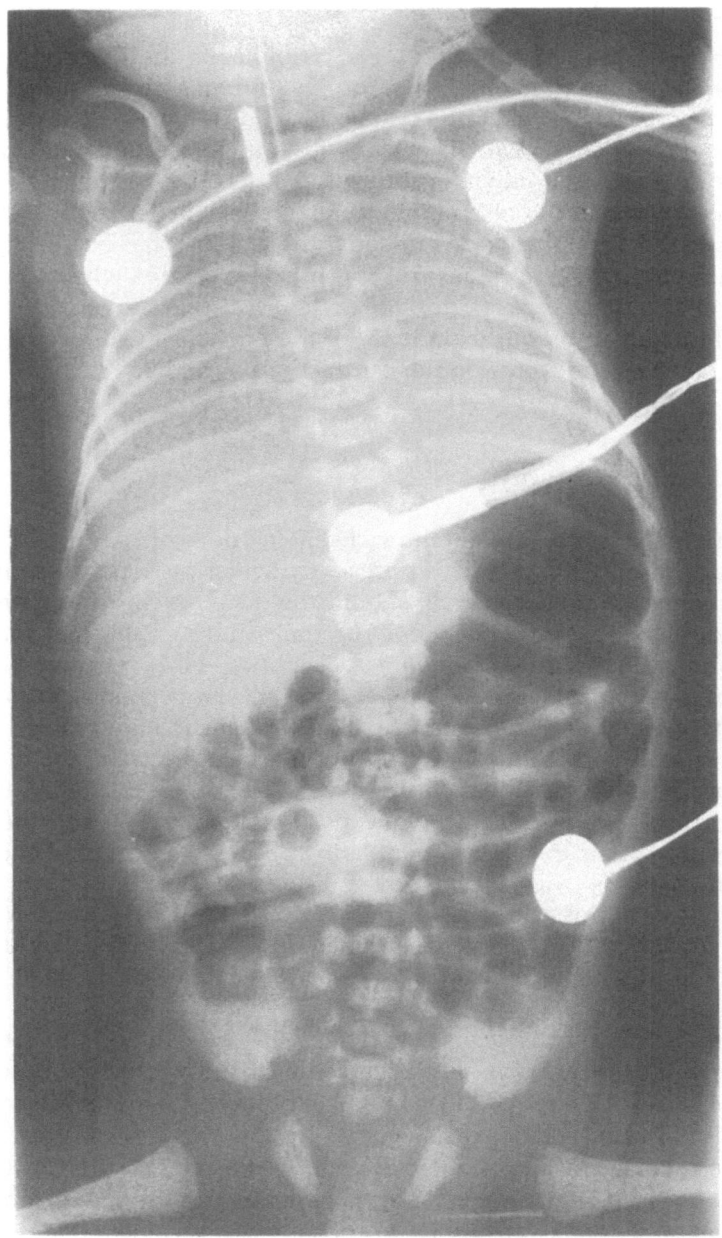

Figure 9.13 Severe hyaline membrane disease in a very premature infant with oesophageal atresia. The infant required endotracheal intubation and assisted ventilation.

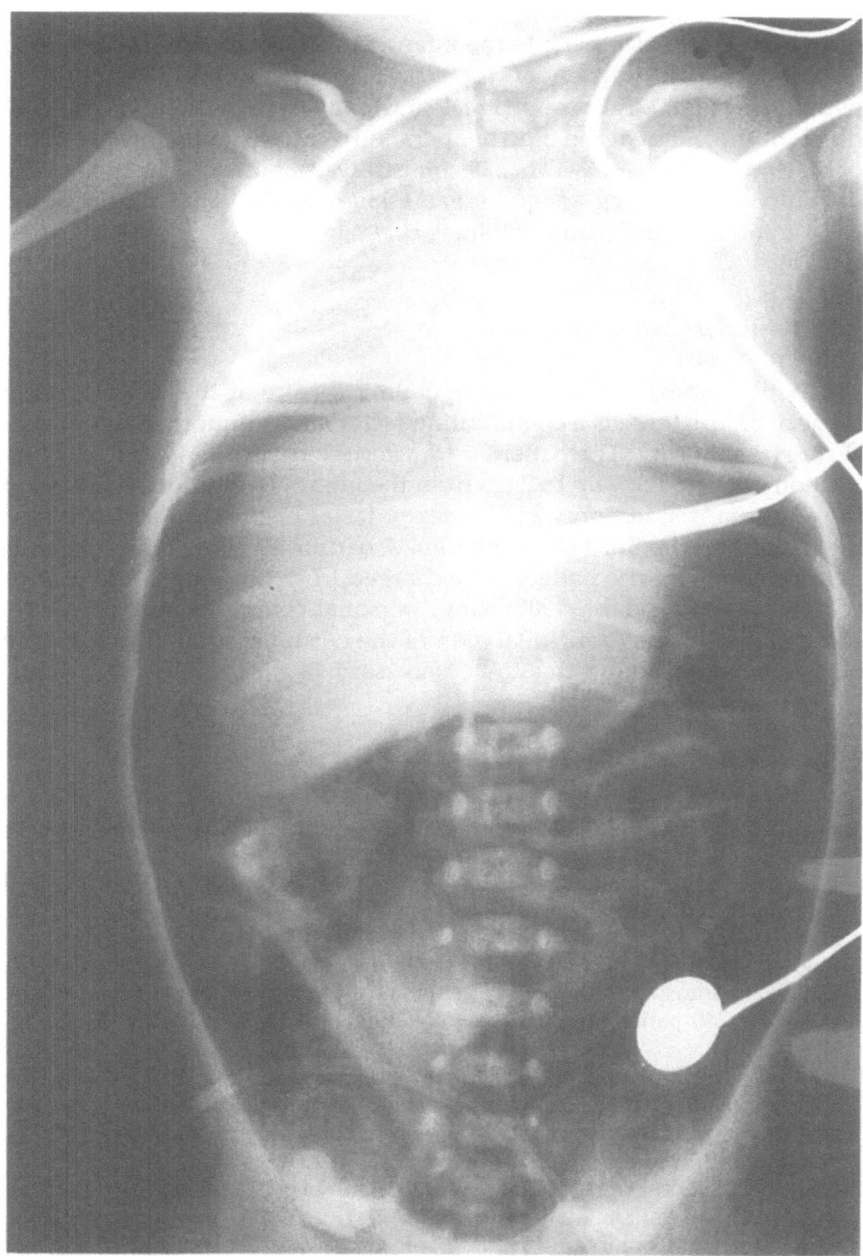

Figure 9.14 Ruptured stomach with gross pneumoperitoneum and elevation of the diaphragm. (Same patient as in Figure 9.13.) This illustrates the danger of failure to control a distal tracheo-oesophageal fistula early in infants likely to develop severe hyaline membrane disease.

complicated and traumatic to the infant. For these reasons, we prefer to undertake early division of the fistula via a thoracotomy (with or without simultaneous oesophageal anastomosis, depending on the condition of the infant at the time of operation) – ideally in the first 12 hours of life and before the HMD has become fully established. The greater the difficulty in achieving adequate gas exchange, the more urgent is the need to occlude the fistula (Holmes *et al.*, 1987).

9.7 Postoperative management

The patient is extubated in the operating theatre at the completion of surgery unless there is a complicating factor such as another anomaly or severe prematurity. The patient is transferred to the Intensive Care Unit. Suction is carried out up to 7 cm from the mouth (well above the level of the anastomosis) but only as necessary. It has been our practice to feed the patient on the third or fourth day. A barium swallow examination is performed before the patient is discharged from hospital. Some centres (Louhimo and Lindahl, 1983; King, personal communication) have recommended prophylactic dilatation of the oesophagus at an early stage but we have not found this to be necessary.

References

Baraka, A. and Slim, M. (1970) Cardiac arrest during IPPV in a newborn with tracheoesophageal fistula. *Anesthesiology*, **32**, 564–5.

Beasley, S. W., Auldist, A. W. and Myers, N. A. (1989) Current surgical management of oesophageal atresia and tracheo-oesophageal fistula. *Aust. N. Z. J. Surg.*, **59**, 707–12.

Bishop, P. J., Klein, M. D., Philippart, A. I., Hixson, D. S. and Hertzler, J. H. (1985) Transpleural repair of esophageal atresia without a primary gastrostomy: 240 patients treated between 1951 and 1983. *J. Pediatr. Surg.*, **20**, 823–8.

Filston, H. C., Chitwood, W. R., Schkolne, B. and Blackmon, L. R. (1982) The Fogarty balloon catheter as an aid to management of the infant with esophageal atresia and tracheoesophageal fistula complicated by severe RDS or pneumonia. *J. Pediatr. Surg.*, **17**, 149–51.

German, J. C., Mahour, G. H. and Woolley, M. M. (1976) Esophageal atresia and associated anomalies. *J. Pediatr. Surg.*, **11**, 299–306.

Haight, C. (1957) Some observations on esophageal atresias and tracheoesophageal fistulas of congenital origin. *J. Thorac. Surg.*, **34**, 141–72.

Holder, T. M., Cloud, D. T., Lewis, J. E. Jr and Pilling, G. P. (1964) Esophageal atresia and tracheoesophageal fistula. *Pediatrics*, **34**, 542–9.

Holmes, S. J. K., Kiely, E. M. and Spitz, L. (1987) Tracheo-oesophageal fistula and the respiratory distress syndrome. *Pediatr. Surg. Int.*, **2**, 16–18.

Jones, T. B., Kirchner, S. G., Lee, F. A. and Heller, R. M. (1980) Stomach rupture associated with esophageal atresia, tracheoesophageal fistula and ventilatory assistance. *Am. J. Radiol.*, **134**, 675–7.

Kadowaki, H., Nakahira, M., Umeda, K., Yamada, C., Takeuchi, S. and Tamate, S. (1982) A method of delayed esophageal anastomosis for high-risk congenital esophageal atresia with additional intra-abdominal anomalies: transgastric balloon 'fistulectomy'. *J. Pediatr. Surg.*, **17**, 230–3.

Karl, H. W. (1985) Control of life-threatening air leak after gastrostomy in an infant with respiratory distress syndrome and tracheoesophageal fistula. *Anesthesiology*, **62**, 670–2.

Leininger, B. J. (1972) Silastic banding of esophagus with subsequent repair of esophageal atresia and tracheoesophageal fistula. *J. Pediatr. Surg.*, **7**, 404–7.

Louhimo, I. and Lindahl, H. (1983) Esophageal atresia: primary results of 500 consecutively treated patients. *J. Pediatr. Surg.*, **18**, 217–29.

Malone, P. S., Kiely, E. M., Brain, A. J. *et al.* (1990) Tracheo-oesophageal fistula and preoperative mechanical ventilation. *Aust. N. Z. J. Surg.*, **60**, 525–7.

Randolph, J. G., Tunnell, W. P. and Lilly, J. R. (1968) Gastric division in the critically ill infant with esophageal atresia and tracheoesophageal fistula. *Surgery*, **63**, 496–502.

Randolph, J. G., Neuman, K. D. and Anderson, K. D. (1989) Current results in repair of esophageal atresia with tracheoesophageal fistula using physiological status as a guide to therapy. *Ann. Surg.*, **209**, 526–31.

Salem, M. R., Wong, A. Y., Lin, Y. H., Firor, H. V. and Bennett, E. J. (1973) Prevention of gastric distension during anaesthesia for newborns with tracheoesophageal fistulas. *Anesthesiology*, **38**, 82–3.

Spitz, L., Kiely, E. and Brereton, R. J. (1987) Esophageal atresia: five year experience with 148 cases. *J. Pediatr. Surg.*, **22**, 103–8.

Strodel, W. E., Coran, A. G., Kirsh, M. M., Weintraub, W. H., Wesley, J. R. and Sloan, H. (1979) Esophageal atresia. A 41-year experience. *Arch. Surg.*, **114**, 523–7.

Waterston, D. J., Bonham Carter, R. E. and Aberdeen, E. (1962) Oesophageal atresia: tracheo-oesophageal fistula. A study of survival in 218 infants. *Lancet*, **ii**, 819–82.

10 Oesophageal atresia without fistula

S. W. BEASLEY

In many respects this anatomical variant (Figure 10.1) represents the most difficult type of oesophageal atresia to manage successfully. The main reason for this is that when a fistula is not present there is almost always a long gap between the oesophageal ends, making oesophageal continuity difficult to achieve. Resort to oesophageal replacement is sometimes necessary, despite the relatively high rate of complications.

Until the 1960s it was generally considered that oesophageal anastomosis in this group was rarely, if ever, possible and survival depended on the establishment of a salivary fistula in the neck (cervical oesophagostomy) and a gastrostomy for feeding. Oesophageal replacement was then undertaken when the child was about 10 kg in weight. These procedures enabled survival in a number of patients who would otherwise have died; but at a cost of considerable morbidity. The concept of staged management which had been introduced originally by Holder *et al.* (1962) and Koop and Hamilton (1965) for oesophageal atresia with distal oesophageal fistula was readily applied to the infant with atresia without fistula. At about the same time, upper pouch bouginage was introduced in the belief that this manoeuvre caused elongation of the upper pouch (Howard and Myers, 1965). Subsequently other techniques were developed to elongate the oesophageal segments such as the 'Olive' technique (Rehbein and Schweder, 1971), electromagnetic bouginage (Hendren and Hale, 1975), electromagnetic traction (Schier *et al.*, 1988), and oesophageal myotomy (Livaditis, 1973; Vizas *et al.*, 1978; Ricketts *et al.*, 1981). We now believe that bouginage was of little value except that it encouraged preservation of the upper pouch in infants who would otherwise have had a cervical oesophagostomy and oesophageal replacement (Myers *et al.*, 1987).

Oesophageal preservation with delayed primary oesophago-oesophageal anastomosis is in fact possible in the majority of patients without fistula, although there are some institutions which still prefer to

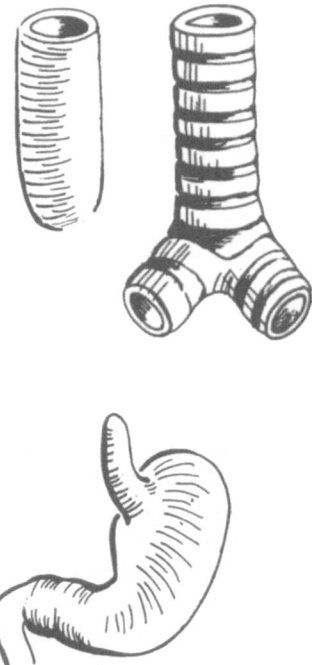

Figure 10.1   Oesophageal atresia without tracheo-oesophageal fistula. The gap between the two oesophageal segments may be extensive, and the stomach is small.

discard the oesophagus and achieve gastrointestinal continuity using stomach, colon or jejunum (Randolph, 1986).

This chapter highlights the clinical features of oesophageal atresia without fistula, the methods by which the gap between the oesophageal segments can be assessed, and the operative technique which in most patients enables direct end-to-end oesophageal anastomosis.

10.1   Incidence

The incidence of oesophageal atresia without fistula ranges from 2–10% in most series (Table 10.1). As a proportion of patients with oesophageal atresia and a gasless abdomen, it ranges from 67–100% (Table 10.2).

Table 10.1 Oesophageal atresia without fistula : incidence

Author (Year)	Total number in series	Isolated oesophageal atresia (%)
Waterston *et al.* (1963)	218	8.7
Holder *et al.* (1964)	1058	7.7
Holder *et al.* (1987)	100	2.0
Louhimo and Lindahl (1983)	500	7.8
Connolly and Guiney (1987)	139	10.0
Strodel *et al.* (1979)	365	7.4
	(353 evaluated)	
German *et al.* (1976)	102	6.0
Haight (1957)	200	10.0
Myers and Aberdeen (1979)	404	7.5
RCH (Melbourne)	584	6.0

10.2 Surgical anatomy

In this variant the gap between the two oesophageal ends is usually extensive. This may make the ends difficult to identify in the chest at operation. Introduction of a catheter into the pouch by the anaesthetist assists in its recognition posterior to the trachea in the superior mediastinum. The lower segment extends a variable distance through the oesophageal hiatus of the diaphragm and is of relatively narrow calibre. It can be identified by dissection of the posterior mediastinum anterior to the descending aorta using the vagal fibres as a guide to its position. Occasionally, the lower segment is so short it does not reach the thorax. This becomes apparent at the time of gastrostomy when an attempt is made to introduce a metal sound into the oesophagus from below (Figure 10.2).

The upper pouch is dilated and thick-walled, and may cause tracheal compression (Gauntlett *et al.*, 1986). The appearance of an intact oesophagus at operation may indicate a membranous interruption of the lumen of the oesophagus with muscular continuity of its wall: this is an extremely rare anomaly and would normally be suspected before thoracotomy.

In the absence of a distal tracheo-oesophageal fistula the stomach is smaller than normal (Figure 10.3). This is the result of inability of the

Table 10.2 The gasless abdomen: proportion of patients with and without proximal fistula

Author (year)	Total number in series	% With airless abdomen	Airless abdomen	
			% With oesophageal atresia alone	% With oesophageal atresia with proximal fistula
Holder et al. (1964)	1058	8.6	90	10
Louhimo and Lindahl (1983)	500	8.0	95	5
German et al. (1976)	102	8.0	75	25
Randolph (1986)	107	9.0	100	0
Spitz et al. (1987)	148	8.8	77	23
Holder et al. (1987)	100	3.0	67	33
RCH Melbourne (1988)	584	8.0	77	23

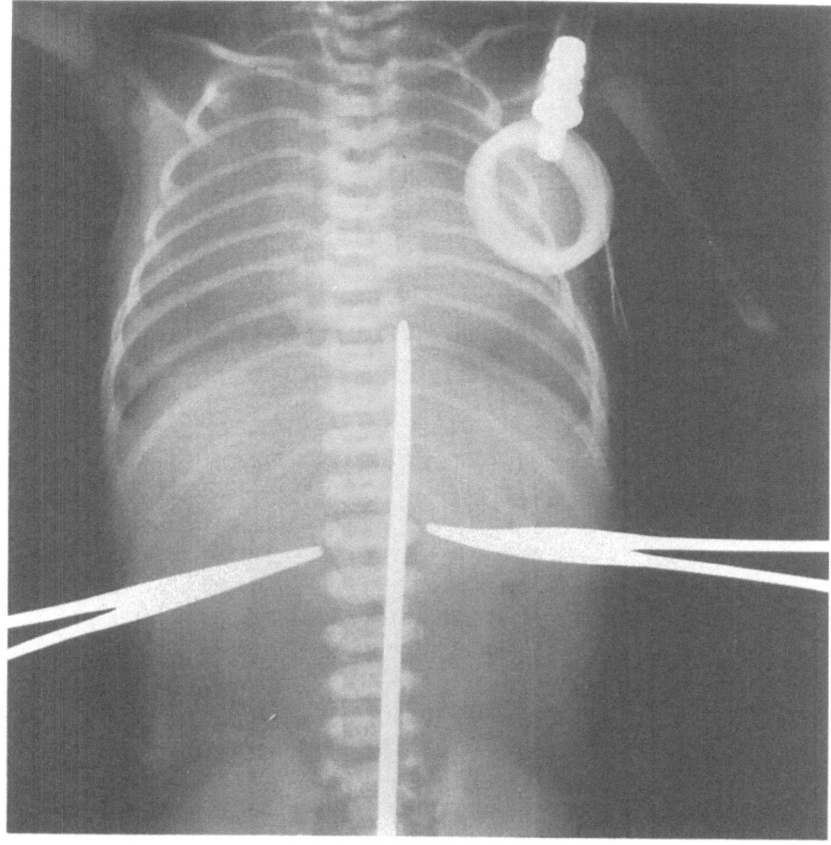

Figure 10.2 In oesophageal atresia without fistula, the lower oesophageal segment is short and may barely reach the thorax.

fetus to swallow amniotic fluid or for fluid to enter the stomach through a distal fistula. The clinical significance relates to the problems a small stomach creates when a gastrostomy is being fashioned without compromising later gastric interposition (if required) or in some patients, when an antireflux operation is required.

10.3 Royal Children's Hospital experience

Oesophageal atresia without fistula was seen in 37 patients (6.4%) of whom 22 had associated congenital anomalies (Table 10.3). Polyhydram-

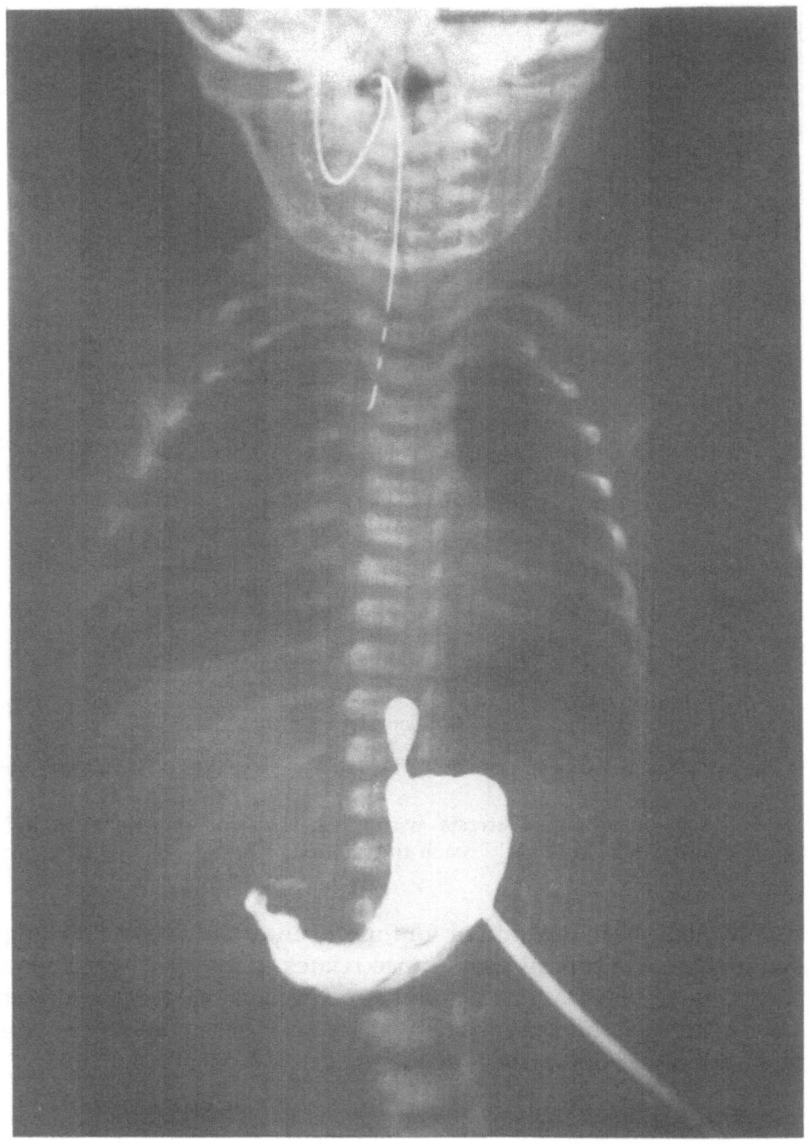

Figure 10.3 When there is no oesophageal continuity or distal tracheo-oesophageal fistula the stomach is smaller than usual. This may create problems when siting the gastrostomy or performing fundoplication.

Table 10.3 Associated congenital abnormalities in 22 of 37 patients with oesophageal atresia without fistula

		No. of cases
Chromosomal aberrations		6
Trisomy 21	5	
Trisomy 18	1	
Gastrointestinal		15
Anorectal	7	
Other	8	
Cardiac (excluding PDA)		8
Genitourinary		6
Skeletal		12
Vertebral	4	
Digital	6	
Other	2	
Miscellaneous: Hydrocephalus, hypospadias, cleft palate, biliary tract abnormality.		

nios was recorded in all but three patients and birth weight ranged from 1.6 to 3.6 kg. Gestation was less than 37 weeks in 18 patients.

Alimentary continuity was achieved in 28 patients. The nine patients who received either no surgery, or gastrostomy and/or oesophagostomy alone, had major associated anomalies which precluded further active measures, or, in the two earliest patients, died before alimentary continuity could be attempted. In the 28 patients in whom alimentary continuity was established 16 had an oesophageal anastomosis, although two of these subsequently required oesophageal replacement as a result of complications. Twelve patients had oesophageal replacement, with no attempt at oesophageal anastomosis, and two had oesophageal replacement following failed oesophageal anastomosis. The overall management and type of replacement are summarized in Figure 10.4. One colonic replacement followed failed gastric tube replacement and one greater curvature gastric tube was constructed after failure of a Rehbein procedure (Rehbein and Schweder, 1971). The patient in whom a polythene prosthetic oesophagus was inserted in 1953 died. Patients in whom oesophageal anastomosis was achieved had less morbidity and have fewer continuing problems than those with oesophageal replacement, although the former group involves most of

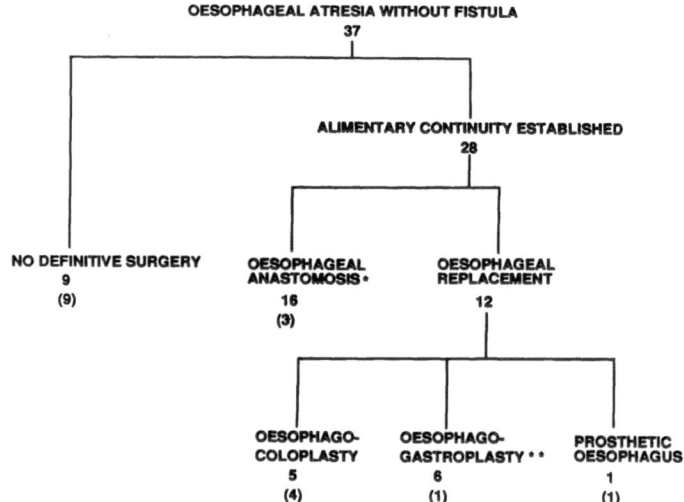

OESOPHAGEAL ATRESIA WITHOUT FISTULA
37

ALIMENTARY CONTINUITY ESTABLISHED
28

NO DEFINITIVE SURGERY
9
(9)

OESOPHAGEAL ANASTOMOSIS *
16
(3)

OESOPHAGEAL REPLACEMENT
12

OESOPHAGO-COLOPLASTY
5
(4)

OESOPHAGO-GASTROPLASTY * *
6
(1)

PROSTHETIC OESOPHAGUS
1
(1)

Figure 10.4 Flow diagram of management of 37 patients with oesophageal atresia without fistula. Number of deaths is indicated in parentheses; *two patients required oesophageal replacement; **one patient required later coloplasty.

the more recent patients. Indeed, oesophageal anastomosis has been successfully achieved in eight of the last 12 patients.

10.4 Diagnosis

The diagnosis of oesophageal atresia without fistula should be considered when an infant with oesophageal atresia proven by failure to pass an orogastric tube into the stomach is noted to have a scaphoid abdomen on clinical examination and no gas in the abdomen on plain X-rays (Figures 10.5 and 10.6). For this reason, every infant with oesophageal atresia should have an X-ray which includes the abdomen. In both the normal child, and the child with a distal tracheo-oesophageal fistula, an abdominal X-ray taken shortly after birth will almost always show some gas below the diaphragm. On the other hand, when there is no communication with the lower oesophagus and stomach the abdomen appears featureless (Figure 10.5).

When a child with oesophageal atresia is shown to have a gasless abdomen the main variant from which oesophageal atresia without fistula has to be distinguished is oesophageal atresia with a proximal tracheo-oesophageal fistula. This latter condition is less common but accounts for 23% of patients with a gasless abdomen in our series

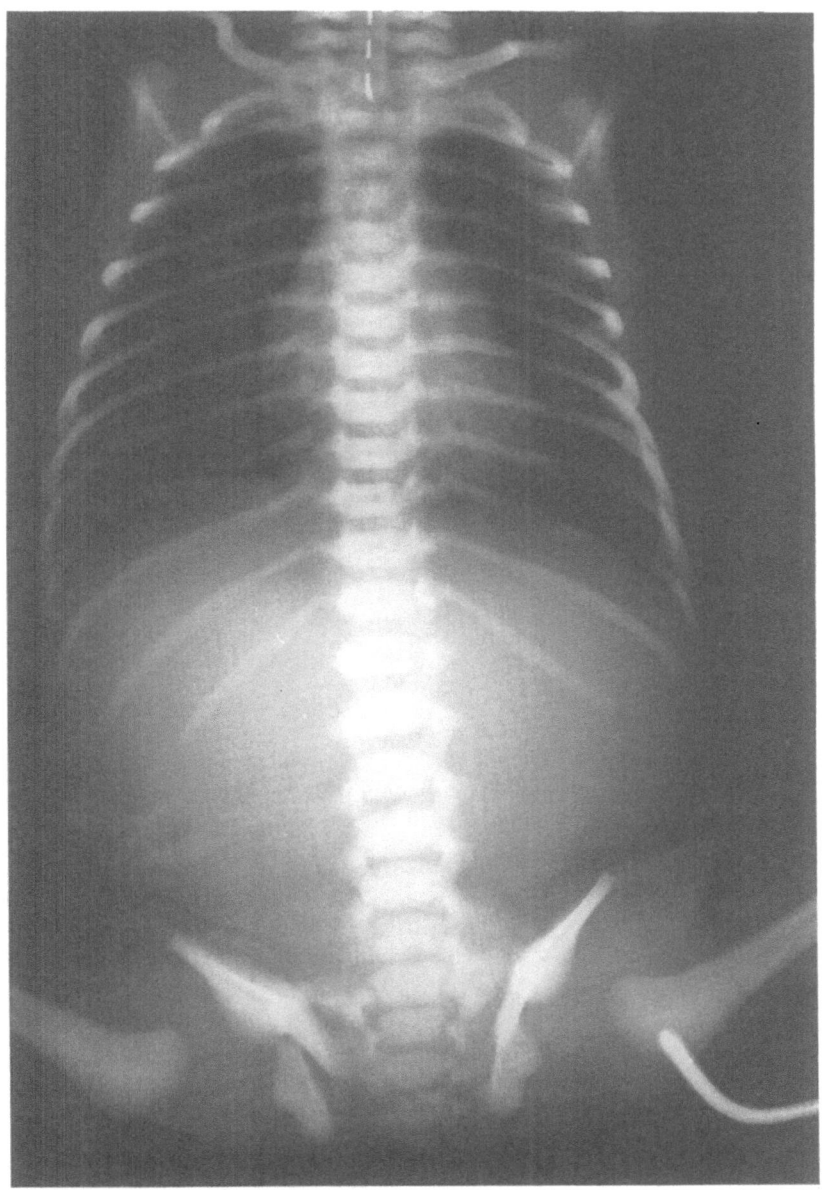

Figure 10.5 Plain X-ray of the chest and abdomen in an infant with oesophageal atresia when there is no distal tracheo-oesophageal fistula.

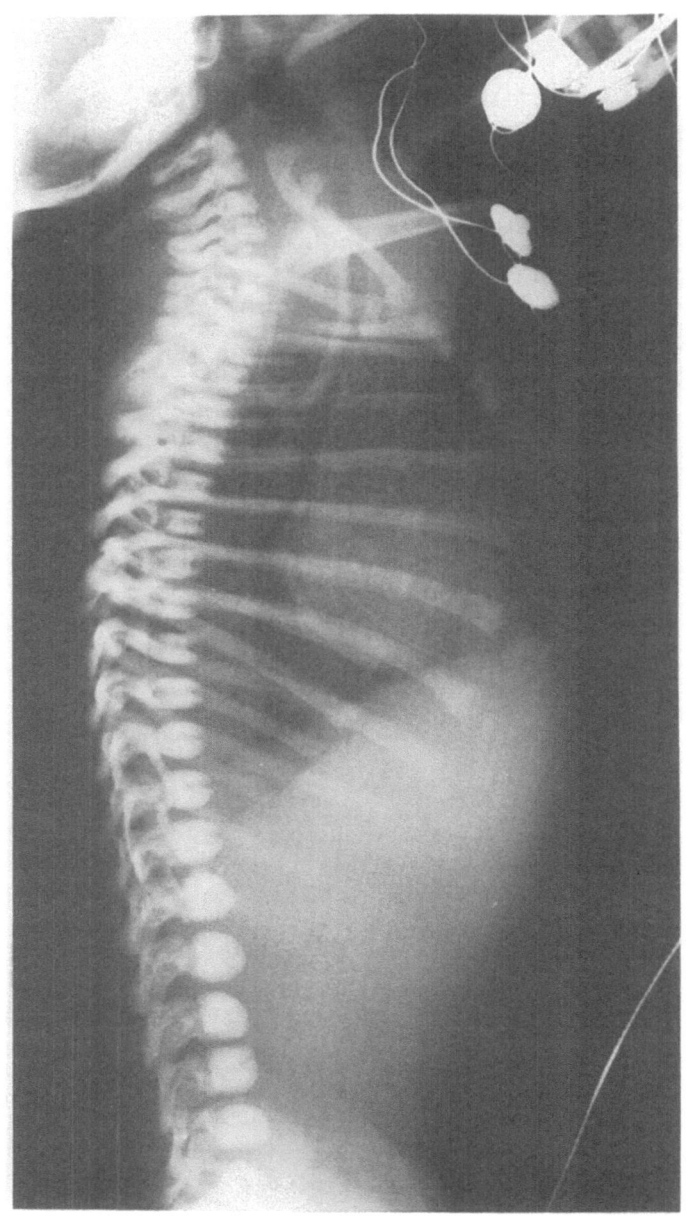

Figure 10.6 Lateral view of gasless abdomen. The length of the upper pouch is clearly evident.

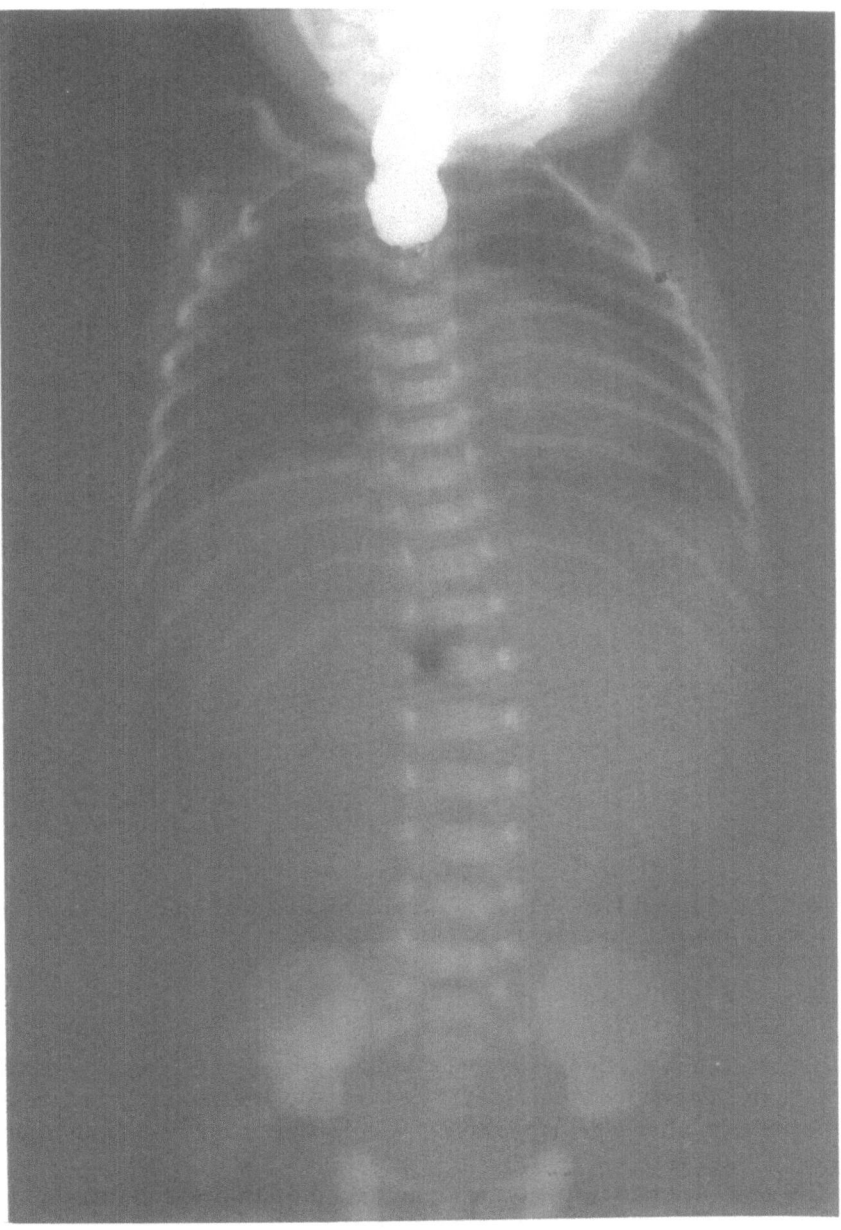

Figure 10.7 Contrast study of upper oesophageal pouch in a baby with an airless abdomen. There is no escape of contrast from the proximal oesophagus through a fistula into the trachea. An upper pouch fistula is excluded.

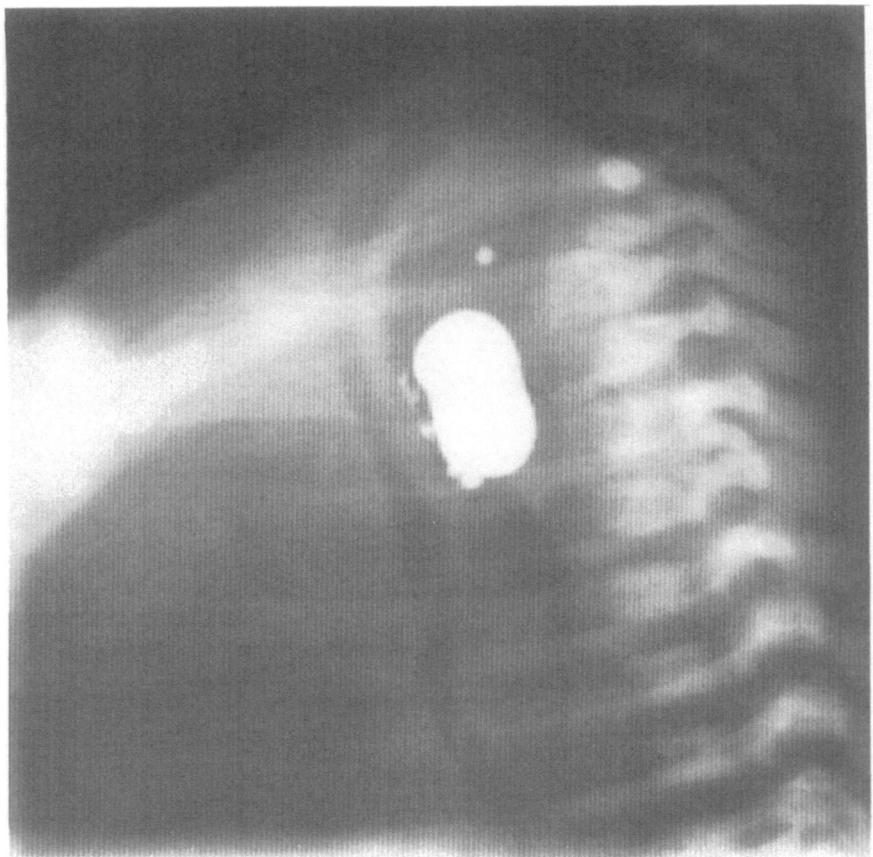

Figure 10.8 Lateral view during an upper pouch contrast study. Normally, a smaller volume of contrast would be used. Care must be taken to avoid spillover and aspiration.

(Chapter 11). Oesophageal atresia with a distal tracheo-oesophageal fistula through which no air has passed into the stomach has been reported (Haight, 1957; Waterston *et al.*, 1963) but this is an extremely unusual situation.

The absence of an upper pouch fistula can be accepted when a careful contrast study of the upper oesophageal pouch fails to demonstrate contrast escaping through a fistula into the trachea (Figures 10.7 and 10.8). When performed by an experienced radiologist using a small volume of contrast and continuous fluoroscopic control 'spillover' and aspiration should be avoided. The other method of excluding an upper pouch fistula is by endoscopy, a procedure which requires general anaesthesia without paralysis and which, despite expertise, may be difficult in a small or premature infant with respiratory embarrassment.

10.5   Assessment of length of gap

Once a diagnosis of oesophageal atresia without fistula is made the length of gap between the oesophageal ends must be established. As a rule the gap between the oesophageal ends is much greater than in patients who have a tracheo-oesophageal fistula. Assessment of the length of gap is essential as it dictates subsequent management.

Preoperatively, the length of the upper segment will have been demonstrated by contrast study (Figure 10.7) but will be confirmed at operation when the anaesthetist passes a metal bougie or a radio-opaque tipped flexible catheter through the mouth into the upper oesophagus.

The lower segment is evaluated at the time of gastrostomy by the introduction of a metal bougie or sound at the same time as a catheter or bougie is placed in the upper segment. Gentle pressure can be exerted on each end to assess how close the segments can be approximated as an indicator of the likelihood of early successful oesophageal anastomosis. If the initial gap is less than two vertebrae in length (Figure 10.9) or if the two ends can be approximated with a force which would not represent unacceptable tension to an anastomosis it is safe to proceed to immediate thoracotomy and primary end-to-end anastomosis. This is an uncommon situation and in our series there has not been such a case.

The more common finding is that the gap between the ends is greater than two vertebrae in length and the two sounds cannot be brought together (Figure 10.10). In these patients, further evaluation can be performed at monthly intervals by simultaneous insertion of radio-opaque sounds into upper and lower segments in the expectation that over the first 3 months some decrease in the length of gap will be observed (Figures 10.11 and 10.12). This decrease, which has previously been attributed to bouginage, occurs predominantly in the upper pouch, and is most likely to represent oesophageal pouch growth, perhaps stimulated by saliva and frequent suction. The lower oesophageal segment may also grow in size, particularly if there is gastro-oesophageal reflux and filling of the lower oesophagus (Figure 10.13) which is the reason for encouraging bolus gastrostomy feeds during the weeks before oesophageal anastomosis (Myers *et al.*, 1987).

As soon as the gap appears small enough to enable primary anastomosis, or at three months, primary anastomosis is attempted via a thoracotomy. Only if this fails would we advocate cervical oesophagostomy and subsequent oesophageal replacement.

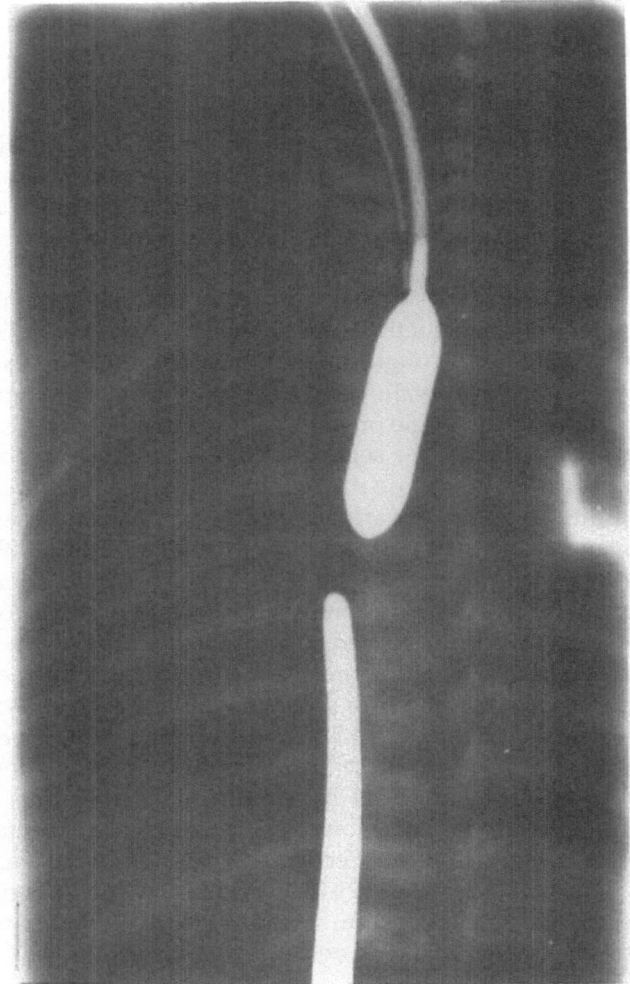

Figure 10.9 An unusually small gap between the oesophageal ends in oesopha-geal atresia without fistula. It is safe to proceed to immediate thoracotomy and primary end-to-end anastomosis.

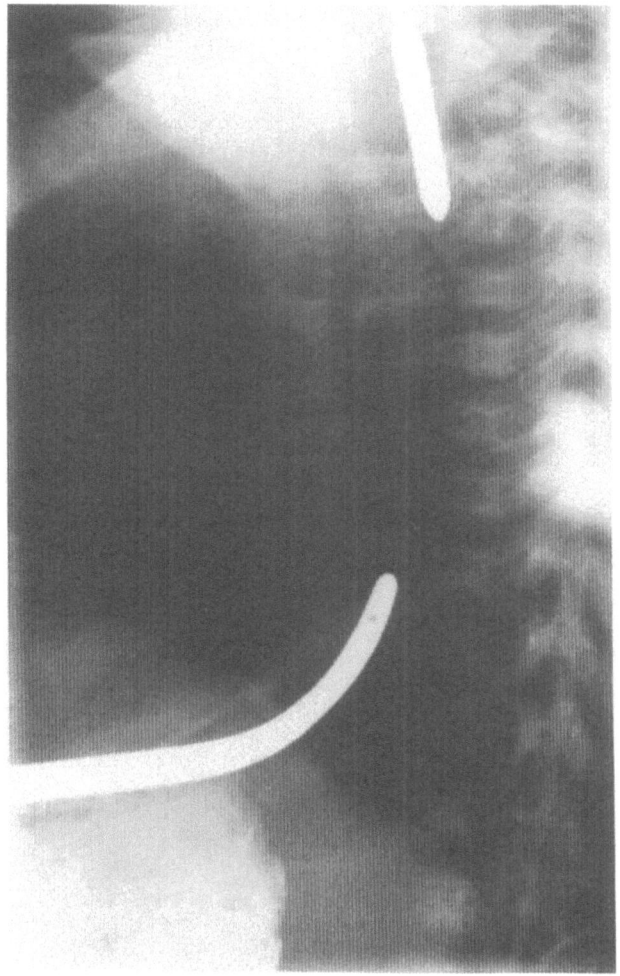

Figure 10.10 Assessment of length of gap between oesophageal ends in oesophageal atresia without a fistula. Sounds are introduced into both oesophageal segments simultaneously. In the absence of a distal fistula the gap between the oesophageal ends is often great.

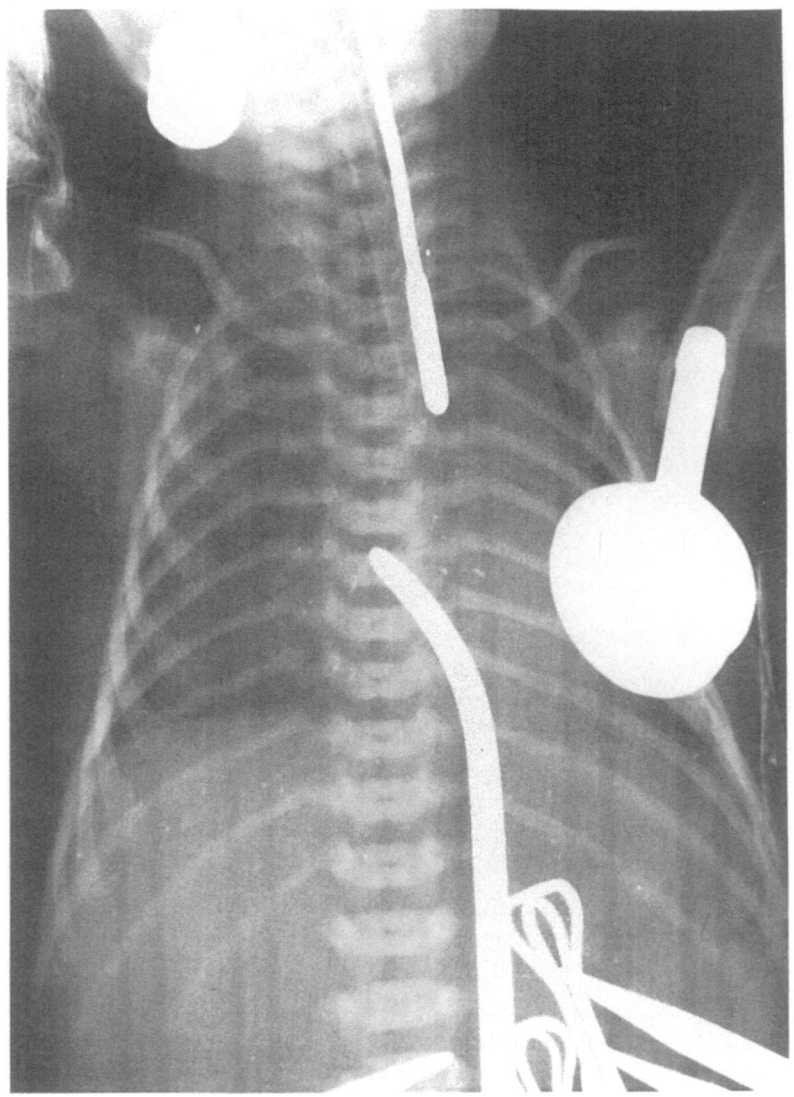

Figure 10.11   Length of gap at time of gastrostomy.

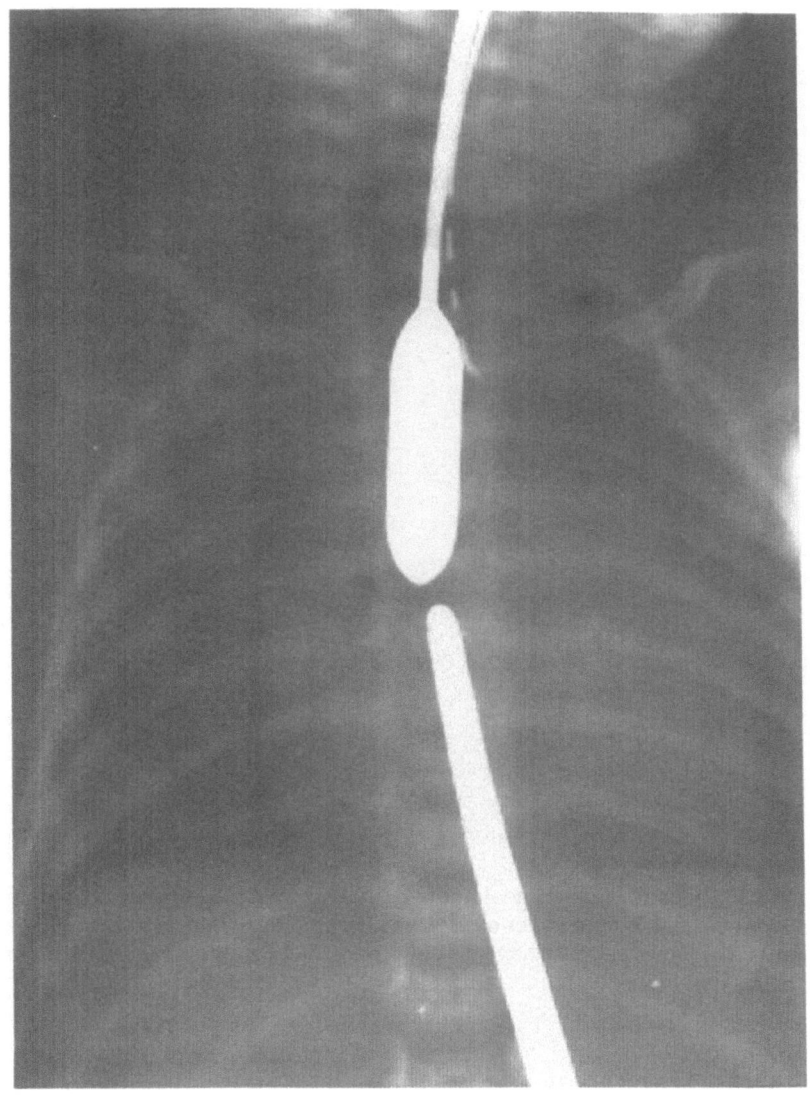

Figure 10.12 Length of gap at 2 months of age (same patients as in Figure 10.11).

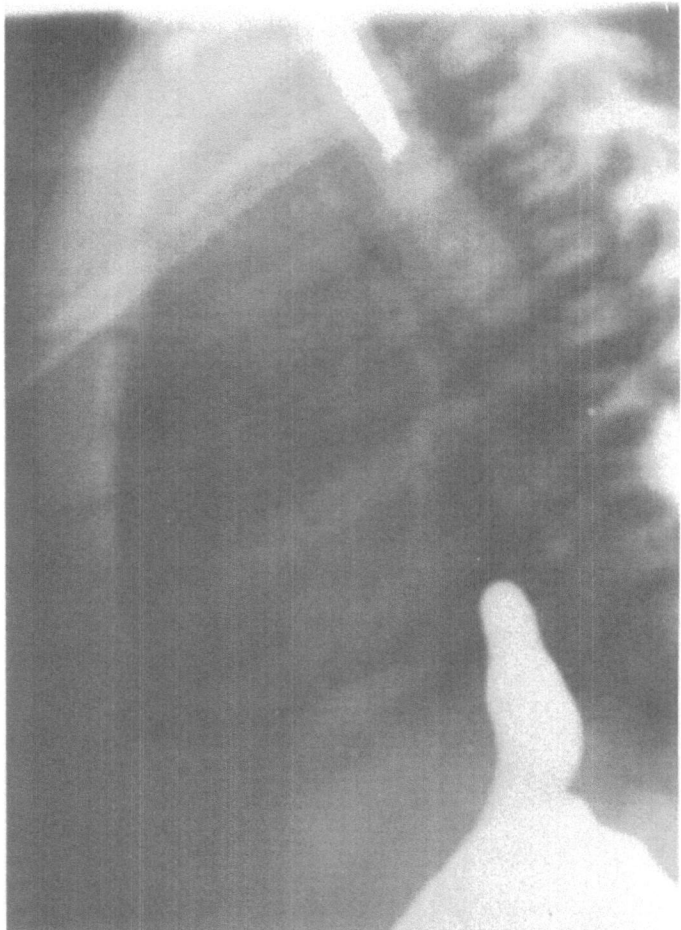

Figure 10.13   Gastro-oesophageal reflux allows contrast introduced through the gastrostomy to outline the lower oesophageal segment. Bolus gastrostomy feeds in infants with gastro-oesophageal reflux may help stimulate growth of the lower segment. Note the Hurst bougie in the upper segment.

10.6   Operative technique

In our institution a patient with oesophageal atresia alone will have had an upper pouch fistula excluded by a contrast study prior to operation. In those centres where this is not performed an initial endoscopy to rule out an upper pouch fistula would be required.

10.6.1 TECHNIQUE OF GASTROSTOMY

A left transverse incision is made and the muscles of the ventral abdominal wall divided to gain access to the peritoneal cavity. The stomach, which is usually small, is identified and a 3/0 polyglycolic acid pursestring suture inserted on the anterior surface of the body of the stomach near the most dependent part of the greater curvature. The choice of position must take into account possible later use of the greater curvature of the stomach for oesophageal replacement if primary oesophageal anastomosis fails. The stomach is opened within the pursestring and a metal sound passed into the lower oesophageal pouch. This is most easily achieved by running the tip of the sound up the lesser curvature to the gastro-oesophageal junction. Simultaneously, the anaesthetist passes a metal-tipped stiff nasogastric catheter through the infant's mouth into the upper pouch. X-rays are taken to demonstrate the length of gap between the oesophageal segments (Figure 10.8).

The metal bougie is removed. A small transverse stab incision is made about 2 cm below the abdominal incision. A number 14 French Malecot catheter is railroaded through this incision on the ventral abdominal wall and placed in the stomach. The pursestring suture is tightened around the catheter and a second similar pursestring suture inserted. Three or four further sutures are placed between the seromuscular layers of the stomach and the peritoneum of the ventral abdominal wall and drawn together to make the anterior surface of the stomach adherent to the abdominal wall. The abdominal incision is closed.

10.6.2 DEFINITIVE OESOPHAGEAL REPAIR

The definitive repair of the oesophagus is performed through a right thoracotomy incision. The incision and approach used are the same as in a thoracotomy for oesophageal atresia with distal tracheo-oesophageal fistula (Chapter 9).

Identification and mobilization of upper pouch

After division of the azygos vein the thin endothoracic fascia of the posterior mediastinum is incised. The upper pouch will usually be obvious but on occasions, particularly if short, its identification can be assisted by the anaesthetist who inserts a catheter into it. This manoeuvre reveals its lowest point through which a 3/0 stay suture is placed. The upper pouch is then mobilized by separating it from its surrounding structures taking care to avoid damage to the trachea, to which it is closely related. This manoeuvre does not significantly damage its blood supply as its vascularity comes from above (Chapter 4). The mobilization can be continued superiorly as far as the cricopharyngeus. Tension on the stay suture enables assessment of the additional oesophageal length obtained.

Assessment of distal segment

The fine white fibres of the vagus nerve can be identified as they run down the posterior mediastinum behind the hilum of the lung and anterior to the aorta. They course towards the lower oesophageal segment. Again, the thin fascia of the posterior mediastinum overlying the oesophagus must be divided. Some clue as to the likely upper limit of the lower segment will have been obtained from previous contrast studies. In most patients the lower oesophageal segment will be identified in the lower part of the thorax, a few centimetres above the diaphragm. It will appear small and insignificant. Once it is identified a polyglycolic acid suture can be placed through its uppermost limit to facilitate its gentle dissection from surrounding structures. Mobilization can be achieved without complete disruption of its vascular supply which appears as a small leash of vessels from the aorta. Approximation of the two stay sutures will indicate whether the oesophageal ends are close enough for primary anastomosis. If they cannot be approximated without undue tension (greater tension than would enable a safe anastomosis) three further manoeuvres can be considered:

1.   More extensive mobilization of the hiatus to allow the intra-abdominal oesophagus to ride up into the thorax, with or without a portion of the stomach
2.   A circular or spiral (Kimura *et al.*, 1987) myotomy of the upper pouch. In recent years we have preferred dissection of the hiatus to a circular myotomy, because of the potential injury to the motility and vascular supply of the upper pouch which a myotomy may cause. Furthermore, the incidence of diverticulum formation is not insignificant (Taylor and Myers, 1989).

Techniques have been described whereby a modified endotracheal tube (de Carvalho *et al.*, 1989) or a Fogarty catheter (Schwartz, 1983) can be used to aid the mobilization of the upper pouch in patients with long gap oesophageal atresia. Such devices have been found to be helpful in the performance of a circular myotomy where this is necessary. Before opening the upper pouch the cuff (or balloon) is inflated to unfold the mucosa without over distension of the muscle layers. The tube described by de Carvalho *et al.* (1989) is a modified 5 mm cuffed Portex endotracheal tube in which the tube distal to the cuff has been removed and the lumen sealed with a rounded smooth obturator. In addition, the technique enables the surgeon to gauge precisely the tension in the upper pouch, and the need for myotomy without risk to trauma to the proximal oesophagus. It maximizes stability during the performance of the myotomy.

3. An anterior muco-muscular flap (Bar-Baor *et al.*, 1989). This method is based on the fact that the atretic upper pouch has an excellent longitudinal blood supply and is 2–3 times wider than the lower pouch. An anterior muco-muscular flap is created and anastomosed to the lower oesophagus. A similar method had previously been described by Gough (1980).

Endoscopic oesophageal anastomosis

An endoscopic technique of achieving oesophageal continuity in long gap oesophageal atresia without thoracotomy has been described (Okmian *et al.*, 1975; Booss *et al.*, 1982). This involves endoscopic introduction via the gastrostomy of a non-absorbable suture attached to a long straight needle into the lower oesophageal segment. The needle is pushed through the upper end of the segment and through the fundus of the upper pouch where it is retrieved by an oesophagoscope passed into the upper oesophageal segment. The exact position of the two endoscopes is controlled by continuous fluoroscopy. Care is taken to avoid pleural and bronchial injury. By using the 'olive method' (Rehbein and Schweder, 1971) oesophageal continuity can then be established.

Complete failure of oesophageal anastomosis

If all these measures fail then a cervical oesophagostomy should be performed as a prelude to oesophageal replacement; this is discussed in detail in Chapter 12. Table 10.4 summarizes the measures which can be undertaken before resorting to cervical oesophagostomy and later oesophageal replacement.

Table 10.4 Intraoperative techniques for gaining oesophageal length in 'long gap' oesophageal atresia

---

Mobilization of upper oesophageal segments as far as cricopharyngeus

Mobilization of lower oesophageal segment:
  to diaphragm with preservation of segmental vascular supply
  oesophageal hiatus

Upper segmental myotomy:
  circular or spiral
  (muco-muscular flap)

References

Bar-Baor, J. A., Shoshany, G. and Sweed, Y. (1989) Wide gap oesophageal atresia: a new method to elongate the upper pouch. *J. Pediatr. Surg.*, **24**, 882–3.

Booss, D., Hollwarth, M. and Sauer, H. (1982) Endoscopic esophageal anastomosis. *J. Pediatr. Surg.*, **17**, 138–43.

Connolly, B. and Guiney, E. J. (1987) Trends in tracheo-esophageal fistula. *Surg. Gynecol. Obstet.*, **16A**, 308–12.

de Carvalho, J. L., Maynard, J. and Hadley, G. P. (1989) An improved technique for *in situ* oesophageal myotomy and proximal pouch mobilisation in patients with oesophageal atresia. *J. Pediatr. Surg.*, **24**, 872–3.

Gauntlett, I., Hochmann, M. and Duncan, A. W. (1986) Tracheal compression by the upper pouch in oesophageal atresia without tracheo-oesophageal fistula. *Pediatr. Surg. Int.*, **1**, 243–5.

German, J. C., Mahour, G. H. and Woolley, M. M. (1976) Esophageal atresia and associated anomalies. *J. Pediatr. Surg.*, **11**, 299–306.

Gough, M. H. (1980) Esophageal atresia: use of an anterior flap in the difficult anastomosis. *J. Pediatr. Surg.*, **15**, 310–11.

Haight, C. (1957) Some observations on esophageal atresias and tracheo-esophageal fistulas of congenital origin. *J. Thorac. Surg.*, **34**, 141–72.

Hendren, W. H. and Hale, J. R. (1975) Electromagnetic bougienage to lengthen esophageal segments in congenital esophageal atresia. *N. Engl. J. Med.*, **293**, 428–32.

Holder, T. M., Cloud, D. T., Lewis, J. E. Jr and Pilling, G. P. (1964) Esophageal atresia and tracheoesophageal fistula. A survey of its members by the surgical section of the American Academy of Pediatrics. *Pediatrics*, **34**, 542–9.

Holder, T. M., Ashcraft, K. W., Sharp, R. J. and Amoury, R. A. (1987) Care of infants with esophageal atresia, tracheoesophageal fistula, and associated anomalies. *J. Thorac. Cardiovasc. Surg.*, **94**, 828–35.

Holder, T. M., McDonald, V. A. Jr and Woolley, M. M. (1962) The premature or critically ill infant with esophageal atresia: increased success with a staged approach. *J. Thorac. Cardiovasc. Surg.*, **44**, 344–58.

Howard, R. and Myers, N. A. (1965) Oesophageal atresia: a technique for elongating the upper pouch. *Surgery*, **58**, 725–7.

Kimura, K., Nishijima, E., Stugawa, C. and Matsumoto, Y. (1987) A new approach for the salvage of unsuccessful esophageal atresia repair: a spiral myotomy and delayed definitive operation. *J. Pediatr. Surg.*, **22**, 981–3.

Koop, C. E. and Hamilton, J. P. (1965) Atresia of the esophagus. Increased survival with staged procedures in the poor risk infant. *Ann. Surg.*, **162**, 389–401.

Livaditis, A. (1973) Esophageal atresia; a method of over-bridging large segmental gaps. *Z. Kinderchir.*, **13**, 298–306.

Louhimo, I. and Lindahl, H. (1983) Esophageal atresia: primary results of 500 consecutively treated patients. *J. Pediatr. Surg.*, **18**, 217–29.

Myers, N. A., Beasley, S. W., Auldist, A. W. *et al.* (1987) Oesophageal atresia without fistula – anastomosis or replacement? *Pediatr. Surg. Int.*, **2**, 216–22.

Myers, N. A. and Aberdeen, E. (1979) Congenital esophageal atresia and tracheoesophageal fistula, in *Pediatric Surgery* (3rd edn.) pp. 446–9.

Okmian, L., Booss, D. and Ekelund, I. (1975) An endoscopic technique for Rehbein's silver olive method. *Z. Kinderchir.*, **16**, 212–15.

Randolph, J. (1986) Esophageal atresia and congenital stenosis. in *Pediatric Surgery* (eds K. J. Welch, M. M. Ravitch, J. A. O'Neill and M. I. Rowe), Year Book Publishing, Chicago, pp. 682–93.

Rehbein, F. and Schweder, N. (1971) Reconstruction of the oesophagus without colon transplantation in cases of atresia. *J. Pediatr. Surg.*, **6**, 746–52.

Ricketts, R. R., Luck, S. R. and Raffensperger, J. G. (1981) Circular esophagomyotomy for primary repair of long-gap esophageal atresia. *J. Pediatr. Surg.*, **16**, 365–9.

Schier, F., Mick, C., Schier, C. and Waldschmidt, J. (1988) Simultaneous bouginage and anastomosis in long gap oesophageal atresia: a new technical device. Presented at 9th Congress of Asian Association of Paediatric Surgeons, Singapore, April.

Schwartz, M. Z. (1983) An improved technique for circular myotomy in long gap esophageal atresia. *J. Pediatr. Surg.*, **18**, 833–4.

Spitz, L., Kiely, E. and Brereton, R. J. (1987) Esophageal atresia: five year experience with 148 cases. *J. Pediatr. Surg.*, **22**, 103–8.

Strodel, W. E., Coran, A. G., Kirsch, M. M., Weintraub, W. H., Wesley, J. R. and Sloan, H. (1979) Esophageal atresia. A 41-year experience. *Arch. Surg.*, **114**, 523–7.

Taylor, R. G. and Myers, N. A. (1989) Management of a post-Livaditis-procedure oesophageal diverticulum. *Pediatr. Surg. Int.*, **4**, 238–40.

Vizas, D., Ein, S. H. and Simpson, J. S. (1978) The value of circular myotomy for esophageal atresia. *J. Pediatr. Surg.*, **13**, 357–9.

Waterston, D. J., Bonham-Carter, R. E. and Aberdeen, E. (1963) Congenital tracheo-oesophageal fistula in association with oesophageal atresia. *Lancet*, **ii**, 55–7.

11 Oesophageal atresia with proximal tracheo-oesophageal fistula

A. W. AULDIST

Oesophageal atresia with proximal tracheo-oesophageal fistula (Figure 11.1) is an uncommon anatomical variant of oesophageal atresia and one with a relatively high incidence of complications. This is the result of a number of factors including diagnostic difficulties in demonstrating the upper pouch fistula, the long gap which may be present between the two oesophageal segments, and the fact that a proximal fistula is more likely to allow soiling of the lung. The management of this anomaly is, therefore, a challenge in both diagnostic and technical terms.

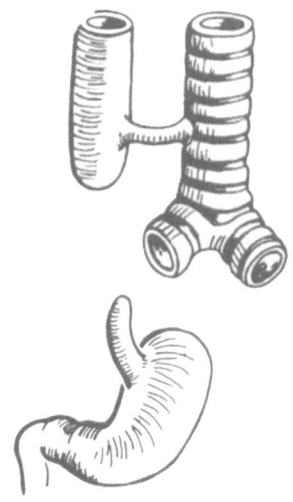

Figure 11.1 Oesophageal atresia with a proximal tracheo-oesophageal fistula.

Oesophageal atresia and proximal tracheo-oesophageal fistula may be associated with a distal tracheo-oesophageal fistula, the so-called 'double-fistula'. In almost all series, including our own, this combination occurs extremely rarely. The presentation of oesophageal atresia and double fistula resembles that of oesophageal atresia and distal tracheo-oesophageal fistula (e.g. gas is observed below the diaphragm) but despite this many authors have preferred to include it for discussion purposes with proximal tracheo-oesophageal fistulae (Dudgeon *et al.*, 1972). The anomaly is considered separately in section 11.6.

11.1 Incidence

In most reports of oesophageal atresia and proximal tracheo-oesophageal fistula, the incidence ranges between 0–3% of all oesophageal atresias (Table 11.1) but the number of patients seen in any one institution is small. At the Royal Children's Hospital there were 11 patients with a single proximal tracheo-oesophageal fistula in association with a blind lower oesophagus.

Table 11.1 Relative incidence of oesophageal atresia with proximal tracheo-oesophageal fistula

Author (year)	*Total number in series*	*Atresia with proximal fistula (%)*
Waterston *et al.* (1962)	218	1.0
Holder *et al.* (1964)	1058	0.8
Louhimo and Lindahl (1983)	100	1.0
Randolph (1986)	500	0.4
Connolly and Guiney (1987)	139	0.7
Hays *et al.* (1966)	108	3.0
Strodel *et al.* (1979)	365	0.0
Waterston *et al.* (1963)	218	0.9
German *et al.* (1976)	102	2.0
Bishop *et al.* (1985)	295	0.0
Haight (1957)	200	0.0
Spitz *et al.* (1987)	148	2.0
RCH Melbourne (1988)	584	1.9

11.2   Surgical anatomy

Although the upper oesophageal pouch may be as capacious as an upper pouch without proximal tracheo-oesophageal fistula, there is a tendency for it to be small. This may be because liquor escapes through the fistula into the trachea, rather than accumulating in the upper pouch and causing it to distend during intrauterine life.

The upper fistula is usually single but there are isolated reports of a double fistula to the upper pouch (Kluth, 1976). The fistula may be angled downward from the trachea towards the oesophagus in the same manner as an isolated 'H' fistula (Dudgeon *et al.*, 1972) (Chapter 13). The

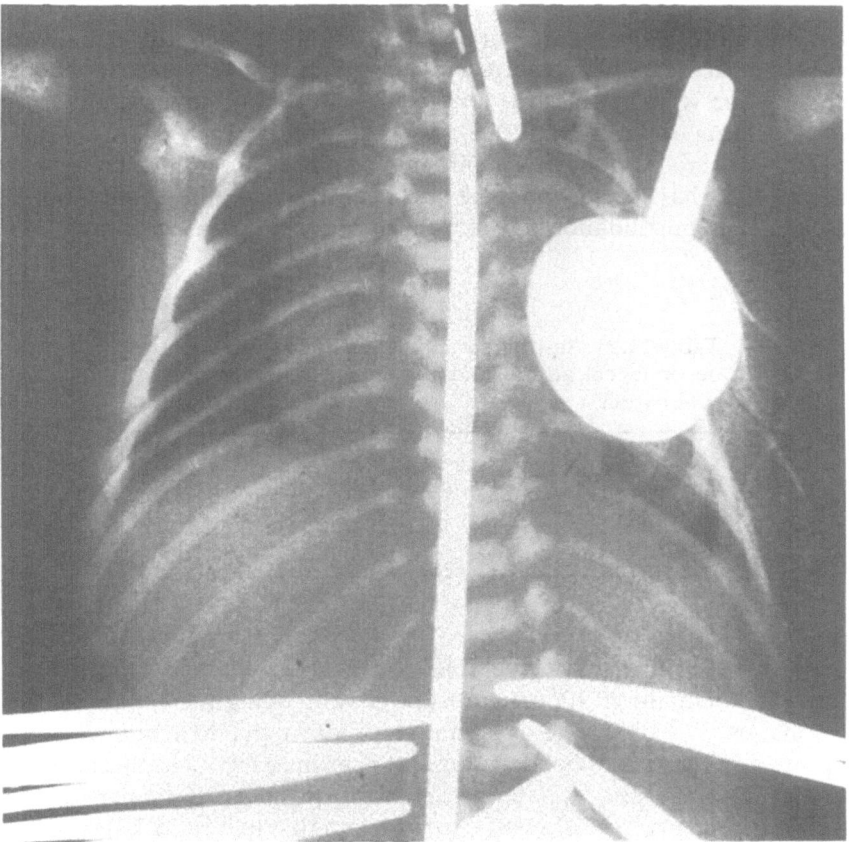

Figure 11.2   Oesophageal atresia with proximal tracheo-oesophageal fistula: operative study showing overlapping oesophageal segments.

oesophageal end of the fistula is usually proximal to the fundus of the upper oesophageal segment and for this reason it is often appropriate to divide it through a cervical approach.

The length of the lower oesophageal segment is variable. In about half our cases, the lower oesophagus extended proximally almost as far as the upper oesophageal segment, allowing anastomosis without tension. Occasionally, the segments may overlap (Figure 11.2). In the remainder, the distal segment commences well below the upper pouch, making primary anastomosis difficult to achieve.

11.3   Royal Children's Hospital experience

There was a history of maternal polyhydramnios in 10 of the 11 patients treated with oesophageal atresia and proximal tracheo-oesophageal fistula. Four were premature, one was small for gestational age, and birth weights ranged from 1.8 to 3.2 kg (mean 2.4 kg). Associated anomalies were present in four infants (Table 11.2). All patients were diagnosed as having oesophageal atresia at the time of delivery, and six had signs of consolidation in the right upper lobe on initial X-ray of the chest.

Table 11.2   Associated anomalies in 11 infants with oesophageal atresia and proximal tracheo-oesophageal fistula

Cardiac	2
Chromosomal	1
Cleft palate	1
Renal	1

One infant with a hypoplastic left heart received no surgical treatment. The remaining 10 patients underwent operative repair of the oesophagus. A wide range of operative procedures and sequences was employed, reflecting the distribution of cases over four decades and the fact that in four of the 10 patients diagnosis of the proximal fistula was delayed (Cass and Auldist, 1987). In two patients, failure of diagnosis of the fistula was due to the assumption that the presence of an airless abdomen was diagnostic of oesophageal atresia without fistula and resulted in the omission of a preoperative contrast study. In another two, there was misinterpretation of the contrast study, the presence of contrast material in the trachea being attributed to 'spill-over', rather than passage of contrast through a fistula. This highlights the importance of continuous fluoroscopic control.

Gastrostomy was performed in all 10 patients. The oesophagus was repaired with an end-to-end anastomosis in seven, one early and six delayed. One anastomotic disruption necessitated cervical oesophagostomy. Four patients had a cervical oesophagostomy which was followed by gastric tube replacement (three) or colonic interposition (one). The proximal tracheo-oesophageal fistula was divided by a thoracic approach in six infants and by a cervical approach in four (Cass and Auldist, 1987).

There were three deaths: one from a chest infection after gastric tube replacement at the age of 14 months in a child in whom the tracheo-oesophageal fistula remained undiagnosed; a second in a retarded child with a colonic interposition who died at 17 months from aspiration; and a third with Down's syndrome who died at 7 months of age from pneumonia. All three had previous major complications including recurrent pneumonia, empyema, gastrostomy leak with peritonitis, or recurrent fistula. One had a temporary recurrent laryngeal nerve palsy after thoracic division of the fistula and another required tracheostomy because of prolonged intubation and subglottic stenosis.

One of the seven survivors has chronic lung problems and persistent dysphagia. Fundoplication was required in three patients with gastro-oesophageal reflux.

The rarity of the anatomical variant, delay in diagnosis of the fistula and lack of a standard protocol for management account for the overall poor results of this group of patients. From the experience at the Royal Children's Hospital a plan for the management of these patients was developed and is described below.

11.4 Diagnosis

Diagnosis is of primary importance if the morbidity of a proximal fistula as described above is to be avoided. Radiological signs of pneumonic changes at presentation should alert the clinician to the possibility of an associated proximal tracheo-oesophageal fistula. All patients with oesophageal atresia and gasless abdomen should have a contrast study of the upper oesophagus or endoscopy to identify a proximal fistula (Figure 11.3). A contrast study of the upper pouch must be done with care to avoid contamination of the lungs: a small volume of contrast is used under continuous fluoroscopic control. Filling of the fistula is best seen in the lateral oblique view. In some centres (Kosloske *et al.*, 1988)

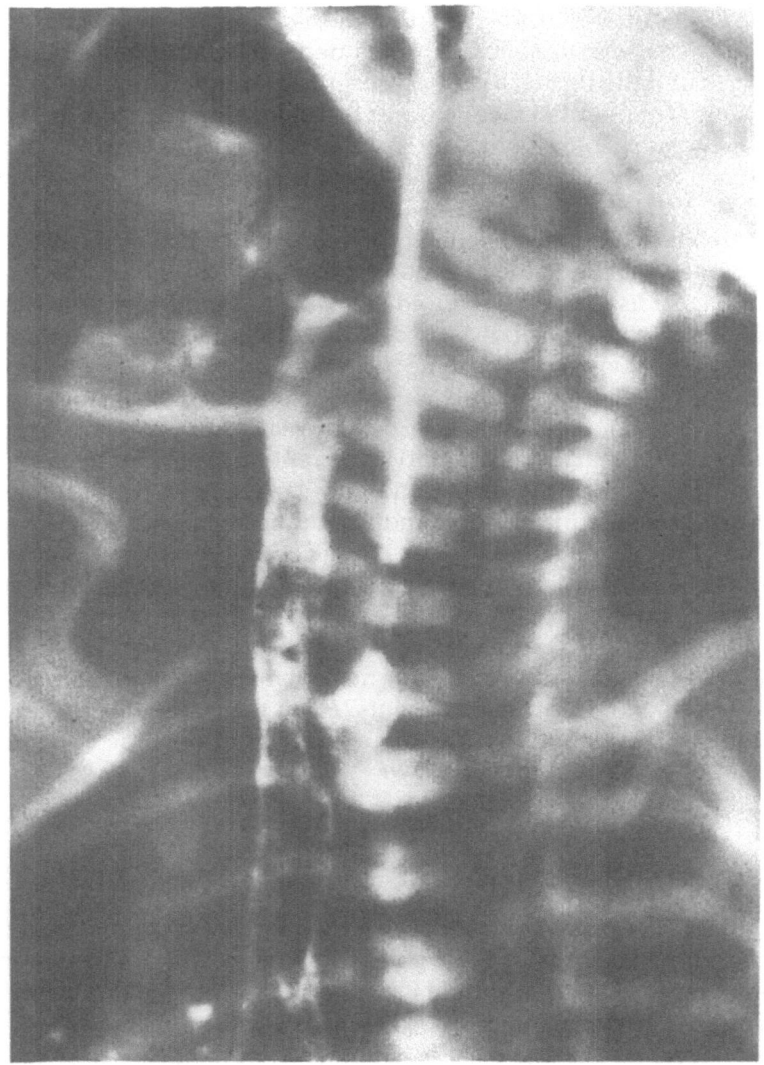

Figure 11.3 Contrast study of a patient with oesophageal atresia and gasless abdomen. Contrast escaping from the oesophagus into the trachea is indicative of an upper pouch fistula. Continuous fluoroscopic control is necessary to ensure that the contrast in the airways is not the result of 'spillover'.

endoscopy is performed in all patients with oesophageal atresia and gasless abdomen: the fistula is most easily seen at its tracheal end.

Occasionally, a proximal fistula will be identified at operation when preoperative investigations have failed to demonstrate one. The anterior aspect of the oesophagus will appear to be adherent to the trachea a variable distance above the fundus of the upper pouch.

11.5 Surgical management

After diagnosis of a proximal tracheo-oesophageal fistula in those patients without gas in the abdomen we recommend that the surgeon proceed to gastrostomy (Figure 11.4). This enables demonstration of the length of the lower oesophagus using a metal sound introduced through the gastrotomy at the time of surgery. An X-ray taken on the table may show a long lower oesophageal segment: if this is found it may be

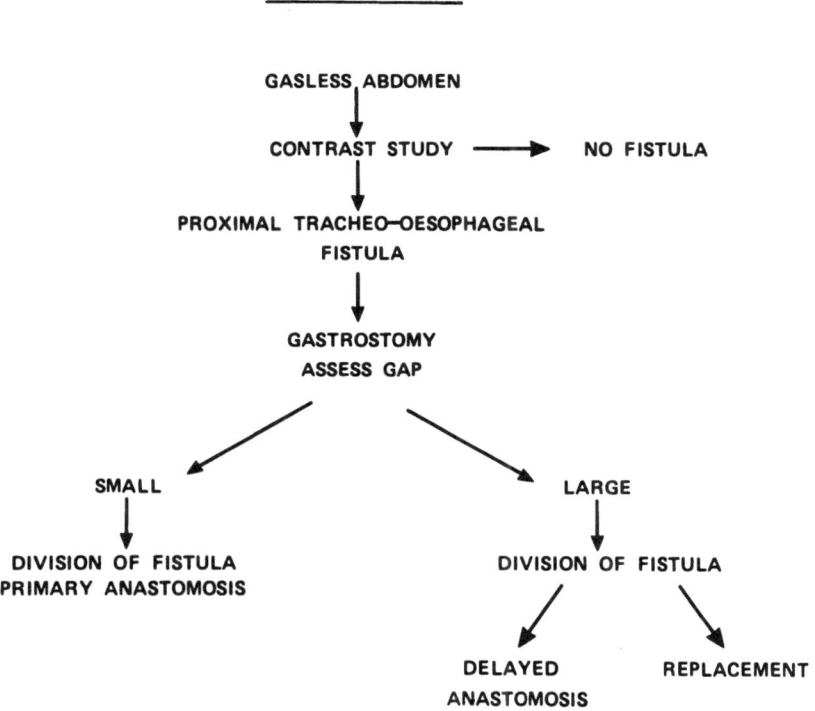

Figure 11.4 Flow diagram of the management of an infant with a proximal tracheo-oesophageal fistula.

appropriate to proceed with thoracotomy, division of the proximal fistula and primary anastomosis of the oesophagus. If the X-ray shows that there is only a short lower oesophagus and a large gap between the oesophageal ends then it is appropriate to divide the fistula, usually through a cervical approach, and proceed with oesophageal anastomosis at a later stage. If this is not possible oesophageal replacement may be required, as in some patients with oesophageal atresia without fistula (Chapter 10).

11.6   Oesophageal atresia with a double fistula

This is a very uncommon anomaly (Figure 11.5; two patients in our series of 584), but in some centres it has been seen more frequently (Table 11.3). The presence of a proximal fistula might be suspected in a patient with gas in the abdomen when there is more respiratory difficulty than would be expected normally. In earlier years, a routine upper pouch study was performed in all patients. Although this was helpful in diagnosing a proximal fistula, the low incidence of double fistula has not encouraged us to continue doing a contrast study in all patients with oesophageal atresia. Routine endoscopy of the trachea before repair of the oesophageal atresia is another method which has been used to diagnose double fistulae (Kosloske *et al.*, 1988).

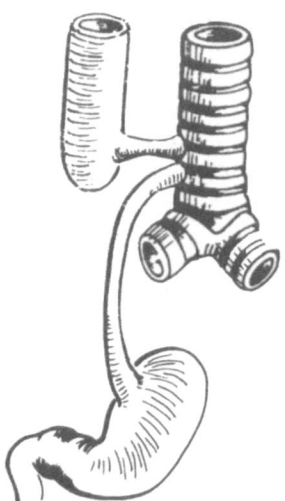

Figure 11.5   Oesophageal atresia with proximal and distal tracheo-oesophageal fistulae.

Table 11.3 Relative incidence of oesophageal atresia with a proximal and distal ('double') tracheo-oesophageal fistula

Author (year)	Total number of patients	% Double fistula
Waterston et al. (1963)	218	1.4
Haight (1969)	288	1.8
Bishop et al. (1985)	295	0.7
Holder et al. (1964)	1058	0.7
Holder et al. (1986)	100	6.0
Louhimo and Lindahl (1983)	500	1.0
RCH Melbourne (1988)	584	0.35

The surgeon may suspect a double fistula if the upper pouch distends in the inspiratory phase of positive pressure ventilation during thoracotomy for oesophageal atresia and distal fistula. During dissection of the oesophagus from the posterior aspect of the trachea a fistula may be found, although dissection is necessary only if additional oesophageal length is required to bridge a gap.

11.7 Conclusion

Though patients in our series, which extends over several decades, were treated by a variety of methods, there has been a gradual rationalization of the therapeutic approach. After demonstration of a proximal fistula with a careful contrast study, a gastrostomy is fashioned, and during this procedure the length of the lower oesophagus should be assessed with a metal sound. In those with a long lower oesophagus thoracotomy should be performed, the fistula divided and anastomosis achieved. If, however the lower oesophagus is short, the fistula should be divided by either a thoracic or cervical approach, and continuity be achieved later by anastomosis or oesophageal replacement.

References

Bishop, P. J., Klein, M. D., Philippart, A. I., Hixson, D. S. and Hertzler, J. H. (1985) Transpleural repair of esophageal atresia without a primary gastrostomy: 240 patients treated between 1951 and 1983. *J. Pediatr. Surg.*, **20**, 823–8.

Conolly, B., Guiney, E. J. (1987) Trends in tracheoesophageal fistula. *Surg. Gynecol. Obstet.*, **164**, 308.

Cass, D. and Auldist, A. W. (1987) Oesophageal atresia with proximal tracheo-oesophageal fistula. *Pediatr. Surg. Int.*, **2**, 212–15.

Dudgeon, D. L., Morrison, C. W. and Woolley, M. M. (1972) Congenital proximal tracheo-oesophageal fistula. *J. Pediatr. Surg.*, **7**, 614–19.

German, J. C., Mahour, G. H. and Woolley, M. M. (1976) Esophageal atresia and associated anomalies. *J. Pediatr. Surg.*, **11**, 299–306.

Haight, C. (1957) Some observations on esophageal atresia and tracheo-esophageal fistulas of congenital origin. *J. Thorac. Surg.*, **34**, 141–72.

Haight, C. (1969) in *Pediatric Surgery* (eds Mustard W. T. *et al.*) vol. 1, 2 edn, Year Book Medical Publishers Inc., Chicago, Ch 28, p. 357.

Hays, D. M., Woolley, M. and Snyder, W. H. (1966) Esophageal atresia and tracheo-oesophageal fistula: management of the uncommon types. *J. Pediatr. Surg.*, **1**, 240–52.

Holder, T. M., Cloud, D. T. and Lewis, J. E. (1964) Esophageal atresia and tracheo-esophageal fistula. A survey of its members by the Surgical Section of the American Academy of Pediatrics. *Pediatrics*, **34**, 542–9.

Holder, T. M., Ashcraft, K. W. and Sharp, R. J. *et al.* (1986) Care of infants with esophageal atresia, tracheoesophageal fistula and associated anomalies. *J. Thorac. Cardiovasc. Surg.*, **94**, 828–35.

Kluth, D. (1976) An atlas of oesophageal atresia. *J. Pediatr. Surg.*, **11**, 901–19.

Kosloske, A. M., Jewell, P. F. and Cartwright, K. C. (1988) Crucial bronchoscopic findings in esophageal atresia and tracheoesophageal fistula. *J. Pediatr. Surg.*, **23**, 466–70.

Louhimo, I. and Lindahl, H. (1983) Esophageal atresia: primary results of 500 consecutively treated patients. *J. Pediatr. Surg.*, **18**, 217–29.

Randolph, J. G. (1986) in *Pediatric Surgery* (eds K. J. Welch, J. G. Randolph, M. M. Ravitch, J. A. O'Neill and M. I. Rowe), Year Book Medical Publishers, Chicago, p. 684.

Spitz, L., Kiely, E. and Brereton, R. J. (1987) Esophageal atresia: five year experience with 148 cases. *J. Pediatr. Surg.*, **22**, 103–8.

Strodel, W. E., Coran, A. G. and Kirsh, M. H. (1979) Esophageal atresia: a 41-year experience. *Arch. Surg.*, 523–7.

Waterston, D. J., Bonham-Carter, R. E. and Aberdeen, E. (1962) Oesophageal Atresia *Lancet*, **1**, 819.

Waterston, D. J., Bonham-Carter, R. E. and Aberdeen, E. (1963) Congenital tracheo-oesophageal fistula in association with oesophageal atresia. *Lancet*, **i**, 55–7.

12 *Oesophageal replacement*

N. A. MYERS, S. W. BEASLEY and A. W. AULDIST

With few exceptions, correction of oesophageal atresia by oesophago-oesophageal anastomosis produces a long-term result superior to any form of oesophageal replacement. Even in the presence of a 'long gap' satisfactory anastomosis of the oesophageal ends can usually be achieved either directly, or with the assistance of one of the various innovative methods described in Chapter 10. However, there is a small group of patients in whom primary anastomosis cannot be achieved or in whom the oesophagus has to be abandoned because of failure of the oesophageal anastomotic technique (Ahmed and Spitz, 1986): in these, oesophageal replacement is needed. Although the size of this group has diminished considerably in recent years the surgeon who accepts responsibility for the care of the baby with oesophageal atresia must still be familiar with at least one of the techniques available.

12.1 Historical perspective

Early in the history of the surgical management of oesophageal atresia it became apparent that some patients would require oesophageal replacement. Even before the role of end-to-end anastomosis had been established, and in a period when indirect methods of providing alimentary continuity were in vogue, ante-thoracic skin tubes were used (Ladd, 1944). The many techniques utilizing a variety of materials which have been used (and frequently discarded) bear testimony to surgical ingenuity. Sweet (1948) was a pioneer in his description of a new method which used the stomach to restore continuity of the alimentary canal in cases not treated by immediate primary anastomosis.

However, in time, the use of colon by one technique or another became the preferred method; and in many centres this is still so (Hendren and Hendren, 1985). In recent years there has been a return to the use of stomach either as a greater curvature tube (gastric interposition) or in its entirety (gastric transposition).

The aim of oesophageal replacement must be to achieve continuity of the alimentary tract with a conduit which provides the best functional substitute for the oesophagus with the fewest complications (Ahmed and Spitz, 1986). Currently, the only practical substitutes for the oesophagus are stomach, jejunum, ileo-colon and colon. Skin tubes are of historic interest only and it is unlikely that conduits made from foreign material will ever be feasible or satisfactory (de Lorimier and Harrison, 1986).

12.2   Indications for replacement

Replacement may be required occasionally for any of the anatomical variants of oesophageal atresia but it is most likely to be necessary in the baby with oesophageal atresia without a fistula (Chapter 10). A few babies with oesophageal atresia and a proximal fistula, and even fewer with a distal fistula may also require replacement. The decision to proceed to replacement is often subjective rather than objective and frequently a reflection of the surgeon's experience and preference, or of the facilities available. The main indications for oesophageal replacement are:

1. In oesophageal atresia (without fistula) when investigation has shown that there is minimal or no intrathoracic component to the lower oesophageal segment.
2. When attempted oesophageal anastomosis at thoracotomy proves impossible (a rare event).
3. Where total anastomotic disruption with sepsis has required a cervical oesophagostomy (in some infants it may still be possible to salvage the oesophagus under these circumstances).

As time has passed, however, it has become clear that the most frequent anomaly can almost always be managed by thoracotomy and primary end-to-end oesophageal anastomosis regardless of the size of the baby, the presence of other anomalies or the period of gestation (Randolph *et al.*, 1989).

In the presence of severe respiratory distress, for instance, it is often better to divide the fistula early and perform an end-to-end anastomosis at the same operation or to defer anastomosis until the HMD is resolving (Beasley and Auldist, 1988). This approach is different from that of earlier years when cervical oesophagostomy was sometimes performed in so-called 'high risk' babies with atresia and a distal fistula.

Except in the situation of an extensive and long-standing non-dilatable stricture, oesophageal replacement almost always follows gastrostomy and cervical oesophagostomy performed at an early stage. For this reason the indications for and technique of cervical oesophagostomy are described.

12.3   Cervical oesophagostomy

12.3.1   INDICATIONS

The indications for cervical oesophagostomy can be summarized as follows:

1.   No distal oesophagus, or very extensive gap: end-to-end oesophageal anastomosis impossible.
2.   Life-threatening anastomotic complications.
3.   Long gap and inadequate facilities for prolonged upper pouch care.

A gap which is so extensive that there is no chance of achieving an oesophageal anastomosis is uncommon but may occur in oesophageal atresia without a fistula. It is extremely unusual in a patient with atresia and a distal fistula.

Life-threatening anastomotic complications are rare, but when complete disruption of an anastomosis results in uncontrolled sepsis, mediastinitis, or abscess formation, cervical oesophagostomy may be indicated.

The patient who has a long gap, for whom there are no immediate plans for anastomosis, in an institution where there are poor facilities for prolonged management of the upper pouch presents a special problem. In the past oesophagostomy was performed quite often as a prelude to oesophageal replacement because of the difficulties involved in long-term suction of the upper pouch, and to prevent soiling of the lungs. The same situation may well apply in those institutions or countries where facilities are inadequate for prolonged care of the upper pouch.

12.3.2   OPERATIVE TECHNIQUE

Cervical oesophagostomy may be performed *de novo* or following thoracotomy: the technique is similar in both circumstances. The patient is supine with the head extended and turned to one side. Cervical oesophagostomy can be performed on either side of the neck, but is often performed on the right side to avoid injury to the thoracic duct, unless the requirements of later replacement make the left side preferable.

An incision is made in the neck just above the clavicle, the same position as is used to approach a tracheo-oesophageal fistula. The incision is deepened in the space between the trachea and the medial edge of the lower end of the sternomastoid muscle. The sternohyoid and sternothyroid muscles are divided or retracted medially to enable mobilization of the oesophagus just below the lobe of the thyroid gland. The recurrent laryngeal nerve is identified. When the operation is being performed following mobilization of the oesophagus from within the thorax it is helpful if a stay suture has already been placed at the bottom end of the upper oesophageal segment: this aids its delivery into the neck. In other situations the oesophagus is mobilized from the neck alone, by blunt dissection which is continued down into the chest. The oesophagus is delivered through the wound, opened and sutured to the skin.

12.4 Replacement of the oesophagus

12.4.1 METHODS AVAILABLE

In choosing the technique to be employed it is necessary to select the viscus to replace the oesophagus, and the anatomical pathway to be used (Table 12.1).

Colon

Historically, oesophagocoloplasty holds pride of place, particularly as a result of the influence of David Waterston of London (Sherman

Table 12.1 Selection of method of oesophageal replacement

1.	Viscus	
	Stomach:	antegrade tube
		retrograde tube
		transposition
	Colon	
	Small bowel	
2.	Route	
	Retrosternal	
	Transpleural	

and Waterston, 1957). The Waterston technique involved the use of transverse colon transplanted in isoperistaltic fashion into the left pleural cavity (Figure 12.1). It was originally performed through separate abdominal and thoraco-abdominal incisions (Howard, 1959) but can be performed entirely through a thoracotomy incision, access to the abdomen being obtained by peripheral division of the diaphragm.

The early results of oesophagocoloplasty were encouraging but long-term follow-up has shown an increasing number of problems. Ahmed and Spitz (1986) reviewed the outcome of colonic replacement in 112 patients who had undergone this procedure at the Hospital for Sick Children, Great Ormond Street, London. The indication was oesophageal atresia in 92 procedures of which 85 were performed within the first two years of life. In 82 the Waterston technique of interposition involved a transthoracic replacement of the oesophagus with proximal anastomosis to the cervical oesophagus. Usually the distal anastomosis was to the blind oesophageal stump and only rarely to the stomach. There were 15 deaths and a high complication rate (Table 12.2). The overall results were:

Excellent: the patients were entirely asymptomatic and could accept a normal diet (43 patients).
Good: the patients were asymptomatic for most of the time but suffered occasional minor disturbances with dysphagia (27 patients).
Fair: the patients suffered significant dysphagia or required frequent dilatations (seven patients).

Lindahl *et al.* (1983) reported operative or gastrointestinal complications in most of their 20 patients with colonic replacement of the

Table 12.2 Complications of colonic replacement of the oesophagus

Necrosis of the interposition
Leakage of an anastomosis
Stricture, particularly at the proximal oesophago-colonic anastomosis
Transient malabsorption (Louhimo *et al.* (1969).
Empyema
Graft-related complications:
  Mild colitis
  Iron deficiency anaemia
  Massive haemorrhage (Stanley-Brown, 1974)
Oesophagocutaneous fistulae
Gastric outlet obstruction
Oesophageal pouch
Diaphragmatic hernia

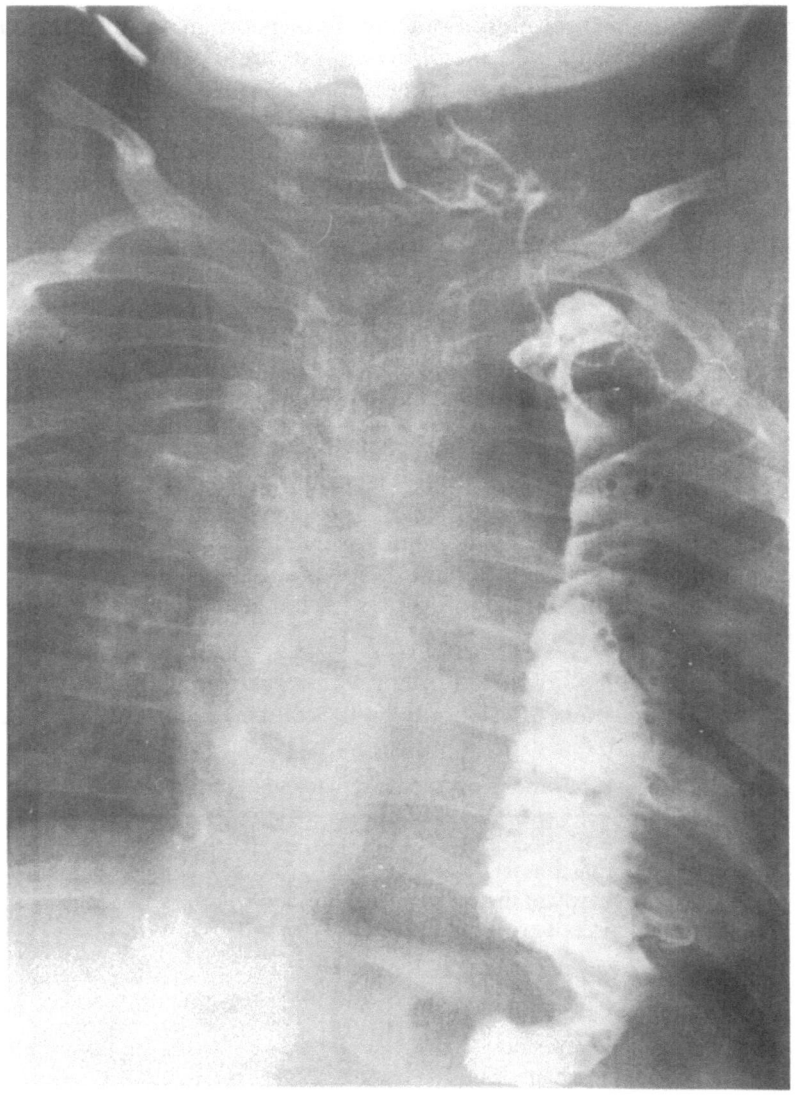

Figure 12.1 The Waterston technique of oesophagocoloplasty: the transverse colon was transplanted in an isoperistaltic fashion into the left pleural cavity.

oesophagus. Eight developed oesophagocutaneous fistulae (seven closed spontaneously), three interpositions became totally necrotic and a fourth was removed at operation. One child died because of an anastomotic leak, and another required exteriorization of both ends.

While some institutions were using the transverse colon with the colonic graft based on the upper left colic artery, others were developing oesophagocoloplasty using right colon or ileo-colon based on the middle colic artery (Martin and Flege, 1964; Martin, 1972).

Stomach

Poor results using the whole stomach as an oesophagus substitute in infancy and early childhood brought the method into disrepute but in recent years there has been increasing interest in the use of stomach as the oesophageal substitute. The most frequently adopted technique is a gastric interposition using a greater curvature tube of the Heimlich–Gavriliu type brought to the neck either via the left pleural cavity or the anterior mediastinum (Heimlich, 1955; Gavriliu, 1975). This tube can be based upon the cardia or on the pylorus.

When the whole stomach is used, the procedure is referred to as gastric transposition.

The recent preference in Melbourne has been to use a pyloric based greater curvature tube replacement sited retrosternally. We have had some experience with oesophagocoloplasty but have not utilized jejunal interposition as recommended by Ring *et al.* (1982) and Foker *et al.* (1982).

Jejunum

The limitation of jejunal transfer may be deduced from the multiplicity of techniques described (Ring *et al.*, 1982; Foker *et al.*, 1982; Jones and Gustavson, 1983; Oesch and Bettex, 1987; Simms *et al.*, 1989). Difficulties in obtaining adequate length of jejunum without compromising its blood supply (May and Samson, 1969) have limited the application of these techniques.

12.5 Surgical techniques

There are many excellent descriptions of the various techniques and their modifications. Several popular techniques using the colon, stomach and jejunum are described below.

12.5.1   OESOPHAGOCOLOPLASTY

Originally this was a three-stage procedure performed when the baby was thriving and aged between six and 12 months. In the first stage the abdomen was opened by a transverse upper abdominal incision and the vascular arrangement of the transverse colon examined. Temporary occlusion of the middle colic and ascending branch of the right colic arteries confirmed that the transverse colon had an adequate marginal arterial blood supply before they were divided. The colon was sectioned at the hepatic flexure and at a point just distal to the splenic flexure (Figure 12.2). After division of the gastrocolic omentum the transverse colon was left as an isolated loop nourished by the left colic and marginal arteries. Colonic continuity was re-established by end-to-end anastomosis (Figure 12.3). The proximal end of the transverse colon loop was closed and attached to the right end of the abdominal incision while the distal end was brought to the surface as a temporary colostomy at the left extremity of the incision.

The second stage was performed one week later; the initial abdominal incision was converted into a thoracoabdominal incision and the left pleural cavity entered. The diaphragm was incised from the costal margin to a point about 2 cm from the oesophageal hiatus. The transverse colonic loop was freed and that part which had formed the colostomy excised. The lower oesophageal segment in the mediastinum was isolated and the colonic loop brought up through the diaphragmatic incision and placed along the posterior mediastinum without tension on its vascular pedicle. The distal end of the colonic loop was anastomosed to the cut end of the thoracic oesophagus and the proximal end was

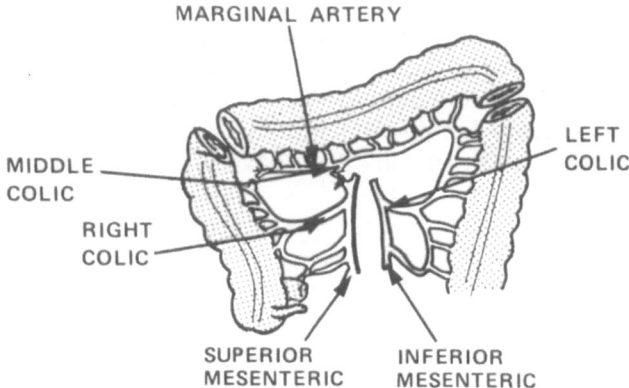

Figure 12.2 The colon is sectioned at the hepatic flexure and at a point just distal to the splenic flexure.

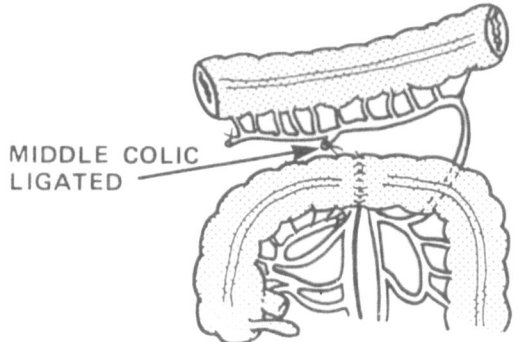

Figure 12.3 Colonic continuity is re-established by end-to-end anastomosis. The proximal end of the transverse colon loop is closed and attached to the right end of the abdominal incision while the distal end is brought to the surface as a temporary colostomy.

passed behind the clavicle and brought forward between the two heads of the left sternomastoid muscle and sutured to the edges of a skin incision made at this point (Figure 12.4). In its thoracic course the loop was anchored to the posterior mediastinum by a series of non-absorbable sutures. The diaphragmatic incision was repaired around the left colic vessels.

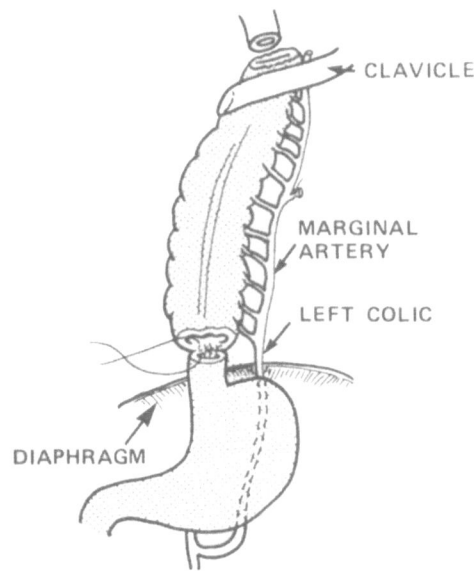

Figure 12.4 The transverse colonic loop is brought up through a diaphragmatic incision and placed along the posterior mediastinum. The distal end of the colonic loop is anastomosed to the cut end of the thoracic oesophagus.

The third stage involved a cervical procedure with anastomosis of the cervical oesophagostomy to the cervical colostomy.

Although Waterston's original technique was modified the principles remained unaltered. The three-stage procedure was reduced to a two-stage procedure and ultimately to a one-stage procedure performed either via a thoracoabdominal incision or via a left thoracotomy through the seventh intercostal space. Peripheral incision of the diaphragm enabled the abdomen to be entered and following preparation of the colonic segment the colonic graft was anastomosed to the distal oesophagus in the posterior mediastinum and to the previously performed oesophagostomy in the neck.

12.5.2   OESOPHAGOCOLOPLASTY USING RIGHT COLON OR ILEOCOLON

The patient is positioned supine and the abdomen opened through a midline incision embracing the gastrostomy stoma and continuing below the umbilicus. The vascular pattern of the colon is inspected and the ascending colon (sometimes with a short segment of distal ileum) used as an isoperistaltic conduit from the neck via a bluntly developed retrosternal tunnel. The right colic and ileocolic arteries are divided, the blood supply to the graft being supplied by the middle colic artery brought up from behind the stomach and through the lesser omentum. The proximal end of the graft is anastomosed to the mobilized oesophagus in the neck and the distal end to the anterior mid-body of the stomach. De Lorimier and Harrison (1986) suggest that reflux can be minimized by anastomosing the colon as cephalad on the stomach as possible.

Advantages claimed for this procedure include the relative simplicity of the operation and a reduced tendency for the conduit to become redundant and kinked.

12.5.3   GREATER CURVATURE TUBE OESOPHAGOPLASTY

This technique can be applied whenever there is an adequate stomach. The gastric tube can be based proximally at the cardia (a 'reverse' tube; Figure 12.5) or distally at the pylorus (an isoperistaltic tube; Figure 12.6) and its position in the chest can be either retrosternal, or in the left chest anterior or posterior to the hilum of the lung. The gastric tube can be placed along the route of the normal oesophagus and joined to an undisturbed upper oesophageal segment. Proponents of the reverse gastric tube (Gavriliu, 1975; Heimlich, 1959, 1972; Cohen *et al.*, 1974; Burrington and Stephens, 1968; Anderson, 1984) claim (1) that the

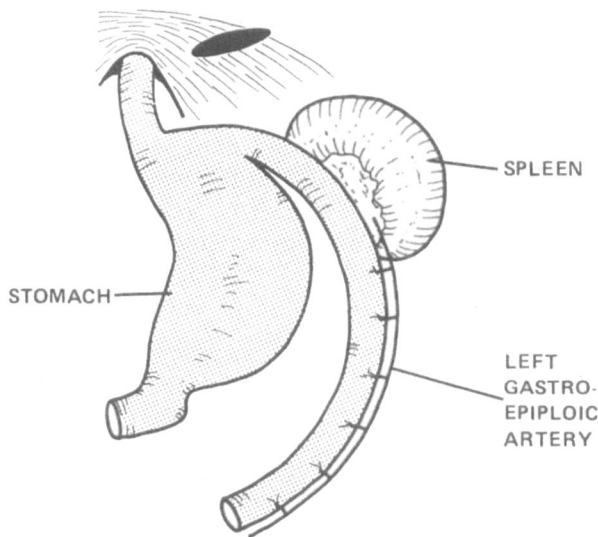

Figure 12.5 The reverse gastric tube is based at the cardia and relies for its blood supply on the left gastroepiploic artery.

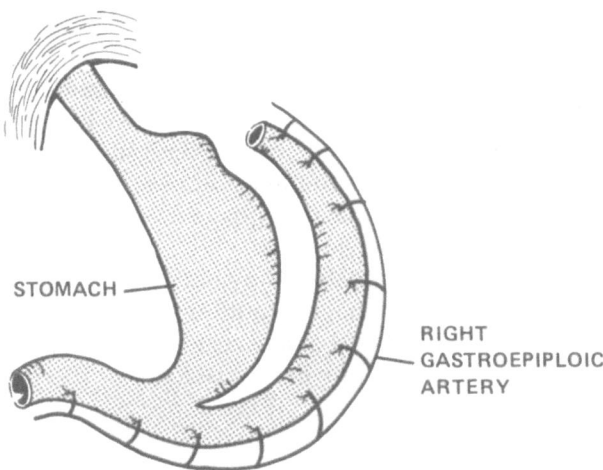

Figure 12.6 The isoperistaltic gastric tube is based at the pylorus and relies for its blood supply on the right gastroepiploic artery.

procedure is technically easier than other methods; (2) that the gastroepiploic arcade is usually complete and of an adequate size; (3) that submucosal collateral vessels are plentiful, ensuring good vascularity of the tube; and (4) that the stomach is at risk of fewer anomalies than the colon and has a natural barrier to acid digestion. Lindahl *et al.* (1983) found that the gastric tube procedure had fewer complications and less mortality than colon replacement. The length of the tube required can be estimated precisely as it is formed and the remaining stomach rapidly grows to reach its preoperative size. It is, moreover, the procedure of choice when there are co-existing anorectal abnormalities (Anderson *et al.*, 1975).

Reverse gastric tube

The original feeding gastrostomy is placed well away from the greater curvature in anticipation of the later gastric tube (Anderson, 1984). The abdomen is opened through a transverse supraumbilical incision and the gastrocolic omentum divided preserving the gastroepiploic arcade. The right gastroepiploic artery is divided at the point of origin of the gastric tube. Care must be taken to avoid narrowing of the pyloric outlet. The GIA stapler is set parallel to the greater curvature approximately 1.5–2 cm from the curvature to create the tube (Anderson, 1984) or it can be constructed by hand around a size 20–26 Bougie (Burrington and Stephens, 1968). The spleen is preserved. The staple line on the gastric tube and remaining stomach can be reinforced simultaneously with interrupted serosal sutures. The gastric tube can be brought up retrosternally or via the left pleural cavity and anastomosed to the oesophagus in the neck after mobilization of the cervical oesophagostomy. (An alternative to immediate oesophagogastric tube anastomosis is to leave the upper end of the tube as a stoma and close it once healing of the tube has occurred.) It is necessary to mobilize the cervical oesophagus as well as the tube to avoid kinking at the anastomosis. Closure of the strap muscles over the surface of the oesophageal anastomosis minimizes bulging of the neck during swallowing.

It is usual to replace the gastrostomy, at an appropriate site, for temporary feeding while oesophageal continuity is established. Creation of a nipple valve at the distal end of a reversed gastric tube in dogs has been shown to be effective in preventing reflux into the tube (Buras *et al.*, 1986).

Isoperistaltic gastric tube

The principles of the isoperistaltic tube based on the pylorus (Figure 12.6) are the same as described above. It relies on the right gastroepiploic artery for its blood supply (Cohen *et al.*, 1974). The location of its base lends itself to the retrosternal route.

12.5.4 GASTRIC TRANSPOSITION

In 1984 Spitz described gastric transposition via the mediastinal route as a procedure appropriate for infants with long-gap oesophageal atresia. Advantages of the procedure included:

1. Good blood supply
2. Adequate length
3. Ease of procedure

Subsequently, Valente *et al.* (1987) reviewed 10 patients managed by this technique. Spitz *et al.* (1987) later described oesophageal replacement by total gastric transposition in 34 infants of whom 32 had oesophageal atresia. Postoperatively, 25 children were entirely asymptomatic and managed a normal diet. The operative procedure consisted of either a transhiatal gastric transposition through the posterior mediastinum without a thoracotomy or a gastric transposition via a thoraco-abdominal approach; the series included eight previously-failed colonic interpositions. Thoracotomy was considered necessary in children with extensive oesophageal strictures and in some of those with failed primary anastomoses where extensive scarring from a leak demanded careful dissection to remove the oesophagus.

When the procedure is performed without thoracotomy the stomach is exposed via an oblique left upper abdominal transverse muscle-cutting incision encompassing the gastrostomy site. Adhesions between the stomach and the left lobe of the liver are divided, and the greater curvature of the stomach mobilized by division of the vessels in the gastrocolic omentum and the short gastric vessels. These vessels are ligated well away from the stomach wall to preserve the vascular arcades of the right gastroepiploic vessels while avoiding damage to the spleen. The lesser curvature of the stomach is freed by incising the lesser omentum from the pylorus to the diaphragmatic hiatus; the right gastric artery is preserved while the left gastric artery is ligated and divided close to the stomach. The lower oesophagus is exposed by dividing the phrenico-oesophageal membrane, and the margins of the oesophageal hiatus and the diaphragm defined. The short blind-ending lower oesophageal stump is dissected out of the posterior mediastinum through the diaphragmatic hiatus. The freed body and fundus of the stomach can now be delivered into the wound. The oesophagus is transected at the gastro-oesophageal junction and the defect closed in two layers (Figure 12.7). A pyloromyotomy is performed and a careful

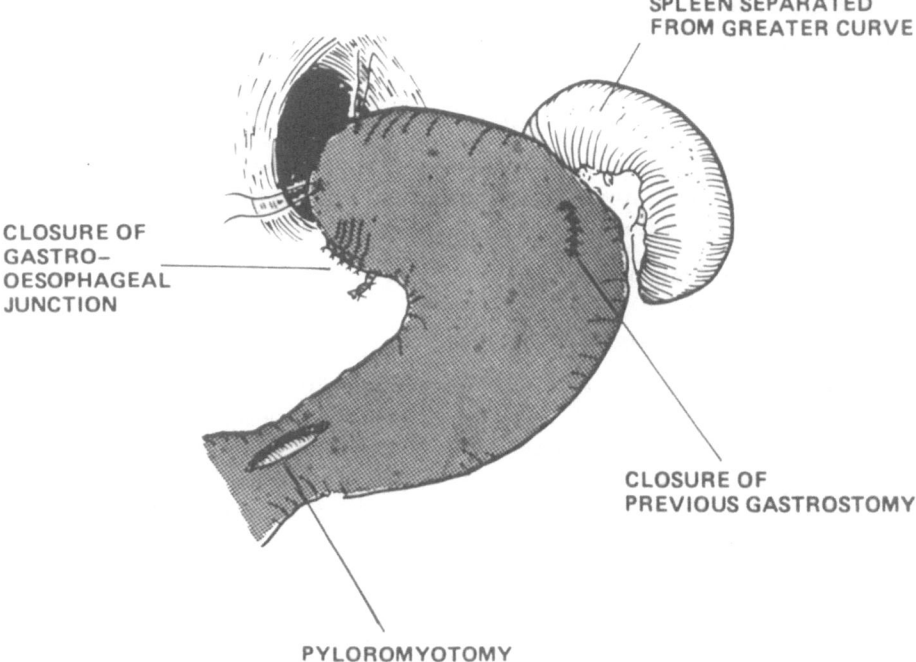

SPLEEN SEPARATED
FROM GREATER CURVE

CLOSURE OF
GASTRO–
OESOPHAGEAL
JUNCTION

CLOSURE OF
PREVIOUS GASTROSTOMY

PYLOROMYOTOMY

Figure 12.7 Gastric transposition: the short gastric vessels are divided to mobilize the spleen from the greater curvature of the stomach; the oesophageal stump is mobilized and the oesophagus is transected at the gastro-oesophageal junction; and a pyloromyotomy performed. (Adapted from Spitz, 1988.)

inspection is made for a mucosal perforation. The second part of the duodenum is 'Kocherized' to obtain maximum mobility of the pylorus (Spitz, 1984).

The previously constructed cervical oesophagostomy is mobilized taking care not to damage the muscular coat of the oesophagus or the recurrent laryngeal nerves. A plane of dissection between the membranous posterior surface of the trachea and the prevertebral fascia is established and by blunt dissection immediately in the midline a tunnel is created into the superior mediastinum.

A similar tunnel is fashioned from below the line of the normal oesophageal route by means of blunt dissection through the oesophageal hiatus in the tissue posterior to the heart and anterior to the prevertebral fascia (Figure 12.8).

When continuity of the superior and inferior posterior mediastinal tunnels has been established, the space to be occupied by the stomach is developed into a two to three finger-breadth tunnel.

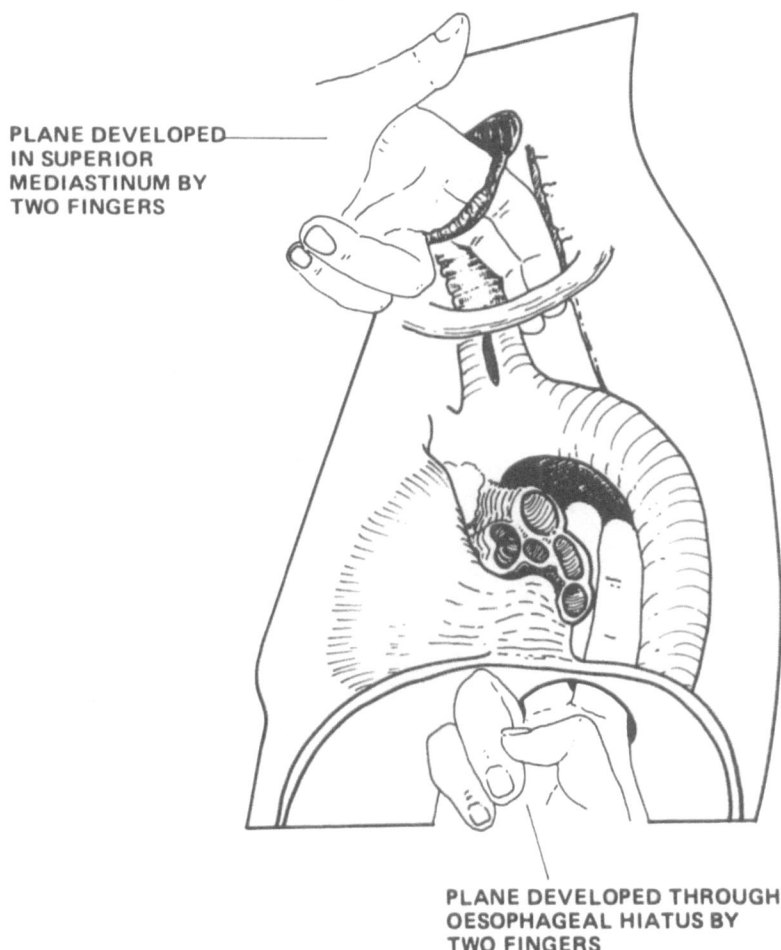

PLANE DEVELOPED
IN SUPERIOR
MEDIASTINUM BY
TWO FINGERS

PLANE DEVELOPED THROUGH
OESOPHAGEAL HIATUS BY
TWO FINGERS

Figure 12.8 Blunt dissection from above and below posterior to the heart and anterior to the prevertebral fascia creates a tunnel through which the stomach can be drawn. (Adapted from Spitz, 1988.)

The stomach is pulled up through the posterior mediastinum into the neck (Figure 12.9) without twisting it, and an oesophagogastric anastomosis constructed.

12.5.5 JEJUNAL INTERPOSITION

The technique of jejunal interposition has been described by Foker *et al.* (1982) and assumes the infant already has a cervical oesophagostomy

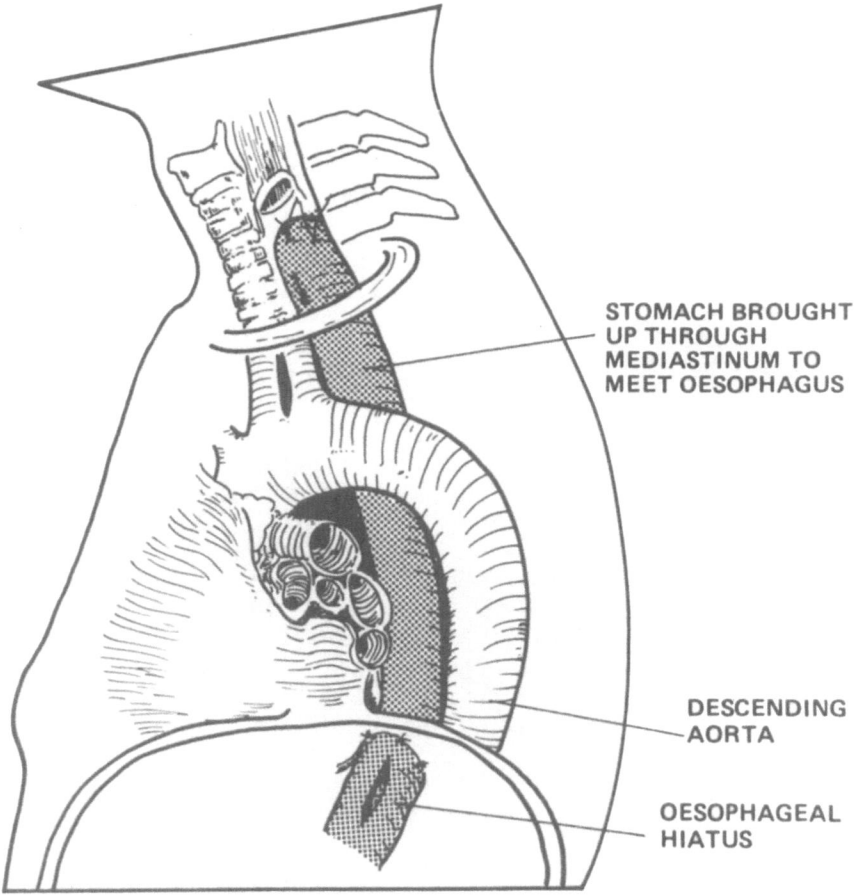

STOMACH BROUGHT UP THROUGH MEDIASTINUM TO MEET OESOPHAGUS

DESCENDING AORTA

OESOPHAGEAL HIATUS

Figure 12.9   The stomach is pulled up through the posterior mediastinum into the neck. (Adapted from Spitz, 1988.)

and gastrostomy. A Roux-en-Y limb of proximal jejunum is created, with preservation of the first major jejunal artery and vein. The next two or three major arterial branches are divided. Division of the base of two secondary arcades and incision of the peritoneum allows the full length of the jejunal limb to be utilized (Figure 12.10). A wide subcutaneous tunnel overlying the sternum is used to bring the jejunum to the neck where it is brought to the surface as a cervical jejunostomy.

The second stage of the interposition involves construction of a cervical anastomosis (oesophagojejunostomy) and jejunoantrostomy (Figure 12.11).

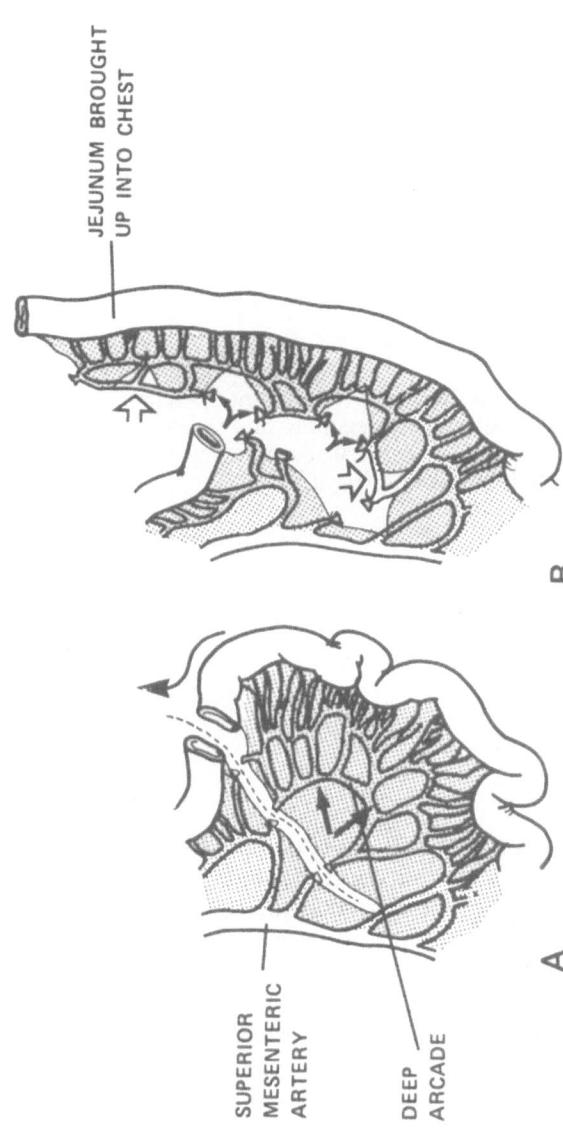

Figure 12.10 Jejunal interposition: mobilization of the vascular arcades during creation of a Roux-en-Y limb of proximal jejunum. The jejunum is divided distal to the first major arterial branch. The length of jejunum is maximized when the base of two secondary arcades is divided (solid arrows) and the peritoneum is incised (open arrows). (Adapted from Foker *et al.*, 1982.)

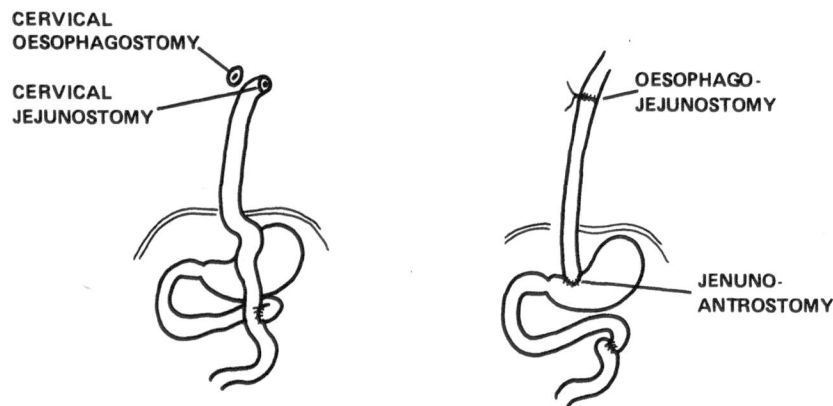

Figure 12.11   The first stage of the Roux-en-Y jejunal interposition (left). The limb has been brought out as a cervical jejunostomy and intestinal continuity restored by a jejunojejunostomy. A cervical oesophagojejunostomy and jejunoantrostomy complete the interposition (right).

Reconstruction of the oesophagus using a free jejunal graft has been described (Jones and Gustavson, 1983; Simms *et al.*, 1989) but has not gained widespread acceptance.

12.6   The future

The aim of oesophageal replacement always has been to achieve continuity of the alimentary tract with a conduit which provides the best function with the fewest complications. All methods have their advantages and disadvantages (Table 12.3) but at present it would appear that the gastric tube procedure has less mortality and fewer complications than colonic interposition (Lindahl *et al.*, 1983). Likewise, the early results of total gastric transposition as an alternative method of oesophageal replacement are encouraging (Spitz *et al.*, 1987).

The final chapter in the story of oesophageal replacement in childhood is yet to be written but one thing is clear; with the passage of time fewer replacements will be required. This is clearly of advantage to the vast majority of patients born with oesophageal atresia, with or without a tracheo-oesophageal fistula. Current experience suggests that the patient's own oesophagus is his best oesophagus.

Table 12.3 Advantages and disadvantages of various types of interposition

Type of interposition	Advantages	Disadvantages
Colon interposition	Adequate length can usually be attained	Blood supply may be precarious. Leaks/strictures from upper or lower anastomosis (25% on average). Redundancy of colon loop. Kinks. Slow transit time.
Gastric tube interposition	Good blood supply. Adequate length. Rapid transit of food.	Long suture line. Leaks from cervical anastomosis (50%) with strictures developing in 25%.
Gastric transposition	Good blood supply. Adequate length. Ease of procedure	Bulk of stomach in mediastinum may cause respiratory problems. Reflux and poor gastric emptying affect growth and development.
Jejunal interposition	Size of intestine appropriate. Good peristaltic activity.	Vascular supply very precarious and adequate length difficult to attain.
Free jejunal graft	Size of intestine appropriate. Good peristaltic activity.	Specialized technique for microvascular anastomosis required.

Adapted from Spitz (1984).

References

Ahmed, D. A. and Spitz, L. (1986) The outcome of colonic replacement of the esophagus in children. *Prog. Pediatr. Surg.*, **19**, 37–54.

Anderson, K. D. (1984) Oesophageal substitution. *Aust. N. Z. J. Surg.*, **54**, 447–9.

Anderson, K. D. and Randolph, J. G. (1973) The gastric tube for esophageal replacement in children. *J. Thor. Cardiovasc. Surg.*, **66**, 333–42.

Anderson, K. D. and Randolph, J. G. (1978) Gastric tube interposition: a satisfactory alternative to the colon for esophageal replacement in children. *Ann. Thorac. Surg.*, **25**, 521–5.

Anderson, K. D., Randolph, J. G. and Lilly, J. R. (1975) Peptic ulcer in children with gastric tube interposition. *J. Pediatr. Surg.*, **10**, 701–7.

Beasley, S. W. and Auldist, A. W. (1988) Current management and distal tracheo-oesophageal fistula. Presented at the International Congress of Paediatric Surgery, Melbourne, November 1988.

Buras, R. R., Jacir, N. N. and Anderson, K. D. (1986) An antireflux procedure for use with reversed gastric tube. *J. Pediatr. Surg.*, **21**, 545–7.

Burrington, J. D. and Stephens, C. A. (1968) Esophageal reconstruction with a gastric tube in infants and children. *J. Pediatr. Surg.*, **3**, 246–52.

Cohen, D. G., Middleton, A. W. and Fletcher, J. (1974) Gastric tube esophagoplasty. *J. Pediatr. Surg.*, **9**, 451–60.

Connolly, B. and Guiney, E. J. (1987) Trends in tracheoesophageal fistula. *Gynec. and Obstet.*, **164**, 308–12.

de Lorimier, A. A. and Harrison, M. R. (1986) Esophageal replacement. In *Pediatric Esophageal Surgery* (eds K. W. Ashcraft and T. M. Holder) pp. 102–36.

Foker, J. E., Ring, W. S. and Varco, R. L. (1982) Technique of jejunal interposition for esophageal replacement. *J. Thorac. Cardiovasc. Surg.*, **83**, 928–33.

Gavriliu, D. (1975) Aspects of esophageal surgery, in *Current Problems in Surgery*. Year Book Medical Publishers, Chicago, pp. 36–64.

Haight, C. (1969) Congenital esophageal atresia, in *Pediatric Surgery* 1 (2nd edn.) (eds W. T. Mustard, M. M. Ravitch, W. H. Snyder, K. J. Welch and C. D. Benson). Year Book Medical Publishers Inc., Chicago, pp. 358–9.

Heimlich, J. H. and Winfield, J. M. (1955) The use of a gastric tube to replace or bypass the esophagus. *Surgery*, **37**, 549–51.

Heimlich, H. J. (1959) Oesophageal replacement with a reversed gastric tube. *Dis. Chest.*, **36**, 478–93.

Heimlich, H. J. (1966) Elective replacement of the oesophagus, *Br. J. Surg.*, **53**, 913–16.

Heimlich, H. J. (1972) Esophagoplasty with reversed gastric tube. *Am. J. Surg.*, **123**, 80–92.

Hendren, W. H. and Hendren, W. G. (1985) Colon interposition for esophagus in children. *J. Pediatr. Surg.*, **20**, 829–39.

Howard, R. N. (1959) Oesophageal atresia; construction of a new oesophagus. *Aust. N. Z. J. Surg.*, **29**, 282–6.

Jones, B. M. and Gustavson, E. H. (1983) Free jejunal transfer for reconstruction of the cervical esophagus in children: a report of two cases. *Br. J. Plastic Surg.*, **36**, 162–7.

Ladd, W. E. (1944) The surgical treatment of esophageal atresia and tracheo-esophageal fistulas. *N. Engl. J. Med.*, **230**, 625–37.

Lindahl, H., Louhimo, I. and Virkola, K. (1983) Colon interposition or gastric tube? Follow up study of colon–esophagus and gastric tube esophagus patients. *J. Pediatr. Surg.*, **18**, 58–63.

Louhimo, I., Pasila, M. and Visakorpi, J. K. (1969) Late gastrointestinal complications in patients with colonic replacement of the esophagus. *J. Pediatr. Surg.*, **4**, 663–73.

Martin, L. W. (1972) The use of colon for oesophageal replacement in children. *Aust. N. Z. J. Surg.*, **42**, 160–3.

Martin, L. W. and Flege, J. B. (1964) Use of colon as a substitute for the esophagus in children. *Am. J. Surg.*, **108**, 69–74.

May, I. A. and Samson, P. C. (1969) Esophageal reconstruction and replacement. *Ann. Thorac. Surg.*, **7**, 249–77.

Oesch, I. and Bettex, M. (1987) Small bowel esophagoplasty without vascular microanastomosis: a preliminary report. *J. Pediatr. Surg.*, **22**, 877–9.

Randolph, J. G., Newman, K. D. and Anderson, K. D. (1989) Current results in repair of esophageal atresia with tracheo-esophageal fistula using physiologic status as a guide to therapy. *Ann. Surg.*, **209**, 526–31.

Ring, W. S., Varco, R. L. and L'Heureaux, P. R. (1982) Esophageal replacement with jejunum in children: an 18 to 33 year follow up. *J. Thorac. Cardiovasc. Surg.*, **83**, 918–27.

Sherman, C. D. and Waterston, D. (1957) Oesophageal reconstruction in children using intrathoracic colon. *Arch. Dis. Child.*, **32**, 11–16.

Simms, M. H., Brearley, S., Watson, D. and Roberts, K. D. (1989) Reconstruction of the esophagus using a free jejunal graft in complicated atresia. *Pediatr. Surg. Int.*, **4**, 159–61.

Spitz, L. (1984) Gastric transposition via the mediastinal route for infants with long gap esophageal atresia. *J. Pediatr. Surg.*, **19**, 149–54.

Spitz, L., Kiely, E. and Sparnon, A. T. (1987) Gastric transposition for esophageal replacement in children. *Ann. Surg.*, **206**, 69–72.

Spitz, L. (1988) Gastric replacement of the oesophagus, in *Rob and Smith's Operative Surgery, Paediatric Surgery* (4th edn.), (eds L. V. Spitz and H. H. Nixon). Butterworths, London, pp. 142–5.

Stanley-Brown, E. G. (1974) Massive haemorrhage after colon interposition: early and late. *J. Pediatr. Surg.*, **9**, 235–7.

Sweet, R. H. (1948) A new method of restoring continuity of the alimentary canal in case of congenital atresia of the esophagus with tracheo-esophageal fistula not treated by immediate primary anastomosis. *Ann. Surg.*, **127**, 757–68.

Valente, A., Brereton, R. J. and Mackersie, A. (1987) Esophageal replacement with whole stomach in infant and children. *J. Pediatr. Surg.*, **2**, 913–17.

Waterston, D. J., Bonham-Carter, R. E. and Aberdeen, E. (1962) Oesophageal atresia; tracheo-oesophageal fistula. A study of survival of 218 infants. *Lancet*, **2**, 819–22.

Waterston, D. J. (1964) Colonic replacement of esophagus (intrathoracic). *Surg. Clin. North Am.*, **44**, 1441–7.

Waterston, D. J. (1979) Colon transplant in long term follow-up in congenital anomalies. *Pediatric Surgical Symposium*, the Children's Hospital of Pittsburgh, p. 7.

13 Tracheo-oesophageal fistula: the 'H' fistula

M. KENT, N. A. MYERS and S. W. BEASLEY

Tracheo-oesophageal fistula without atresia (Figure 13.1) presents a different clinical spectrum from the congenital oesophageal anomalies already described because the oesophagus is intact and patent. By common usage, it has become known as the 'H' fistula although the apparent obliquity of the fistula on X-ray has encouraged some to use the term 'N' fistula (Figure 13.2). The embryology is discussed in Chapter 3.

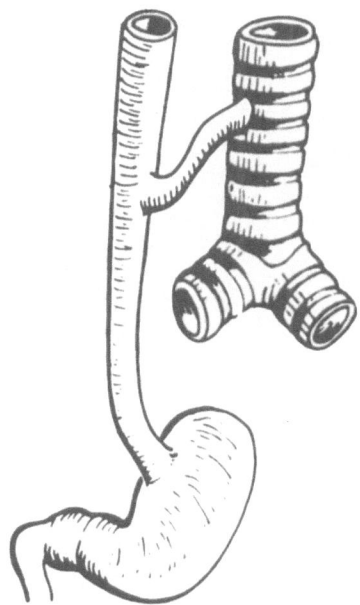

Figure 13.1 Tracheo-oesophageal fistula (the 'H' fistula).

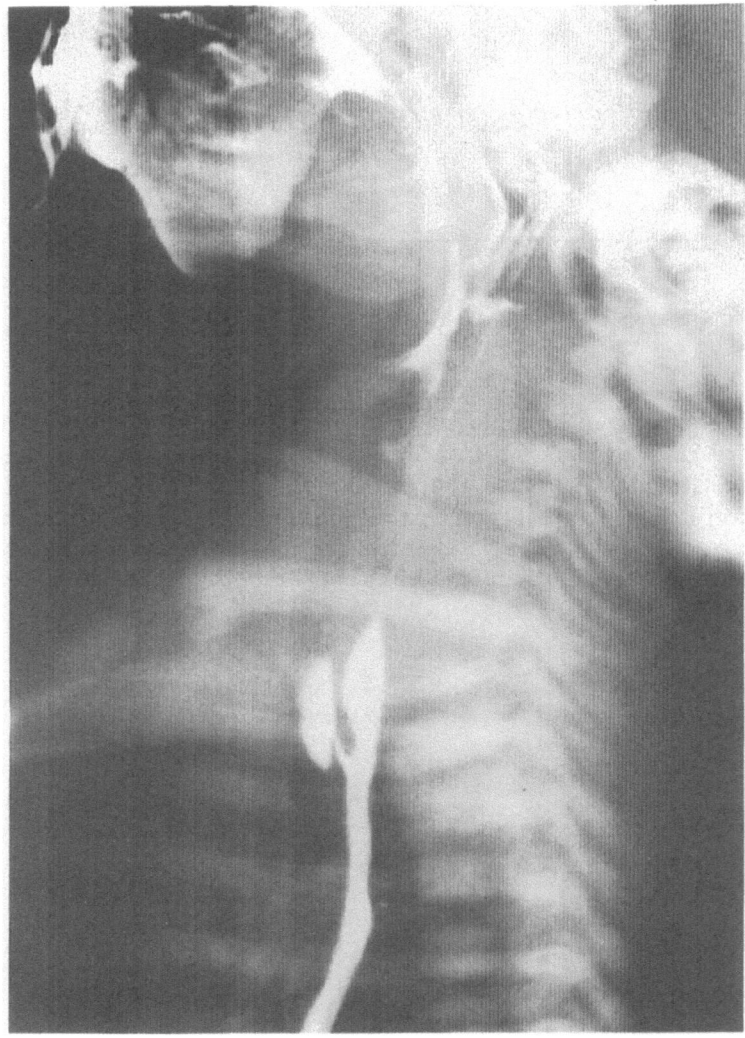

Figure 13.2   On lateral cervical X-ray the 'H' fistula appears to run in an oblique direction from the trachea proximally to the oesophagus distally.

Although the anomaly was recognized as early as 1873 (Lamb, 1873), the first successful surgical repair was not reported until 1939 (Imperatori, 1939). Since then, the surgical management of the 'H' fistula has become well established. The main areas of ongoing concern and controversy relate to problems in the early clinical diagnosis of the fistula and the best methods by which the diagnosis can be confirmed.

Apart from gastro-oesophageal reflux, which has been documented in about 10% of cases, other structural anomalies of the trachea or oesophagus in the absence of oesophageal atresia are unusual. Similarly, congenital anomalies in other organ systems are not as common as in patients with oesophageal atresia.

13.1 Surgical anatomy

The epithelium-lined fistula passes from the trachea in a caudal direction to enter the oesophagus at a slightly lower level. The obliquity of the fistula, and the close apposition of the trachea and oesophagus mean that for much of the time the fistula is occluded. Pressure changes in either structure and upward movement of the oesophagus during swallowing may open the fistula and allow air from the trachea to enter the oesophagus, or the oesophageal contents to enter the trachea (Figures 13.3 and 13.4).

Variants of tracheo-oesophageal fistula have been encountered. These include multiple fistulae (Eckstein and Somarsundaram, 1966)

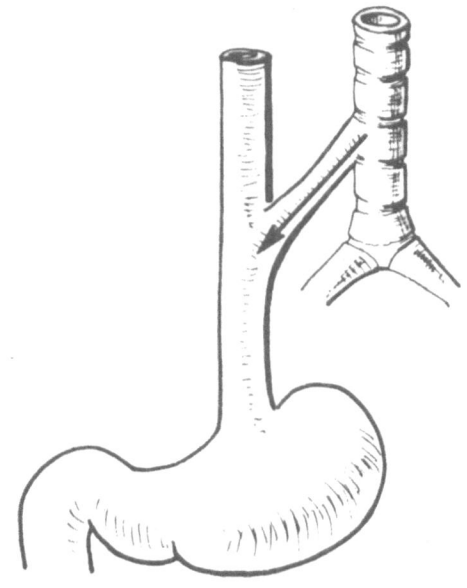

ABDOMINAL DISTENSION

Figure 13.3 Air may escape the trachea and enter the oesophagus through the tracheo-oesophageal fistula causing abdominal distension.

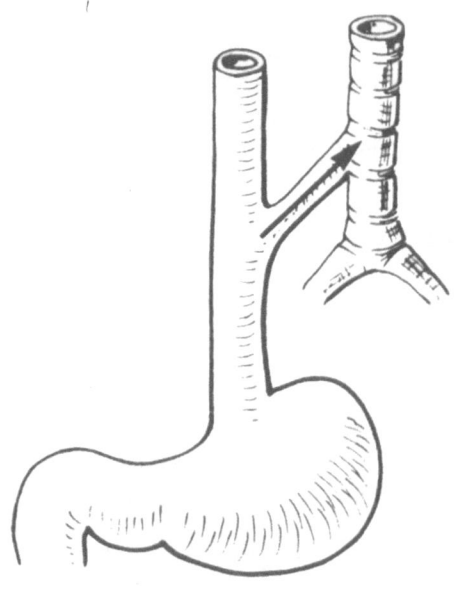

CHOKING & CYANOSIS

PNEUMONIA

Figure 13.4   Oesophageal contents, e.g. saliva, milk or gastric juice, may pass through the fistula into the trachea and contaminate the airways.

and an association of tracheo-oesophageal fistula with other oesophageal abnormalities such as oesophageal stenosis (Dunbar, 1958; Stephens, 1970) and oesophageal duplication (Wolf *et al.*, 1965).

The majority of the fistulae are in the root of the neck, above the level of the second thoracic vertebra. The surgical implication of this is that a cervical approach can almost always be used and thoracotomy is rarely required (Table 13.1). The recurrent laryngeal nerves, which at this level lie in the groove between the oesophagus and the trachea, are closely related to the fistula and are vulnerable to damage during operative dissection unless care is taken.

13.2   Incidence

In the Royal Children's Hospital series 36 patients had an isolated tracheo-oesophageal fistula, representing 6% of the total series. This compares with an incidence in other series which ranges from 1.0% to 11.0% (Table 13.2).

Table 13.1 Level of fistula and surgical approach*

Level of fistula	Total no.	Cervical approach	Thoracotomy
T1 or above	26	25	1
T2	6	5	1
T3	3	1	2
T4	1	—	1
Total	36	31	5

*Most of the thoracotomies were performed in the early years of the series, before it was appreciated that the fistula could be divided through a cervical approach. In retrospect, it is likely that virtually all could have been approached through the neck.

Table 13.2 Incidence of 'H' fistula in various series

Author	Year	Incidence (%)
Swenson	1962	2.0
Haight	1962	3.5
Waterston *et al.*	1963	1.7
Killen and Greenlee	1965	2–3
Hays *et al.*	1966	11.1
Holden and Wooller	1970	1.0
Eckstein *et al.*	1970	4.0
Bedard *et al.*	1974	< 1.0
Sundar *et al.*	1975	8.3
Cumming	1975	6.0
Ashcraft and Holder	1976	4.0
Louhimo and Lindahl	1983	2.4
RCH Melbourne	1988	6.0

13.3 Clinical features and diagnosis

In the 36 patients there was a slight male predominance (19:17). Polyhydramnios was not recorded and almost without exception the babies were born at 37 weeks' gestation, or later, unlike oesophageal atresia where prematurity is common.

Birthweight ranged between 2040 and 4770 g (mean 3085 g). Thirty patients were diagnosed in the neonatal period; the others were diagno-

Table 13.3 Major associated malformations in 11 of 36 patients

Cardiac malformation	5
VSD	2
Aortic arch anomaly	2
Fallot's tetralogy	1
Digital anomaly	4
Chromosomal abnormality	2
Duodenal atresia	1
Renal anomaly	3
Vertebral anomaly	1

sed between 39 days and three years. Associated congenital malformations were present in 11 patients (Table 13.3).

The symptoms produced by 'H' fistulae result from the 'two way
traffic' through the fistula (Figures 13.3 and 13.4). It is predictable,
therefore, that the three cardinal features are:

1. Choking and cyanotic attacks with feeds, usually relieved by gavage
    feeding
2. Pneumonia
3. Abdominal distension with air

Excessive drooling is another feature which is often seen, i.e. the baby
is 'mucousy'. In oesophageal atresia this is a result of oesophageal
obstruction and accumulation of saliva, whereas with the 'H' fistula, the
cause is irritation of the respiratory tract from the passage of saliva and/
or milk through the fistula. Vomiting, a hoarse cry and failure to thrive
are less common features. The frequency with which the four main
symptoms occur is summarized in Table 13.4.

The predominant symptom, choking with or without cyanotic episodes, is frequently attributed to other causes and its alleviation by gavage
feeding may lead to further diagnostic delay. The other symptoms may

Table 13.4 Symptomatology of 'H'
fistula in 36 patients

Choking and cyanotic attacks	35
Pneumonia	28
Abdominal distension	27
'Mucousy'	13

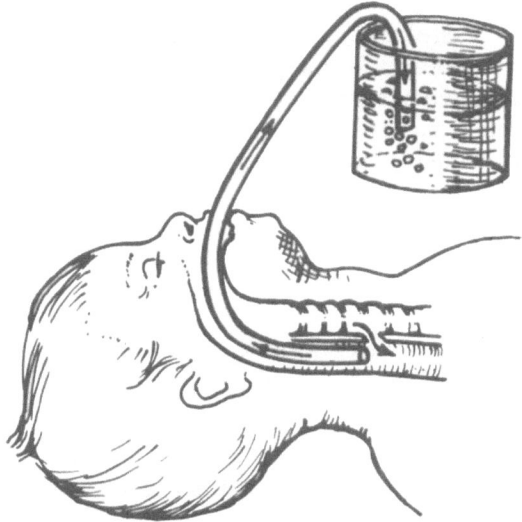

Figure 13.5 The 'catheter test'; bubbling occurs when the oesophagus catheter lies opposite the fistula. (Reproduced with kind permission Myers and Egami, 1987.)

be present in various combinations and permutations (Myers and Egami, 1987), but it is rare for all four features to occur together.

Physical examination may reveal few abnormal signs unless established pneumonia is present or abdominal distension is obvious. The degree of respiratory distress should be noted, as should persistent or intermittent cyanosis. One interesting physical sign may be elicited by performing the 'catheter test' (Myers and Egami, 1987). A catheter is passed into the oesophagus and the end placed under water (Figure 13.5). When a tracheo-oesophageal fistula is present, vigorous bubbling may occur from the proximal end of the catheter. However, a negative 'catheter test' does not exclude a fistula in an infant with suspicious symptomatology, and false positive tests also occur.

Other congenital abnormalities should be sought even though they are less common than in oesophageal atresia.

13.4 Investigation

Although the diagnosis may be suspected on clinical grounds, it is essential to confirm the diagnosis by appropriate investigation. There is no place for exploration of the neck when clinical findings raise the strong suspicion of tracheo-oesophageal fistula, but diagnostic man-oeuvres are unsuccessful, as some have advocated in the past (Lynn and Davis, 1961; Moncrieff and Randolph, 1966).

Investigation has two objectives: to confirm the diagnosis of a tracheo-oesophageal fistula; and to establish the site of the fistula. The former will indicate the need for operative treatment and the latter aids the operative identification of the fistula and may occasionally influence the approach.

13.4.1 RADIOLOGY

The main controversy centres around the relative roles of radiology and endoscopy. Our preference has been for radiological investigation because:

1. The success rate has been high (Table 13.5). The initial study was positive in 75%, and in all patients the diagnosis was confirmed by the third study.
2. Radiology accurately establishes the level of the fistula.
3. Radiology may establish an alternative or additional diagnosis, including nasopharyngeal inco-ordination and gastro-oesophageal reflux, both of which may present with symptoms similar to those of a fistula.

In recent years, the success of radiological confirmation of the fistula has improved to such an extent that in the last ten patients, none has required a second study. This has been attributed to meticulous atten-tion to detail, including recording the entire study on video to allow play-back; and the use of a mid-oesophageal tube (Figure 13.2). Where an initial barium swallow is negative, or where barium appears in the trachea but the route is obscure, we now repeat the examination and introduce the barium through a catheter placed in the mid-oesophagus (Beasley and Myers, 1988) (Figure 13.6). Confirmation of the diagnosis enables surgery to proceed without preliminary bronchoscopy. It is our belief that should diagnostic doubt persist despite an adequate mid-

Table 13.5   Radiological diagnosis of 'H' fistula

	No. performed	Positive
First study	36	27
Second study	9	7
Third study	2	2

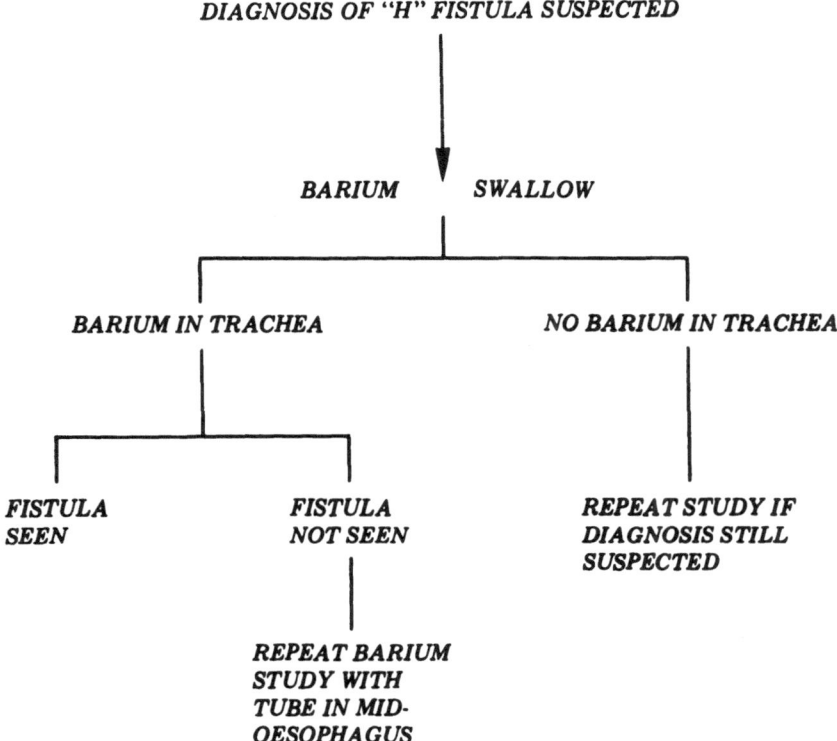

Figure 13.6 Algorithm of the radiological investigation of an infant with a suspected 'H' fistula.

oesophageal radiological investigation, bronchoscopy should be performed. There is no role for oesophagoscopy (Bedard *et al.*, 1974) or the introduction of dyes, such as methylene blue, to identify the fistula.

13.4.2 BRONCHOSCOPY

The other method of investigation is bronchoscopy which has its strong advocates (Gans and Johnson, 1977) and usually identifies a fistula, if present. Preliminary cannulation of the fistula (Filston *et al.*, 1982) to aid its operative localization is not always easy and is probably unnecessary provided the fistula is approached through a cervical incision (Beasley and Myers, 1988).

Both contrast radiology and endoscopy have a place in the diagnosis of tracheo-oesophageal fistulae, and with appropriate expertise, one is not clearly superior to the other.

13.5   Differential diagnosis

Although many conditions enter into the differential diagnosis, it is particularly important to recognize the following:

1. Other causes of a 'mucousy' baby, e.g. oesophageal atresia (with or without fistula), and oesophageal stricture;
2. Other causes of aspiration pneumonia, e.g. nasopharyngeal inco-ordination, gastro-oesophageal reflux;
3. Other causes of abdominal distension, e.g. Hirschsprung's disease. There are now several reports of infants with 'H' fistulae being investigated or treated as suspected Hirschsprung's disease (Myers and Egami, 1987; Hays *et al.*, 1966; Sieber and Girdany, 1956).
4. Acquired tracheo-oesophageal fistula.

Delay in diagnosis of tracheo-oesophageal fistula is common (Figure 13.7) and highlights the importance of a high index of suspicion.

13.6   Management

The steps in the management of confirmed tracheo-oesophageal fistula are summarized in Table 13.6.

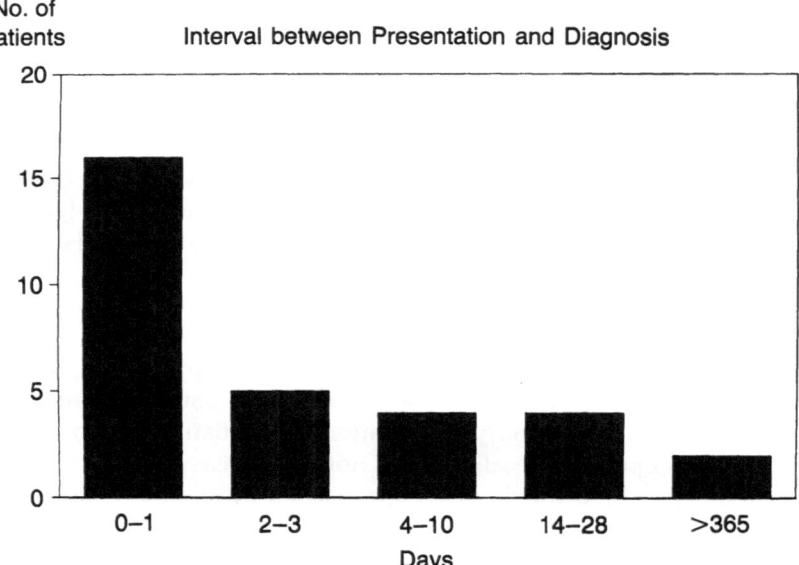

Figure 13.7 Delay in diagnosis: the interval between presentation and diagnosis.

Table 13.6 Summary of management of 'H' fistula

1. Preoperative management
   (a) Cessation of feeds
   (b) Commencement of antibiotics
   (c) Observation and monitoring of vital signs,
       particularly respiratory rate and temperature

2. Surgical ablation of the fistula
   (a) Cervical approach
   (b) Division of fistula

3. Postoperative management
   (a) Inspect vocal cords
   (b) Commence oral feeds day 3.

Surgical closure of the fistula should proceed as soon as possible but in some patients the severity of established pneumonia may necessitate one or several days of antibiotic treatment. Preoperatively, fluids and antibiotics will be given by the intravenous route. Endotracheal intubation may be required before surgery if severe pneumonia or respiratory distress is present.

13.6.1 OPERATIVE PROCEDURE

With few exceptions, the fistula is best approached via a supraclavicular approach. Our preference is for a right-sided incision to reduce the likelihood of injury to the thoracic duct. The incision is made 1–1.5 cm above the clavicle, and is deepened through platysma to expose the right sternomastoid muscle. Exposure is usually quite adequate without division of the sternomastoid. The strap muscles are retracted medially and the dissection is continued medial to the carotid sheath. Determination of the exact position of the oesophagus may be facilitated by the introduction of a naso-oesophageal tube by the anaesthetist, while the trachea can be recognized by its rings. The fistula is found in the groove between the trachea and oesophagus. It is short and runs obliquely upwards from the oesophagus to the trachea. Care must be taken to avoid injury to the recurrent laryngeal nerves which also run between the oesophagus and trachea. We no longer place catheter slings around the oesophagus above and below the fistula because the increased dissection involved is more likely to cause recurrent laryngeal nerve injury. A vascular sling is placed around the fistula itself to assist in its control during division. Each end of the fistula is closed using 4/0 or 5/0

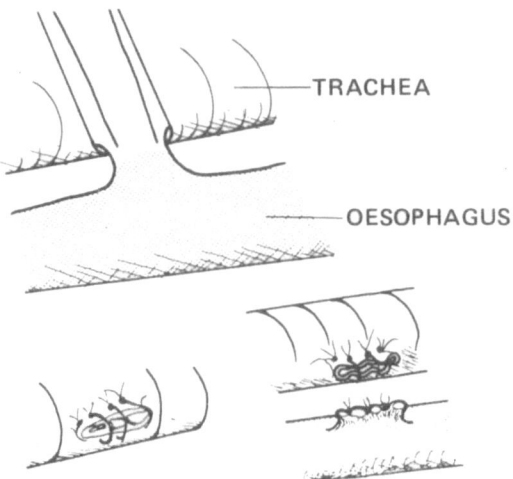

Figure 13.8 After the fistula has been identified it is divided and each end closed with interrupted sutures. Care is taken to avoid narrowing of either lumen.

polyglycolic acid interrupted sutures, leaving a suture line on both trachea and oesophagus (Figure 13.8). Drainage of the wound is not normally necessary, and the interposition of a muscle flap from the neck to separate the trachea and oesophagus is quite difficult to achieve.

In the few patients where thoracotomy was adopted, a right transpleural approach to the mediastinum was followed by dissection of the oesophagus at the appropriate level with identification of the fistula and division as described above.

13.6.2 THE ROLE OF GASTROSTOMY

We do not now advocate routine gastrostomy. In the early years gastrostomy was performed routinely and, for a time, it was combined with a transpyloric jejunal feeding-tube. Over recent years, however, as in oesophageal atresia with a distal fistula (Chapter 9), gastrostomy has been found to be unnecessary and liable to increase morbidity.

13.6.3 POSTOPERATIVE MANAGEMENT

At the completion of operation, the anaesthetist inspects the vocal cords to determine whether there has been any injury to the recurrent laryngeal nerves. If this is unilateral, special measures will not be required, but care must be taken when oral feeding is commenced. The baby is fed by the intravenous route for three or four days before commencing oral feeds.

13.7 Complications

In recent years, complications of closure of 'H' fistulae (Table 13.7) have become less common, but recurrent laryngeal nerve palsy and recurrence of the fistula may still occur. There were six recurrences in the 36 patients treated.

In the surgical management of recurrence, correction of possible contributing factors should be considered (Table 13.8): delay in re-

Table 13.7 Complications of repair of 'H' fistula

Recurrent laryngeal nerve palsy
  Unilateral
  Bilateral

Leak at site of closure
  Mediastinitis
  Recurrent fistula
  Oesophago-cutaneous fistula

Recurrent tracheo-oesophageal fistula

Miscellaneous
  Pneumothorax
  Tracheal obstruction
  Pneumonia
  Postoperative aspiration

Table 13.8 Factors which may contribute to recurrence of the tracheo-oesophageal fistula

1. Poor nutritional status preoperatively
2. Preoperative pulmonary infection or septicaemia
3. Failure to divide the fistula (ligation alone inadequate)
4. Leak at the suture lines
5. Juxtaposition of the two suture lines
6. Infection at the site of fistula closure
7. Septicaemia and mulnutrition in the postoperative period
8. Traumatic and/or repeated endotracheal tube manipulations after operation
9. Non-absbable suture material

operation may allow control of infection and correction of malnutrition; fistula closure should be achieved in healthy viable tissue without tension and (ideally) with separation of suture lines; and postoperative care should be meticulous in relation to control of the airway, infection and nutrition.

13.8 Summary

1. The clinical picture is confused by the fact that at times, the patient may have periods of being completely asymptomatic.
2. The step from suspicion to diagnosis is difficult (Bivins) as no type of roentgenographic contrast study of the oesophagus or endoscopic manoeuvre is infallible in making the diagnosis.
3. Surgical division of the fistula can usually be via the cervical route, and can be accomplished simply and without gastrostomy or drainage.

References

Ashcraft, T. M. and Holden, K. W. (1976) Esophageal atresia and tracheo-oesophageal fistula malformations. *Surg. Clin. North Am.*, **56**, 299–315.

Beasley, S. W. and Myers, N. A. (1988) Diagnosis of congenital tracheo-oesophageal fistula. *J. Pediatr. Surg.*, **23**, 415–7.

Bedard, P., Girvan, D. P. and Shandling, B. (1974) Congenital H-type tracheo-oesophageal fistula. *J. Pediatr. Surg.*, **9**, 663–8.

Cumming, W. A. (1975) Esophageal atresia and tracheoesophageal fistula. *Radiol. Clin. North Am.*, **13**, 277–95.

Dunbar, J. S. (1958) Congenital oesophageal stenosis. *Pediatr. Clin. North Am.*, **5**, 443–55.

Eckstein, H. B., Aberdeen, E., Chrispin, A., Nixon, H. H., Waterston, D. H. and Wilkinson, A. (1970) Tracheoesophageal fistula without esophageal atresia. *Z. Kinderchir.*, **9**, 43–9.

Eckstein, H. B. and Somasundarum, K. (1966) Multiple tracheoesophageal fistulas without atresia. Report of a case. *J. Pediatr. Surg.*, **1**, 381–3.

Filston, H. C., Rankin, J. S. and Kirks, D. R. (1982) The diagnosis of primary and recurrent tracheo-esophageal fistulas; value of selective catheterisation. *J. Pediatr. Surg.*, **17**, 144–8.

Gans, S. L. and Johnson, R. D. (1977) Diagnosis and management of 'H' type tracheo-esophageal fistula in infants and children. *J. Pediatr. Surg.*, **12**, 233–6.

Haight, C. (1962) in *Pediatric Surgery*, (eds C. D. Benson, W. T., Mustard, M. M. Ravitch, W. H. Snyder and K. J. Welch), Year Book Medical Publishers, Chicago, pp. 266–7.

Hays, D. M., Woolley, M. M. and Snyder, W. H. (1966) Esophageal atresia and tracheo-esophageal fistula; management of the uncommon types. *J. Pediatr. Surg.*, **1**, 240–52.

Holden, M. P. and Wooler, G. H. (1970) Tracheo-oesophageal fistula and oesophageal atresia: result of 30 years' experience. *Thorax*, **25**, 406–12.

Imperatori, C. J. (1939) Congenital tracheo-esophageal fistula without atresia of the esophagus. Report of a case with plastic closure and cure. *Arch. Otolaryngol.*, **30**, 352–9.

Killen, D. A. and Greenlee, H. B. (1965) Transcervical repair of H-type congenital tracheo-esophageal fistula. Review of the literature. *Ann. Surg.*, **162**, 145–50.

Lamb, D. S. (1873) A fatal case of congenital tracheo-esophageal fistula. *Philadelphia Med. Times*, **3**, 705.

Louhimo, I. and Lindahl, H. (1983) Esophageal atresia. Primary results of 500 consecutively treated patients. *J. Pediatr. Surg.*, **18**, 217–29.

Lynn, H. and Davis, L. (1961) Tracheo-esophageal fistula. *Surg. Clin. North Am.*, **41**, 871–83.

Moncrieff, J. D. and Randolph, J. G. (1966) Congenital tracheo-esophageal fistula without atresia of the esophagus. *J. Thorac. Cardiovasc. Surg.*, **51**, 434–42.

Myers, N. A. and Egami, K. (1987) Congenital tracheo-esophageal fistula. 'H' or 'N' fistula. *Pediatr. Surg. Int.*, **2**, 198–211.

Sieber, W. K. and Girdany, B. R. (1956) Tracheo-esophageal fistula without esophageal atresia – congenital and recurrent. *Pediatrics*, **18**, 935–42.

Stephens, H. B. (1970) H-type tracheo-oesophageal fistula complicated by esophageal stenosis. *J. Thorac. Cardiovasc. Surg.*, **59**, 325–9.

Sundar, B., Guiney, E. J. and O'Donnell, B. (1975) Congenital H-type tracheo-esophageal fistula. *Arch. Dis. Child.*, **50**, 862–3.

Swenson, O. (1962) in *Pediatric Surgery*, Appleton-Century-Crofts, New York, p. 155.

Waterston, D. J., Bonham-Carter, R. E. and Aberdeen, E. (1963) Congenital tracheo-esophageal fistula in association with esophageal atresia. *Lancet*, **ii**, 55–7.

Wolf, R. Y., Duncan, L. and Pate, J. W. (1965) Tracheo-esophageal fistula associated with esophageal duplication. *Surgery*, **58**, 728–30.

PART FIVE
Associated Anomalies

14   Associated anomalies

N. A. MYERS, S. W. BEASLEY and A. W. AULDIST

Reference to associated anomalies in oesophageal atresia started with its first description in 1670 when Durston documented oesophageal atresia in one of conjoined twins (Durston, 1670). Later, Hill (1840) reported the association between oesophageal atresia and anorectal anomalies.

In the 1940s the significance of associated anomalies was largely overlooked or ignored. For example, Humphreys (1944) wrote that associated anomalies are relatively infrequent and unimportant! In the same year Cameron Haight commented: 'other congenital anomalies usually do not contra-indicate operation as the anomalies that are most likely to be encountered are ones that are compatible with life' (Haight, 1944). By 1969, however, Haight had clearly recognized the significance of associated anomalies, reporting a 31.6% association in a series of 288 patients (Haight, 1969).

14.1   Incidence

In one of the first extensive surveys of associated anomalies in oesophageal atresia, Holder et al. (1964) found that 48% of 1058 patients with oesophageal atresia had another anomaly. They identified 849 anomalies in 505 patients (Table 14.1) and recognized four main groups: congenital heart disease, gastrointestinal anomalies including imperforate anus, genito-urinary anomalies and musculo-skeletal anomalies (particularly vertebral).

In his report of 143 patients of whom 65 had 128 anomalies, Hertzler (1965) recognized the prognostic significance of associated anomalies. The survival rate of those 65 infants with anomalies was 29% compared with a survival rate in those infants with oesophageal atresia alone of 45%. Three years earlier, Waterston et al. (1962) acknowledged the importance of associated anomalies by incorporating them into his classification of risk groups.

Since then there have been numerous contributions to the literature reviewing the incidence of associated anomalies (Table 14.2). Multiple anomalies occur more frequently in oesophageal atresia without tracheo-oesophageal fistula (Chittmittrapap *et al.*, 1989) and less frequently in 'H' fistula (Myers and Egami, 1987). In recent years, the incidence of associated anomalies appears to have increased (Louhimo and Lindahl, 1983); this is almost certainly due to more thorough and effective investigation in the neonatal period (Beasley *et al.*, 1989).

Table 14.1 Associated congenital anomalies in 1058 patients with oesophageal atresia

Congenital heart disease	201
Gastrointestinal	134
Genito-urinary	109
Imperforate anus	99
Musculoskeletal	91
Central nervous system	63
Face	53
Other	99

From Holder *et al.* (1964).

14.2 Royal Children's Hospital experience

Table 14.3 summarizes the type of anomalies identified in the 584 patients reviewed. Three or more anomalies coexisted in 81 patients. Post-mortem examinations were performed in the majority of patients who died and 86% of survivors have been reviewed as part of a long-term follow-up study (Chapter 25). Therefore, it is likely that the incidence and types of congenital anomalies described is fairly accurate. In our experience, associated anomalies are slightly more common in association with oesophageal atresia without fistula (Table 14.4) (Chapter 10) and in oesophageal atresia with a proximal fistula (Chapter 11) and less common in patients with an 'H' fistula (Chapter 13).

Table 14.2 Reported incidence of associated anomalies in oesophageal atresia

Series	Total number of patients	Patients with congenital abnormalities (%)	Type of abnormality					
			Cardiac (%)	Urinary* (%)	Orthopaedic (%)	Gastrointestinal (%)	Chromosomal (%)	Other (%)
Holder et al. (1964)	1058	52	19	10.3	8.5	22	2.6	20
Holder et al. (1987)	100	> 50	25	8	15	15	3	?
Spitz et al. (1987)	148	47	21.5	12.2	11	23	2	14
Chittimittrapap et al. (1989)	253	48	29	14	10	27	4	?
Ein et al. (1989)	97	53	29	8	12.3	17	8	12.5
Strodel et al. (1979)	365	31.6	26	16	15	25	?	18
Louhimo and Lindahl (1983)	500	40.6	13.2	12	11	15.8	3.2	12.2
	200	51	19.5	13.5	15.5	14.5	4	19
RCH (Melbourne)	584	58	20	22	15.5	22.5	4.8	18

*In some series genital abnormalities have been included.

Table 14.3 Breakdown of associated anomalies in 584 patients with oesophageal atresia and/or tracheo-oesophageal fistula*

	Number
Cardiac	119
Urinary tract	127
Anorectal	65
Other gastrointestinal	68
Orthopaedic:	
Structural vertebral	59
Limb	33
Central nervous system	19
Eye	.7
Chromosomal	28
Miscellaneous	82

*607 anomalies were identified in 339 (58%) patients.

Table 14.4 Associated congenital anomalies in 22 of 37 patients with oesophageal atresia without fistula

Chromosomal defect		6
Trisomy 21	5	
Trisomy 18	1	
Gastrointestinal		12
Anorectal	7	
Other	5	
Cardiac (excluding PDA)		8
Genitourinary		6
Skeletal		12
Vertebral	4	
Digital	6	
Other	2	

Miscellaneous: hydrocephalus, hypospadias, cleft palate, biliary tract abnormality

Table 14.5 Relevance of associated anomalies for oesophageal atresia

Relevance of associated anomaly to oesophageal atresia	*Examples*
A. Interesting but not relevant in relation to management	Meckel's diverticulum duplex kidney
B. Relevant because of frequency of association (treatment may be required)	Vertebral anomalies
C. Demand treatment, but not urgently, and oesophageal atresia takes undisputed priority	Pelvi-ureteric junction obstruction
D. Demand early treatment	
1. Needs to be co-ordinated with treatment of oesophageal atresia	Duodenal atresia and anorectal anomaly
2. Does not need to be co-ordinated with treatment of oesophageal atresia	Congenital dislocation of the hip
3. May take priority over complete repair of oesophageal atresia	Occasional cardiac malformation
E. Incompatible with survival	Trisomy 18 Bilateral renal agenesis

14.3 Classification of anomalies according to their significance

Not all associated anomalies affect the management of oesophageal atresia; and not all require treatment with the same urgency. In Table 14.5 associated anomalies are classified according to their management requirements in relation to those of the oesophageal atresia. From a practical point of view those that require treatment (Groups C, D and E) are best diagnosed early and should be detected in the first days of life.

14.4 The VATER association

In 1973 Quan and Smith proposed the acronym 'VATER' to denote the commonly encountered spectrum of associated anomalies:

V — Vertebral
A — Anorectal
TE — Tracheo-esophageal
R — Radial and renal

The concept of the so-called 'VATER association' gained rapid and widespread acceptance, even when all the components of the spectrum were not present. It was soon realized that the most important of the associated anomalies, cardiac defects, were omitted, leading to the introduction of the acronym 'VACTER', and then when the frequency of radial and other limb anomalies was appreciated the acronym was

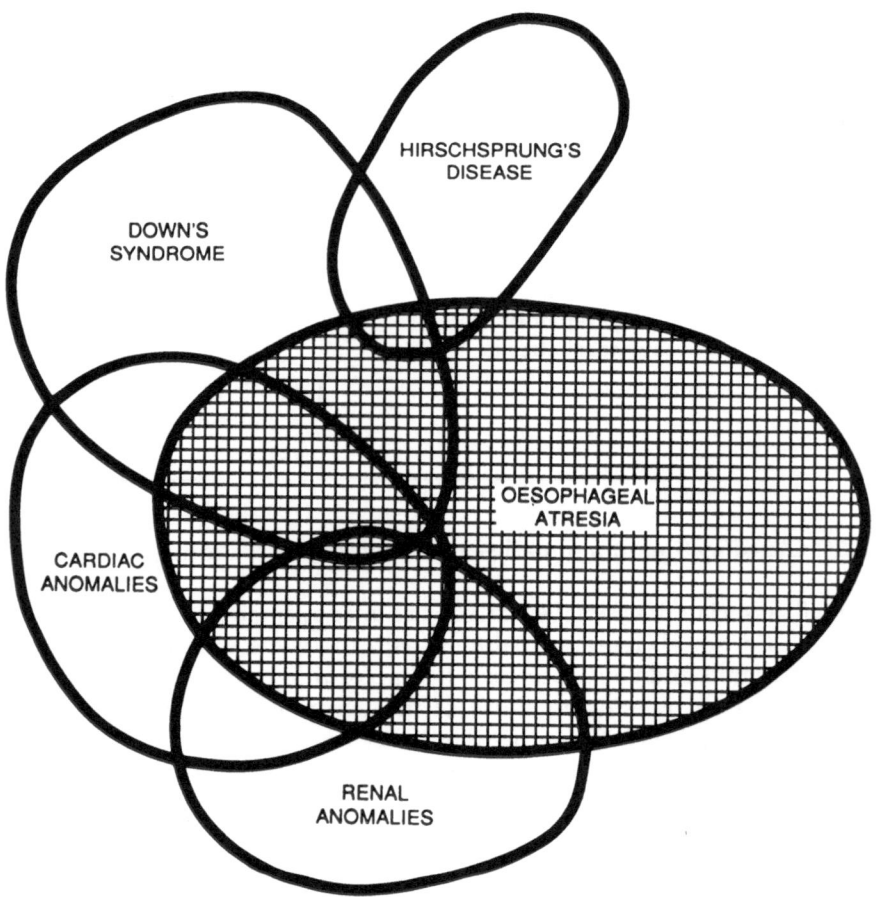

Figure 14.1 Schematic representation of the interrelationship of some of the congenital abnormalities seen in oesophageal atresia.

modified yet again to become 'VACTERL'. Another variation offered has been VACTEL (Nora and Nora, 1973). The acronym VATER (VACTER, VACTEL or VACTERL) is of limited usefulness other than to highlight the most frequently occurring anomalies that must be excluded. Suffice to say oesophageal atresia occurs often in association with one or more of the anomalies referred to above, but it is rare that any of the three suggested acronyms are fulfilled completely. It is more appropriate, perhaps, to regard the VATER association as one end of a spectrum of anomalies that ranges from the occurrence of any one of the defects singly to the full set of VATER anomalies, including congenital heart disease (Barry and Auldist, 1974). At the present time, the reason for the co-existence of the anomalies is not known.

A number of other anomalies, e.g. Trisomy 21 and Hirschsprung's disease, appear to occur in conjunction with oesophageal atresia more frequently than would be anticipated, and it may be that they form another part of the spectrum (Figure 14.1). In short, the occurrence of any one of the set of defects, including lesser degrees of radial dysplasia in a baby, should alert the paediatrician to look carefully for other components of the VATER association.

14.5 CHARGE association

There have been several reports of patients with oesophageal atresia and the CHARGE association (Pagon *et al.*, 1981; Valente and Brereton, 1987). Likewise, recent reviews of oesophageal atresia have identified a high incidence of the CHARGE association: Chittimittrapap *et al.* (1989) recognized the combination in five of 253 infants (2%); and in our series, since the association was first described by Hittner *et al.* (1979) we have identified it in four infants (3%). Occasionally, patients with oesophageal atresia have been described as having both the CHARGE and VATER associations (Weaver *et al.*, 1986; Chittimittrapap *et al.*, 1989); this is not surprising because they have a number of anomalies in common.

Recent reports (Oley *et al.*, 1988) and our own experience suggest that the outlook in children with the CHARGE association is better than previously suspected, with about a third being mentally normal or only mildly retarded.

14.6 Gastrointestinal abnormalities

Gastrointestinal anomalies are common in infants with oesophageal atresia: there were 133 gastrointestinal anomalies identified in 118 pa-

Table 14.6 Gastrointestinal anomalies (133 anomalies in 118 patients)

Anorectal (including cloacal)	65
Duodenal:	16*
atresia 13	
stenosis 3	
Pyloric atresia	1
Oesophageal stricture due to tracheo-bronchial remnant[†]	3
Pyloric stenosis	9
Hirschsprung's disease	1
Miscellaneous	38

*Six had anorectal anomaly + duodenal atresia.
[†]Only one proved histologically.

Table 14.7 Gastrointestinal anomalies in oesophageal atresia without fistula ($n = 37$)

Anorectal anomalies	7
Biliary tract anomaly	1
Cleft palate	1
Meckel's diverticulum	1
Exomphalos	1
Duodenal diverticulum	1
Total	12*

*One patient had two abnormalities.

tients (Table 14.6). The most frequent and important abnormalities were anorectal and duodenal. Six infants with an anorectal abnormality also had duodenal atresia. These groups are discussed separately.

Patients with oesophageal atresia without fistula have a particularly high incidence of gastrointestinal anomalies: 11 of 37 (30%) had an abnormality identified (Table 14.7).

14.6.1 ANORECTAL ANOMALIES

All babies with an anorectal anomaly should have the oesophageal patency confirmed by passing an oro-oesophageal tube into the stomach (Chapter 6). Likewise, all babies with oesophageal atresia should have their perineal region examined carefully (Stephens and Smith, 1971). Gross abnormalities are obvious, particularly in the male (Figure 14.2)

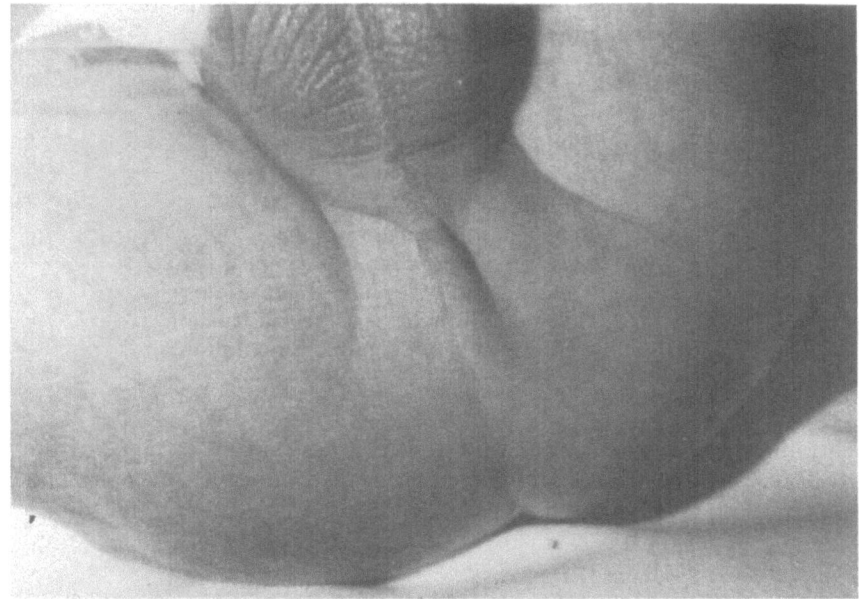

Figure 14.2 High imperforate anus in the male. A micturating cystourethrogram will reveal the presence of a rectovesical or rectourethral fistula. A plain X-ray will identify sacral abnormalities and an invertogram will show the level of the anorectal abnormality. Colostomy is constructed immediately following repair of the oesophageal atresia.

but more subtle abnormalities, such as an anteriorly placed anus or anal stenosis may be overlooked. The anorectal anomaly may be of an unusual type, e.g. 'H'-type rectourethral fistula without atresia (Stephens, personal communication).

The discovery of an anorectal anomaly demands careful physical inspection and radiology to determine whether it is a high or low lesion. The initial management of a high lesion usually involves construction of a colostomy, and a low lesion a perineal cutback anoplasty. When an anorectal anomaly occurs in conjunction with oesophageal atresia priorities in management need to be established. The following situations may arise.

Oesophageal atresia with distal tracheo-oesophageal fistula and a high anorectal anomaly

The tracheo-oesophageal fistula should be divided and the oesophageal atresia repaired before the infant is repositioned and a colostomy

Table 14.8   Management of oesophageal atresia and anorectal anomaly

1.	Assess level of anorectal anomaly
2.	Look for other anomalies:
	clinical examination
	echocardiography
	renal ultrasound
3.	Repair oesophageal atresia
	division of tracheo-oesophageal fistula
	end-to-end oesophageal anastomosis
4.	Colostomy to relieve bowel obstruction.
5.	Definitive repair of anorectum at later date.

fashioned under the same anaesthetic (Table 14.8). The colostomy effectively relieves the bowel obstruction. Definitive repair of the anorectal anomaly is planned as an elective procedure at the usual time.

Oesophageal aresia without fistula and a high anorectal anomaly

An upper pouch study excludes a proximal tracheo-oesophageal fistula. At the time of gastrostomy the duodenum is inspected (to exclude duodenal atresia) and a colostomy is fashioned. Definitive repair of the high anorectal anomaly is performed electively.

Oesophageal atresia, anorectal anomaly and intraluminal calcification

The combination of oesophageal atresia and anorectal anomalies may produce intraluminal calcification which is evident on plain X-rays of the abdomen at birth (Selke and Cowley, 1978; Berger and Bar-Maor, 1980; Beasley and de Campo, 1986). Intraluminal calcification must be distinguished from the calcification of meconium peritonitis, since the latter almost always represents a surgical emergency and implies significant intra-abdominal pathology (Beasley and de Campo, 1986). The radiological features of intraluminal calcification are summarized in Table 14.9. The oesophageal atresia should be repaired and a colostomy fashioned at the same procedure; when the meconium is passed it contains calcific densities which appear radio-opaque on X-ray.

14.6.2   DUODENAL OBSTRUCTION

Although duodenal atresia is the most common lesion causing duodenal obstruction, duodenal stenosis may occur as well. Occasionally duodenal obstruction will result from malrotation with volvulus and

Table 14.9 Radiological features of intraluminal calcification and calcification of meconium peritonitis

	Intraluminal calcification	Meconium peritonitis
Appearance	Small, punctate, discrete flecks, nodular	Linear or plaquelike, along the surface of viscera, e.g. liver
Distribution	Within distribution of bowel only	Anywhere within peritoneal cavity, scrotal
Localization	May be localized to one part of bowel or widespread	Frequently has localized area of predominance, even when widespread
Movement	Position alters with movement of bowel and bowel contents	Constant position
Resolution	With passage of meconium	Often removed at laparotomy
Other	Meconium calcified on X-ray	Meconium not calcified on X-ray

From Beasley and de Campo (1986).

when this combination occurs the outcome is frequently poor, due mostly to delay in diagnosis (Dibbins, 1970).

All babies with oesophageal atresia have an X-ray of the abdomen in addition to that of the chest. In duodenal atresia the typical 'double bubble' is present on the erect film (Figures 14.3 and 14.4), but the findings in duodenal stenosis may be less obvious. Particular note should be taken of excessive gastric distension with minimal distal gas. On occasions, the combination of oesophageal atresia and duodenal atresia can be recognized on antenatal ultrasound, particularly if there is no distal fistula (Figure 14.5). The management of oesophageal atresia and duodenal obstruction is described below.

Oesophageal atresia and 'double bubble'

If there is no distal bowel gas the infant almost certainly has duodenal atresia, although occasionally a small amount of gas does enter the bowel distal to the duodenal atresia via the common bile duct which

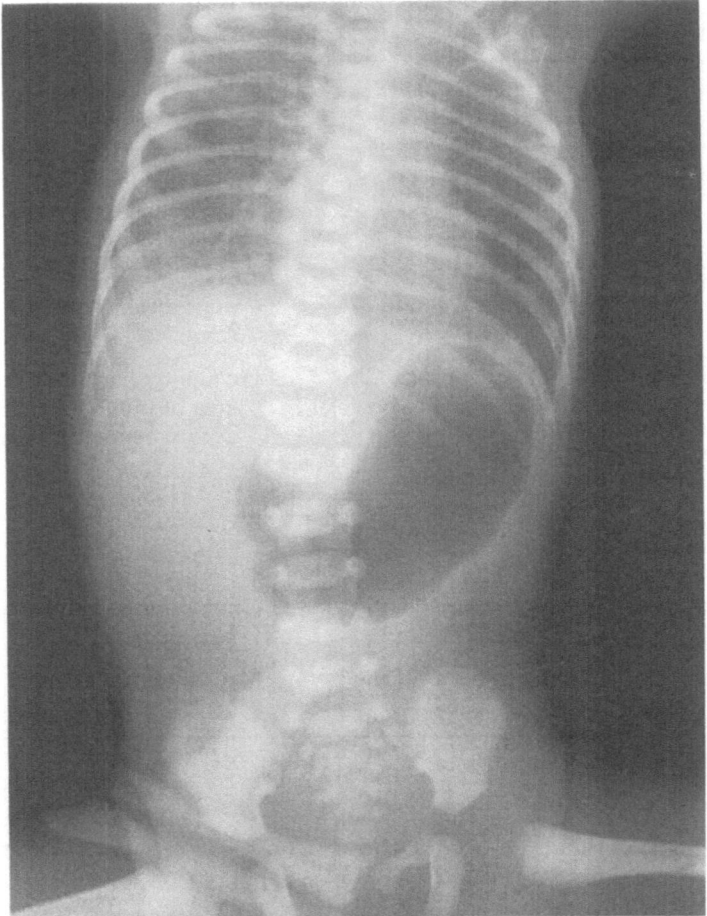

Figure 14.3   Oesophageal atresia, distal tracheo-oesophageal fistula and duodenal atresia, supine view.

may communicate with the duodenum on both sides of the atresia. The infant must be examined carefully for evidence of Down's syndrome. Routine preoperative investigation includes echocardiography (Chapter 15) and renal ultrasound (Chapter 16). The oesophageal atresia is repaired first and the duodenal atresia second (Spitz *et al.*, 1981; Kawana *et al.*, 1989) (Table 14.10). Gastrostomy is not required. The oesophageal atresia is repaired first to prevent difficulties in ventilation and respiratory complications occurring in the presence of a patent tracheo-oesophageal fistula during laparotomy. The duodenoduodenostomy may be performed under the same anaesthetic or delayed several days

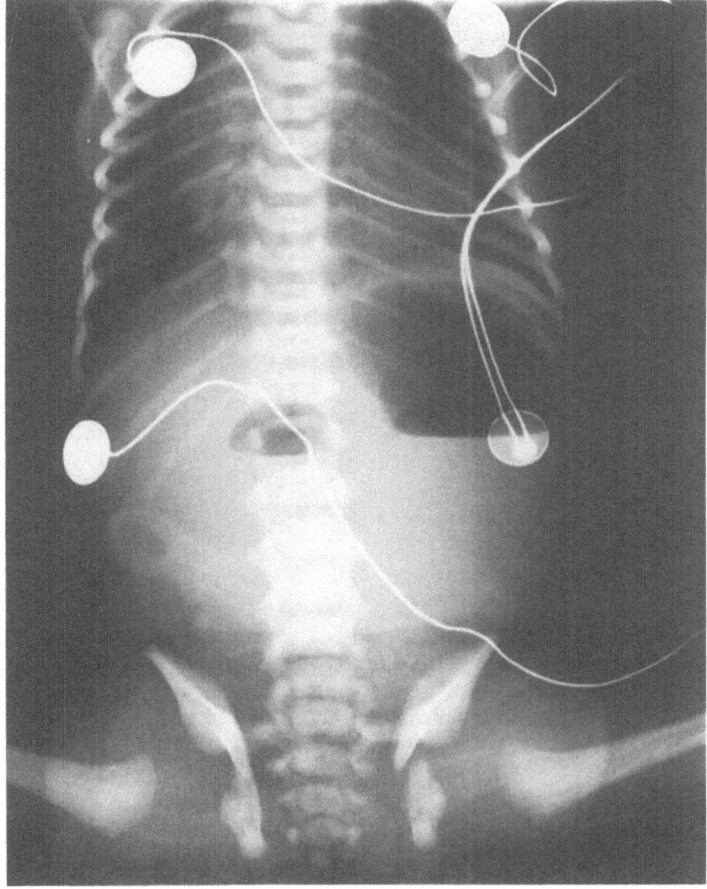

Figure 14.4 Oesophageal atresia, distal tracheo-oesophageal fistula and duodenal atresia: the classical 'double bubble' is clearly evident on the erect view.

according to the condition of the infant. If the duodenoduodenostomy is
delayed a transanastomotic tube should be passed at the time of thoracotomy to allow decompression of the stomach.

Oesophageal atresia, high anorectal anomaly and duodenal atresia

This combination occurred in six infants reviewed. The radiological
appearance of the abdomen was the same as for duodenal atresia alone.
When all three abnormalities coexist the oesophageal atresia is best
corrected first, followed by repair of the duodenal atresia and construction of a colostomy (Kawana *et al.*, 1989) (Table 14.11).

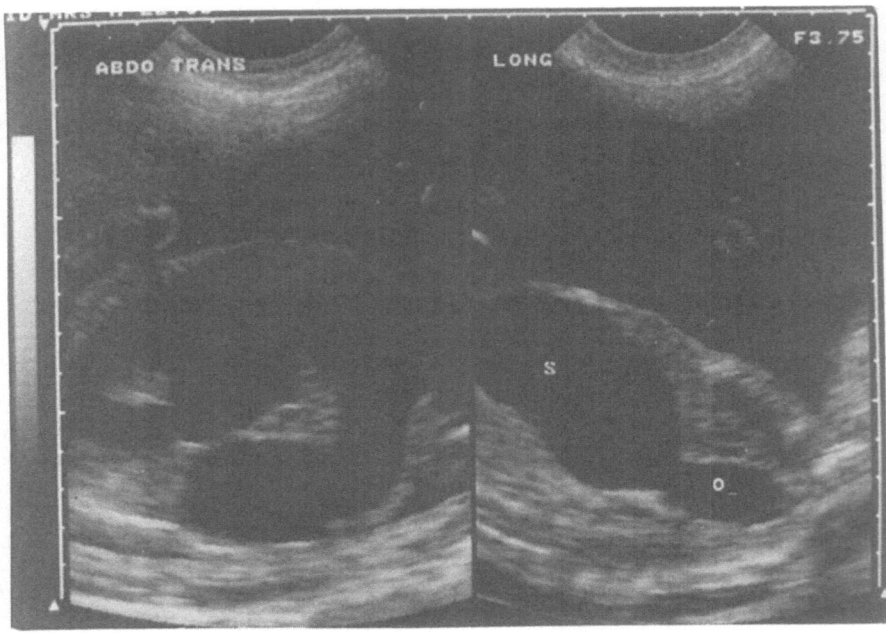

Figure 14.5 Antenatal diagnosis of oesophageal atresia and duodenal atresia: distension of the lower oesophageal segment (O) can be seen as it enters the stomach (S). There was no distal fistula. (Courtesy of E. Simpson.)

14.6.3 PYLORIC STENOSIS

There appears to be more than a coincidental association between oesophageal atresia and hypertrophic pyloric stenosis (Glasson *et al.*, 1973; Czernik and Raine, 1982): in our series, pyloric stenosis occurred in nine patients; of these, six were diagnosed at post mortem (early in the series) and three were managed successfully by pyloromyotomy.

Diagnosis may not be easy: the presence of a gastrostomy tube and abdominal wall scarring may make it difficult to palpate the tumour; and gastro-oesophageal reflux, common in babies with oesophageal atresia, may cause confusing symptomatology and lead to diagnostic delay.

14.7   Chromosomal abnormalities

Trisomy 18 and trisomy 21 are common in oesophageal atresia. In a series of 97 newborns treated between 1979 and 1985, Ein *et al.* (1989)

Table 14.10 Management of oesophageal atresia with distal fistula
and duodenal atresia

1. Look for other anomalies: e.g. Down's syndrome, congenital heart
    disease, imperforate anus
        clinical examination
        echocardiography
        ultrasound

2. Repair oesophageal atresia:
        division tracheo-oesophageal fistula
        end-to-end oesophageal anastomosis
        gastrostomy NOT required

3. Duodenoduodenostomy

Table 14.11 Sequence of surgery in
oesophageal atresia with distal fistula,
duodenal atresia and high imperforate anus

1. Thoracotomy:
        division of tracheo-oesophageal fistula
        oesophageal anastomosis

2. Laparotomy:
        duodenoduodenostomy
        colostomy
        no gastrostomy

identified trisomy 18 in seven and Down's syndrome in one. In our
series 28 (5%) infants had chromosomal aberrations of which 14 were
trisomy 18 and ten were Down's syndrome (Table 14.12).

It is important to recognize Trisomy 18 early because its poor prognosis does not justify active surgical intervention (Chapter 20). If the
diagnosis is suspected clinically, analysis of the chromosomes should be
undertaken immediately and surgery postponed until the results are
available.

Down's syndrome may be difficult to detect clinically in the immediate neonatal period, especially in the premature. However, if there are
features suggestive of Down's syndrome, the possibility of duodenal
atresia, cardiac disease and Hirschsprung's disease must be considered
as well.

226 *Associated anomalies*

Table 14.12 Chromosomal abnormalities

Trisomy 21 (Downs)		10
Oesophageal atresia with distal fistula	5	
Oesophageal atresia without fistula	5	
Trisomy 18		14
Others		4
Inversion long arm chromosome 15, mosaic G trisomy, Group D, 4p trisomy		
Total		28

References

Barry, J. E. and Auldist, A. W. (1974) The Vater association: one end of a spectrum of anomalies. *Am. J. Dis. Child.*, **128**, 769–71.

Beasley, S. W. and de Campo, M. (1986) Intraluminal calcification in the newborn: diagnostic and surgical implications. *Pediatr. Surg. Int.*, **1**, 249–51.

Beasley, S. W., Shann, F. A., Myers, N. A. and Auldist, A. W. (1989) Developments in the management of oesophageal atresia and tracheo-oesophageal fistula. *Med. J. Aust.*, **150**, 501–3.

Berger, J. and Bar-Maor, J. A. (1980) Intraluminal intestinal calcifications in a newborn with atresia of the oesophagus and imperforate anus. *Clin. Pediatr.*, **19**, 770–2.

Bishop, P. J., Klein, M. D., Philippart, A. I., Hixson, D. S. and Hertzler, J. H. (1985) Transpleural repair of esophageal atresia without a primary gastrostomy: 240 patients treated between 1951 and 1983. *J. Pediatr. Surg.*, **20**, 823–8.

Chittmittrapap, S., Spitz, L., Kiely, E. M. and Brereton, R. J. (1989) Oesophageal atresia and associated anomalies. *Arch. Dis. Child.*, **64**, 364–8.

Czernik, J. and Raine, P. A. M. (1982) Oesophageal atresia and pyloric stenosis – an association. *Z. Kinderchir.*, **35**, 18–20.

Dibbins, A. (1970) Discussion of paper by J. Raffensperger: Gastrointestinal tract defects associated with esophageal atresia and tracheo-esophageal fistula. *Arch. Surg.*, **101**, 241–4.

Durston, W. (1670) A narrative of a monstrous birth in Plymouth October 22 1670: together with the anatomical observations taken thereupon by William Durston, Doctor of Physick and communications to Dr Tim Clerk. *Phil. Trans. Royal. Soc.*, **V**, 2096.

Ein, S. H., Shandling, B., Wesson, D. and Filler, R. M. (1989) Esophageal atresia with distal tracheoesophageal fistula: associated anomalies and prognosis in the 1980s. *J. Pediatr. Surg.*, **24**, 1055–9.

German, J. C., Mahour, G. H. and Woolley, M. M. (1976) Esophageal atresia and associated anomalies. *J. Pediatr. Surg.*, **11**, 299–306.

Glasson, M. J., Bandrevics, V. and Cohen, D. H. (1973) Hypertrophic pyloric stenosis complicating esophageal atresia. *Surgery*, **74**, 530–5.

Haight, C. (1944) Congenital atresia of the esophagus with tracheo-esophageal fistula. *Ann. Surg.*, **120**, 623–55.

Haight, C. (1969) Congenital esophageal atresia. in *Pediatric Surgery*, vol. 1, 2nd edn. (eds W. T. Mustard, M. M. Ravitch, W. H. Snyder, K. J. Welch and C. D. Benson), Year Book Medical Publishers Inc., Chicago, pp. 358–9.

Hertzler, J. H. (1965) Congenital esophageal atresia: problems and management. *Am. J. Surg.*, **109**, 780–7.

Hill, T. P. (1840) Congenital malformation. *Boston Med. Surg. J.*, **21**, 320.

Hittner, H. M., Hirsch, N. J., Kreh, G. M. and Rudolph, A. J. (1979) Colobomatous micropthalmia, heart diseaes, hearing loss and mental retardation – a syndrome. *J. Pediatr. Ophthalmol.*, **16**, 122–8.

Holder, T. M., Ashcraft, K. W., Sharp, R. J. and Amoury, R. A. (1987) Care of infants with esophageal atresia, tracheoesophageal fistula, and associated anomalies. *J. Thorac. Cardiovasc. Surg.*, **94**, 828–35.

Holder, T. M., Cloud, D. T., Lewis, J. E. and Pilling, G. P. (1964) Esophageal atresia and tracheoesophageal fistula. A survey of its members by the surgical section of the American Academy of Pediatrics. *Pediatrics*, **34**, 542–9.

Humphreys, G. H. (1944) The surgical treatment of congenital atresia of the esophagus. *Surgery*, **15**, 801–23.

Kawana, T., Ikeda, K., Nakagawara, A., Kajiwara, M., Fukazawa, M. and Haia, K. (1989) A case of VACTEL syndrome with antenatally diagnosed duodenal atresia. *J. Pediatr. Surg.*, **24**, 1158–60.

Louhimo, I. and Lindahl, H. (1983) Esophageal atresia. Primary results of 500 consecutively treated patients. *J. Pediatr. Surg.*, **18**, 217–29.

Myers, N. A. and Egami, K. (1987) Congenital tracheo-oesophageal fistula. 'H' or 'N' fistula. *Pediatr. Surg. Int.*, **2**, 198–211.

Nora, J. J. and Nora, A. H. (1973) Birth defects and oral contraceptives. *Lancet*, **i**, 941–2.

Oley, C. A., Baraitser, M. and Grant, D. B. (1988) A re-appraisal of the CHARGE association. *J. Med. Genet.*, **25**, 147–56.

Pagon, R. A., Graham, J. M., Zonana, J. and Yong, S. L. (1981) Coloboma, congenital heart disease and choanal atresia with multiple anomalies: CHARGE association. *J. Pediatr.*, **99**, 223–7.

Selke, A. C. and Cowley, C. E. (1978) Calcified intraluminal meconium in a female with imperforate anus. *Am. J. Radiol.*, **130**, 786–8.

Spitz, L., Ali, M. and Brereton, R. J. (1981) Combined esophageal and duodenal atresia: experience of 18 patients. *J. Pediatr. Surg.*, **16**, 4–7.

Stephens, F. D. and Smith, E. D. (1971) *Anorectal Abnormalities in Children*, Year Book Medical Publishers, Chicago, pp. 282–3.

Strodel, W. E., Coran, A. G., Kirsch, M. M., Weintraub, W. H., Wesley, J. R. and Sloan, H. (1979) Esophageal atresia. A 41-year experience. *Arch. Surg.*, **114**, 523–7.

Valente, A. and Brereton, R. J. (1987) Oesophageal atresia and the CHARGE association. *Pediatr. Surg. Int.*, **2**, 93–4.

Waterston, D. J., Bonham-Carter, R. E. and Aberdeen, E. (1962) Oesophageal atresia: tracheo-oesophageal fistula. A study of survival of 218 infants. *Lancet*, **i**, 819–22.

Waterston, D. J., Bonham-Carter, R. E. and Aberdeen, E. (1963) Congenital tracheo-oesophageal fistula in association with oesophageal atresia. *Lancet*, **ii**, 55–7.

Weaver, D. D., Mapstone, C. L. and Yu, P. (1986) The VATER association: analysis of 46 patients. *Am. J. Dis. Child.*, **140**, 225–9.

15 *Congenital heart disease*

R. B. B. MEE

In this chapter, the influence of congenital heart disease (CHD) on the investigation and management of oesophageal atresia infants is described. Physiological and anatomical implications of the associated CHD affect the urgency of investigation and the timing of surgery. Despite this, the most important determinant of prognosis has become the presence of major chromosomal or non-cardiac, non-oesophageal defects.

15.1 Incidence

One in 4500 births has oesophageal atresia, whereas about one in 100 live births manifests congenital heart disease (CHD). However, between 13 and 29% of patients born with oesophageal atresia are found to have CHD (Table 15.1). In addition, 70% of patients with oesophageal atresia and CHD have other congenital structural and/or chromosomal abnormalities.

CHD was present in 119 of the 584 patients presenting to the Royal Children's Hospital with oesophageal atresia and/or tracheo-oesophageal fistula (Table 15.2). In 52 of the 584 patients, operation was not performed: 21 of these had CHD.

15.2 Significance of associated cardiac anomalies

15.2.1 ANTENATAL ULTRASOUND

The ultrasonographer should be aware of the association between oesophageal atresia and CHD. Cardiac lesions are much more likely to be detected on antenatal ultrasound than oesophageal obstruction; so the finding of the former should stimulate the ultrasonographer to look

Table 15.1 Incidence of congenital heart disease in oesophageal atresia infants

	Number of patients	% Cardiac anomalies
Holder *et al.* (1964)	1058	19.0
Louhimo and Lindahl (1983)	500	13.2
	last 200	19.5
Bishop *et al.*		
1951–1983	271	22.5
1974–1983	65	29.2
Holder *et al.* (1987)	100	25.0
Chittmittrapap *et al.* (1989)	235	29.0
Ein *et al.* (1989)	97	29.0
RCH Melbourne	584	20.0

carefully for a distended upper pouch, disturbance of oesophageal motility and a small stomach. About 0.5% of patients with CHD will have oesophageal atresia and/or tracheo-oesophageal fistula.

15.2.2   INVESTIGATION AT BIRTH

Once the diagnosis of oesophageal atresia has been established, the cardiac status must be evaluated. This involves careful clinical assessment and preoperative echocardiography. A cardiac catheter study is most unlikely to be required at this stage. Echocardiography will define any associated CHD and determine the position of the aortic arch. Complex management decisions may need to be made soon after presentation. Such decisions are assisted if they are based on definitive or near-definitive knowledge. From the respiratory point of view, there is advantage in early repair of the oesophageal atresia. A rapid analysis of other organ systems in a multidisciplinary fashion should be organized in a way that minimizes delay of the oesophageal repair. Suspicion of a severe chromosomal abnormality, however, may justify delaying surgical management until genetic corroboration is obtained.

The finding of a right aortic arch may influence the surgical approach, and encourage the surgeon to perform a left, rather than right, thoracotomy. Likewise, if the CHD *per se* requires early surgical palliation through a thoracotomy, a decision must be made as to which hemithorax will be used for each procedure.

Table 15.2 Types of congenital heart disease associated with oesophageal atresia and/or tracheoesophageal fistula (119 patients)

1.	Isolated intracardiac septation defects (VSD, ASD, CAVC)					
	[( ) = Mortality]					
	ASD	10	(3)			
	VSD	33	(16)			
	CAVC	3	(2)		Total 46	(21)
2.	Intracardiac septation defects + Great Vessel Defects					
	HLHS	2	(2)			
	HRHS	1	(1)			
	Tetralogy of Fallot	15	(10)			
	Truncus arteriosus	3	(3)			
	TGA.VSD	3	(3)			
	VSD (+/−ASD) + CoA or IAA or ANOM. SCA	4	(4)			
	SV + TGA or DOV	2	(2)			
	Other	3	(3)		Total 33	(28)
3.	Isolated great vessel defects					
	Patent ductus arteriosus	16	(11)			
	Coarctation aorta	5	(2)			
	Anom. SCA	6	(3)			
	Right aortic arch	1	(1)			
	Vascular ring	1	(1)			
	Caval	4	(3)		Total 33	(21)
4.	Unknown	7	(3)		Total 7	(3)
					Total 119	(73)

15.2.3 PROGNOSIS

In the past congenital heart disease has had a major impact on the overall morbidity and mortality of oesophageal atresia (Figure 15.1, Table 15.3). In the last decade improvements in intensive care support and the surgical treatment of CHD has essentially nullified this impact in those patients who undergo repair (Figure 15.2). Furthermore, in the last six years only two of 22 patients with combined oesophageal atresia and CHD did not undergo repair, compared with seven of 65 patients without CHD (Table 15.4).

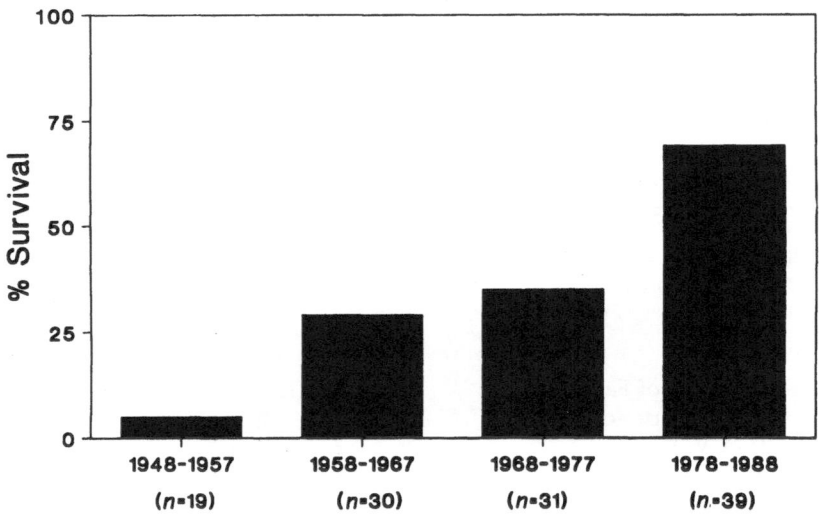

Figure 15.1 Overall effect of congenital heart disease on survival in oesophageal atresia.

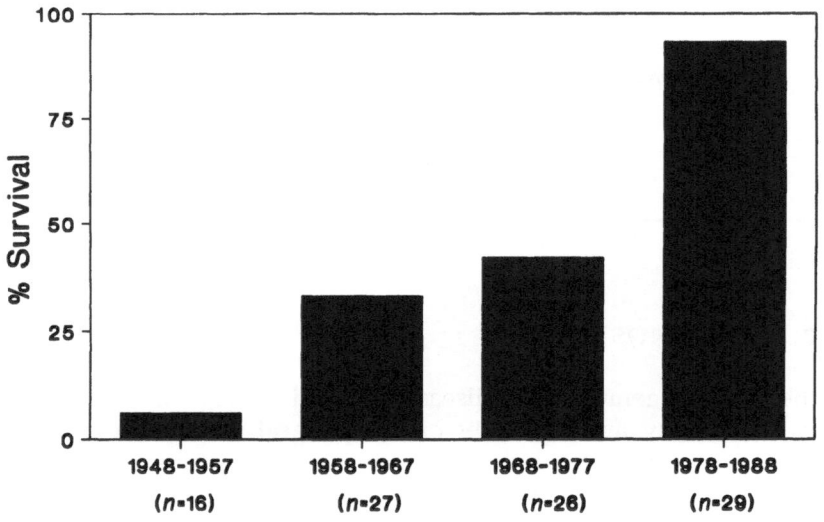

Figure 15.2 Survival of oesophageal atresia patients with congenital heart disease receiving definitive treatment.

Table 15.3 The changing impact of congenital heart disease (CHD) on survival in oesophageal atresia (OA) and/or tracheo-oesophageal fistula undergoing treatment: early and late postoperative mortality in patients with oesophageal atresia and congenital heart disease

Years	OA without CHD		OA + CHD with no, or mild/moderate other abnormalities		OA + CHD with severe other abnormalities	
	No.	% mortality	No.	% mortality	No.	% mortality
1948–1962	114	32	21	95	7	100
1963–1977	197	10	22	41	19	63
1978–1988	119	5	19	0	10	20

15.2.4 TIMING OF SURGERY

The complex management decisions that may need to be made at an early stage require knowledge of the exact nature of the CHD which can usually be determined on echocardiography. The physiological and anatomical significance of the CHD needs to be considered against the background that the tracheo-oesophageal fistula should be divided and the oesophageal atresia repaired early. With few exceptions, repair of the oesophageal atresia precedes the cardiac surgery.

15.2.5 CASE SELECTION

Patients with cardiac and oesophageal abnormalities frequently have other major organ defects and chromosomal defects (Chapter 14), and recognition of these is now the most common reason that no active treatment is initiated. It is rare that CHD alone will contraindicate operative repair of the oesophageal atresia. This has not always been so. In the earlier years of oesophageal atresia surgery little could be offered to infants with a wide variety of CHD, the repair of which has since become routine.

15.3 Physiological significance

Cardiac defects with potential for increased lung blood flow are generally unlikely to pose significant physiological problems in the first 3–4

Table 15.4 Oesophageal atresia and congenital heart disease

| Years | Oesophageal atresia and congenital heart disease | | | | Total |
| | With no, or mild/moderate other organ system defects | | With severe other organ system defects | | |
	Oesophagus not repaired	Oesophagus repaired*	Oesophagus not repaired	Oesophagus repaired*	
1948–1952	0	3 (3)	1	1 (1)	5 (5)
1953–1957	0	10 (9)	2	2 (2)	14 (13)
1958–1962	0	8 (8)	2	4 (4)	14 (14)
1963–1967	0	10 (2)	1	5 (4)	16 (7)
1968–1972	0	7 (4)	1	6 (5)	14 (10)
1973–1977	0	5 (3)	4	8 (3)	17 (10)
1978–1982	0	5 (0)	8	4 (1)	17 (9)
1983–1988	0	14 (0)	2	6 (1)	22 (3)
Total	0	62 (29)	21	36 (21)	119 (71)
1948–1977	0	43 (29)	11	26 (19)	80 (59)
1978–1988	0	19 (0)	10	10 (2)	39 (12)

*Numbers of deaths are given in parentheses.

days of life. The majority will not delay or interfere with early oesophageal repair.

The reason for this is that CHD comprising large septation defects and anatomically unrestricted egress to the pulmonary arteries and aorta are unlikely to manifest as congestive heart failure initially because pulmonary resistance remains high in the first few days of life. Instead they tend to become symptomatic towards the end of the first week. Being prepared and forewarned by early echocardiography of the type of lesion is most useful in planning the timing of repair of the oesophageal atresia and predicting progress in the postoperative period.

On the other hand, patients with congenital heart disease associated with severe right or left heart obstructive lesions in whom either the pulmonary or systemic circulation is duct dependent, will deteriorate rapidly when the duct closes. Many of these patients present in the first day of life *in extremis* because of their CHD *per se*. In others, rapid deterioration may occur during oesophageal atresia repair or in the early postoperative period. Awareness of this possibility is valuable in their perioperative assessment and management.

15.4 Anatomical significance

When the nature of the CHD is known, decisions regarding the necessity for, and the timing of, their repair can be made. These decisions are modified by the degree of physiological disturbance produced. Three groups of anomalies are encountered:

1. Isolated intracardiac septation defects
2. Intracardiac septation defects plus great vessel defects
3. Isolated great vessel defects (Table 15.2)

Transposition of the great vessels in association with oesophageal atresia is less common than would be expected (1%) when compared with a cohort of CHD patients without oesophageal atresia where it accounts for 7–8% of cardiac lesions. The incidence of aortic arch anomalies in this series (particularly anomalous origin of subclavian artery) is higher than expected, as is that of Tetralogy of Fallot (12.5% as opposed to about 8%). The incidence of truncus arteriosus was 2.5% compared to less than 1% in non-oesophageal atresia patients with CHD. The reasons for these differences is unknown.

15.5   Principles of management

In terms of management, patients with oesophageal atresia and congenital heart disease can be divided into those who are not duct-dependent and those who are. Patients who are not duct-dependent for systemic or pulmonary blood flow can proceed safely to early repair of the oesophageal atresia (Figure 15.3).

Patients with a duct-dependent pulmonary or systemic circulation can generally be divided into two groups: (1) infants in good condition with the duct patent; and (2) infants in poor condition in whom the duct is closing or has closed.

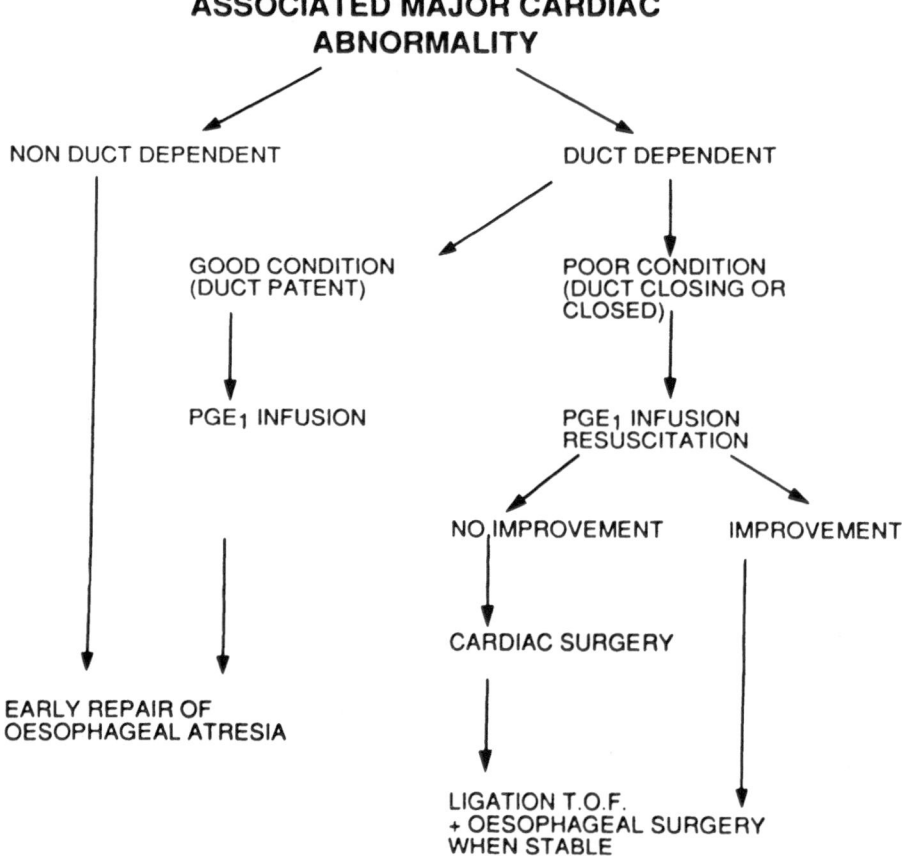

Figure 15.3   The early management of oesophageal atresia infants with congenital heart disease.

In those who are in good condition with the duct still patent, it is recommended that a PGE_1 infusion is commenced and oesophageal repair undertaken early. In the remaining infants who are in poor condition with a closed or closing duct, PGE_1 infusion and resuscitation is implemented and surgery delayed. Occasionally, gastrostomy may be required if there is significant gastric distension, but this may make ventilation more difficult. When improvement occurs or stability is achieved, the patient should proceed to oesophageal repair. If the patient remains acidotic from inadequate pulmonary or systemic blood flow, or if the patient remains anuric from poor lower compartment perfusion, then urgent appropriate palliative or reparative cardiac surgery should be performed first. This procedure may be combined with division of the tracheo-oesophageal fistula, gastrostomy or insertion of a peritoneal dialysis catheter for persistent anuria or hyperkalaemia. Oesophageal repair can be timed according to the subsequent status of the patient. In practice, this is an unusual situation and it has been rare that the cardiac surgical procedure has preceded the oesophageal atresia repair.

15.5.1 MANAGEMENT OF CONGENITAL HEART DISEASE FOLLOWING REPAIR OF OESOPHAGEAL ATRESIA

Duct-dependent conditions

After stability has been achieved on PGE_1 infusion and the oesophageal atresia repaired, there is time to allow the patient to recover from the oesophageal surgery before proceeding with major palliative or reparative cardiac surgery. When the pulmonary circulation is dependent on duct flow, a 4 or 5 mm polytetrafluoroethylene (PTFE) systemic to pulmonary shunt should be performed on the side that best suits the cardiac anatomy (for example, the right side in infants with viscero atrial situs solitus) and the condition of the hemithorax through which the oesophagus has been repaired. If there has been disruption of the anastomosis the shunt may be made on the other side. An arch obstruction with a duct-dependent systemic circulation needs to be repaired from the relevant side, and critical aortic stenosis is best repaired from the front. After palliative shunting, patients with Tetralogy of Fallot should undergo complete repair by 12–18 months of age, with an expected early mortality (30 days) of about 1%. Those with non-septatable hearts (single ventricle or persistent hypoplastic right heart) should be considered for a modified Fontan procedure at 2–5 years of age with an expected early mortality of 8%. Patients with pulmonary atresia and ventricular septal defect who require an external conduit undergo repair at 2–3 years of age and have an expected mortality of less than 5%.

Non-duct-dependent conditions

These are principally those conditions which are likely to produce high pulmonary blood flow when pulmonary resistance falls. In each individual, the management of the cardiac anomaly must be judged according to the patient's progress.

1. If cardiac failure becomes severe and can be managed only by ICU support, surgery should proceed. In general, the surgical options involve intracardiac septation with or without great vessel repair, or pulmonary artery banding as the initial procedure.
2. If the patient becomes independent of the intensive care unit but remains hospital bound, with congestive heart failure and failure to thrive, then intracardiac repair or main pulmonary artery banding are indicated.
3. In patients whose congestive heart failure is controlled sufficiently to permit discharge from hospital, those with anatomically unseptatable hearts should undergo main pulmonary artery banding within the first month of life, and the rest should be electively repaired at 2–3 months of age.
4. In those patients who thrive, and in whom congestive heart failure is not a major problem, and unless the septation defect is small, there should be a high index of suspicion that pulmonary vascular resistance is already elevated. These patients must be fully investigated before 2–3 months of age to measure pulmonary vascular resistance. Complete repair should be performed early despite their apparently thriving state. Good weight gain in this group may falsely reassure both physicians and the patient's parents that all is well.

In our experience the current expected early mortalities for complete repair in truncus arteriosus as an emergency in the neonatal period is 20%. As an elective procedure at 2–3 months the mortality is about 3–5%. In complete atrioventricular canal (CAVC) about 3–5%; for a single VSD, 1–2%; for coarctation of the aorta and VSD in the absence of left ventricular hypoplasia, 2–3%; for patent ductus arteriosus and atrial septal defect, less than 1%; and for transposition of the great arteries and a ventricular septal defect, less than 5%. The decline in mortality of cardiac surgery in infants under six months of age is shown in Table 15.5.

Table 15.5 Cardiac surgery under 6 months of age: 30 day mortality

	1978		*1988*	
Open	8	(63%)	129	(8%)
Closed	48	(10%)	148	(2.7%)
Total	56	(18%)	277	(5%)

15.6 Summary

In handling the complex clinical problems of combined oesophageal atresia and CHD, sound management plans can be formulated only after the anatomical type and physiological consequences of the cardiac anomaly are understood.

Patients with non-duct-dependent conditions usually have the oesophageal atresia repaired early, while pulmonary vascular resistance is high, and have their cardiac condition treated definitively later.

Patients with duct-dependent conditions can usually be supported haemodynamically with PGE_1 infusions, have the oesophageal atresia repaired and then proceed to major palliative or reparative cardiac surgery.

References

Bishop, P. J., Klein, M. D., Philippart, A. I., Hixson, D. S. and Hertzler, J. H. (1985) Transpleural repair of esophageal atresia without a primary gastrostomy: 240 patients treated between 1951 and 1983. *J. Pediatr. Surg.*, **20**, 823–8.

Chittmittrapap, S., Spitz, L., Kiely, E. M. and Brereton, R. J. (1989) Oesophageal atresia and associated anomalies. *Arch. Dis. Child.*, **64**, 364–8.

Ein, S. H., Shandling, B., Wesson, D. and Filler, R. M. (1989) Esophageal atresia with distal tracheoesophageal fistula: associated anomalies and prognosis in the 1980s. *J. Pediatr. Surg.*, **24**, 1055–9.

Holder, T. M., Ashcraft, K. W., Sharp, R. J. and Amoury, R. A. (1987) Care of infants with esophageal atresia, tracheoesophageal fistula and associated anomalies. *J. Thorac. Cardiovasc. Surg.*, **94**, 828–35.

Holder, T. M., Cloud, D. T., Lewis, J. E. Jr and Pilling, G. P. (1964) Esophageal atresia and tracheoesophageal fistula. A survey of its members by the surgical section of the American Academy of Pediatrics. *Pediatrics*, **34**, 542–9.

Louhimo, I. and Lindahl, H. (1983) Esophageal atresia: primary results of 500 consecutively treated patients. *J. Pediatr. Surg.*, **18**, 217–29.

16 Urinary tract abnormalities

E. PHELAN, J. H. KELLY and S. W. BEASLEY

The primary aim of early investigation of the urinary tract in patients with oesophageal atresia and tracheo-oesophageal fistula is to prevent long-term complications of renal disease. Now that advances in the surgical perioperative care of infants with oesophageal atresia have resulted in improved survival and reduced morbidity, the less life-threatening associated congenital anomalies, including urinary tract abnormalities, have assumed greater importance in long-term survival.

Most urinary tract abnormalities are not life-threatening and may not be symptomatic in the immediate neonatal period. When they do present later in life, irreversible damage to the kidneys may have occurred already. This is particularly so in the case of reflux associated nephropathy which occurred in 5% of patients in our series.

16.1 Incidence

The incidence of renal anomalies reported in the literature has been low because in most series only those patients with obvious abnormalities or symptoms referrable to the genitourinary tract have been investigated. The reported incidence of urinary tract abnormalities has ranged between 10 and 19% (Table 16.1). However, in one series in which all patients had genitourinary investigations or post-mortem examination 50% had an abnormality (Atwell and Beard, 1974). The experience of the Royal Children's Hospital, Melbourne falls between these figures with an overall incidence of 24% (Phelan and Chetcuti, 1991). After cardiac abnormalities, renal abnormalities are the next most common associated congenital abnormalities.

Table 16.1 Incidence of urinary tract abnormalities

Author (year)	Number of cases	% with abnormality
Holder *et al.* (1964)	1058	10.3
Romsdahl *et al.* (1966)	42	12.0
Weigel and Kaufman (1976)	83	19.25
Bishop *et al.* (1985)	27	14.0
Louhimo and Lindahl (1983)	500	12.0 (13.5 in last 200 patients)
Atwell and Beard (1974)	38	50
RCH Melbourne (1989)	584	24

16.2 Significance of urinary tract abnormalities

It is convenient to classify urinary abnormalities into four groups according to their impact on management (Table 16.2). Group I includes abnormalities that have no clinical significance in their own right. Group II includes conditions that require no treatment but their existence should be documented because they may become significant later in life, e.g. renal trauma in a patient with unilateral renal agenesis. Group III consists of conditions likely to require treatment (either medical or surgical) and includes conditions that predispose to urinary tract infection or secondary disease; vesicoureteric reflux is the most common condition in this group. Group IV includes conditions likely to lead to early renal failure or death irrespective of treatment.

The impact of concomitant urinary tract abnormalities on the investigation, management and prognosis of a patient with oesophageal atresia depends on the frequency, type and severity of the anomalies.

16.3 Frequency and types of urinary tract abnormalities

Assessment of the urinary tract was possible in 499 of 584 patients (85%) with oesophageal atresia and/or tracheo-oesophageal fistula reviewed. Information was obtained by post-mortem in 147, and radiological examination in 352 survivors. Urinary tract abnormalities were identified in 120 of 499 patients, an overall incidence of 24% and were more common in those who died (Table 16.3). The frequency and types of urinary tract abnormality are summarized in Tables 16.4 and 16.5.

Table 16.2 Clinical significance of urinary tract abnormalities*

Group I: Abnormalities of no clinical significance

Uncomplicated ureteric duplication
Uncomplicated horeshoe kidney
Uncomplicated crossed renal ectopia
Renal malrotation

Group II: Abnormalities requiring no treatment

Unilateral agenesis
Unilateral multicystic dysplastic kidney
Unilateral hypoplasia
Simple renal cyst
Pelvic kidney

Group III: Abnormalities likely to require treatment

Vesico-ureteric reflux
Urinary tract obstruction
Bladder diverticula
Ectopic ureter
Renal scarring

Group IV: Abnormalities likely to lead to early renal failure or death

Bilateral agenesis/hypoplasia
Bilateral cystic kidneys

*Where more than one abnormality is present, the most severe determines the classification.

Table 16.3 Urinary tract abnormalities in oesophageal atresia and/or tracheo-oesophageal fistula

Urinary tract assessed	499	
Urinary tract abnormal	120	(24%)
Survivors	352	
Urinary tract abnormal	75	(23%)
Deaths	147	
Urinary tract abnormal	45	(31%)

Table 16.4 Clinical classification of urinary tract abnormalities in oesophageal atresia according to urinary outcome in 75 survivors

	Frequency	Additional abnormalities	Frequency
Group 1: Abnormalities of no clinical significance			
Horseshoe	12	Duplication	1
Ureteric duplication	3		
Crossed ectopia	3		3
Malrotation	3		
Group 2: Abnormalities likely to require no treatment			
Unilateral agenesis	11	Malrotation	1
Unilateral hypoplasia	2		
Pelvic kidney	2	Duplex	1
		Bilateral	1
Renal cyst	1		
Multicystic dysplastic kidney	1		
Group 3: Abnormalities likely to require treatment			
Vesico-ureteric reflux	21	Renal scars	9
		Contralateral multicystic dysplastic kidney	1
		Vesico-ureteric junction obstruction	1
		Bladder diverticulum	3
		Crossed renal ectopia	3
		Contralateral agenesis	1
		Horseshoe	1
Pelvic-ureteric junction obstruction	3	Contralateral megaureter	1
Vesico-ureteric junction obstruction	3	Reflux	1
Bladder diverticulum	5	Bilateral reflux	1
		Contralateral reflux	1
		Ipsilateral reflux	1
		Contralateral agenesis	1
Ectopic ureter	1	Malrotation, double urethra	1
Double urethra	1	Ectopic ureter	1
Renal scars	18	Malrotation	1
		Vesico-ureteric reflux	9

Table 16.5 Classification of urinary tract abnormalities in 44 patients who died*

Abnormality			Associated abnormality ipsilateral kidney		Associated abnormality contralateral kidney	
1.	Horseshoe	2	Hydronephrosis	1	Hypoplasia	1
			Hypoplasia and megaureter	1	Megaureter	1
2.	Crossed ectopia	2				
3.	Duplication	1			Bilateral	1
4.	Malrotation	2				
5.	Agenesis	15			Hypoplasia	5
					Multicystic dysplastic kidney	3
6.	Hypoplasia	12			Bilateral	3
					Horseshoe	2
					Cystic kidney	1
7.	Cystic kidney	4	Megaureter	1		
			Duplication	1		
					Hydronephrosis and Hydroureter	1
8.	Multicystic dysplastic kidney	1			Bilateral	1
9.	Hydronephrosis	2			Bilateral	2
10.	Bilateral renal agenesis	4				

*Inadequate information in 45th patient.

Where a patient has more than one type of urinary tract abnormality it should be classified according to the most severe abnormality.

A micturating cystourethrogram (MCU) was performed in 39 of the 352 survivors: 21 had vesicoureteric reflux (54%) and nine of these (23%) had renal scars. The incidence of reflux in the remaining 313 patients is unknown as they did not have an MCU, but nine of these children showed renal scars (3%) on other tests. Thus, while the overall incidence of vesicoureteric reflux is unknown, it occurs in at least 21 of 352 (6%), and is almost certainly much more frequent. The overall incidence of renal scarring among the 352 survivors of all ages was 5%. Vesicoureteric reflux was probably present in a similar or increased proportion of patients who died, but because it cannot be identified on post-mortem examination its true frequency remains unknown.

16.4 Investigation and management of the urinary tract

The aim of screening all neonates with oesophageal atresia and tracheo-oesophageal fistula for urinary tract abnormalities is to prevent the long-term morbidity associated with undetected abnormalities, particilarly vesicoureteric reflux and reflux-associated nephropathy.

Covert renal abnormalities must be looked for because, unlike the other congenital anomalies in patients with oesophageal atresia and tracheo-oesophageal fistula, these may not manifest themselves clinically in the neonatal period (Barnes and Smith, 1978). The abnormalities can be grouped according to their impact on management.

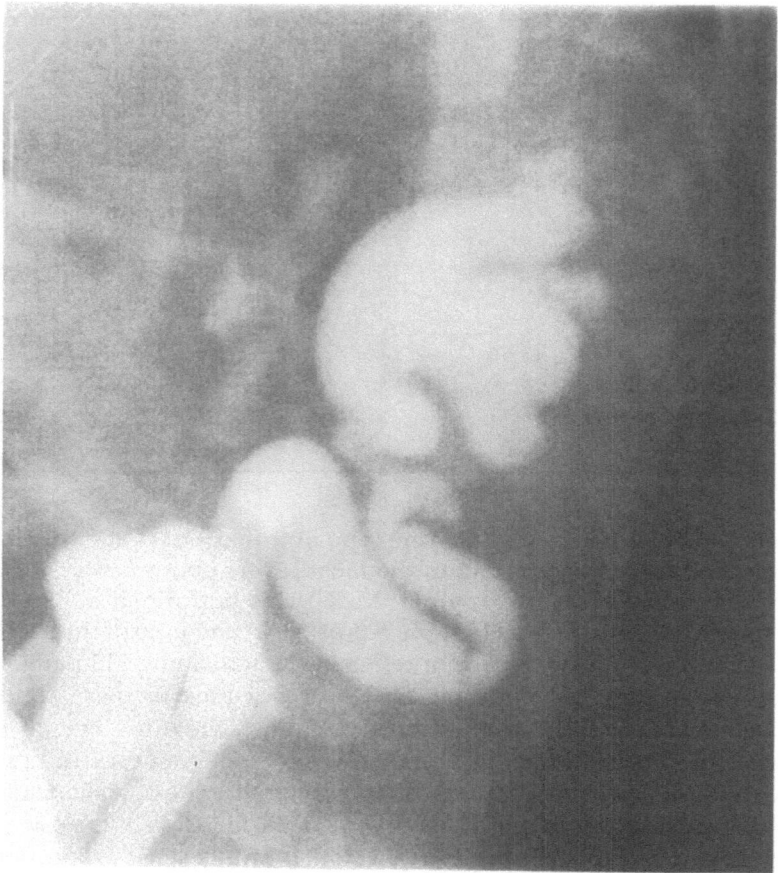

Figure 16.1 Gross left-sided vesicoureteric reflux demonstrated on MCU in an infant with oesophageal atresia.

16.4.1 VESICOURETERIC REFLUX

The overall incidence of vesicoureteric reflux is difficult to estimate accurately because only 39 of the 352 survivors had an MCU. However, the incidence of renal scarring was 5%. This implies that a much higher incidence of reflux would be evident had all patients had an early MCU (Smellie and Normand, 1979). Early detection of vesicoureteric reflux enables prophylactic antibiotics to be commenced immediately, thus reducing the likelihood of renal damage occurring from unrecognized urinary tract infections.

16.4.2 INVESTIGATION IN THE NEONATAL PERIOD

The high incidence of urinary tract abnormalities which require treatment highlights the importance of early investigation of the renal tract in all patients with oesophageal atresia. Micturating cystourethrography (MCU) and renal ultrasound in the neonatal period will detect most significant abnormalities so that appropriate management can be implemented at an early stage (Figure 16.1). This is our current practice, although it will be some time before the cost-effectiveness and benefit to the patient of this policy can be firmly established.

Unless the infant has been observed to pass urine, a renal ultrasound should be performed before repair of the oesophageal atresia (Figure 16.2). The ready availability of ultrasonography and its non-invasive nature enables it to be done as a routine procedure preoperatively. If no kidneys can be found on renal ultrasound examination, a nuclear renal

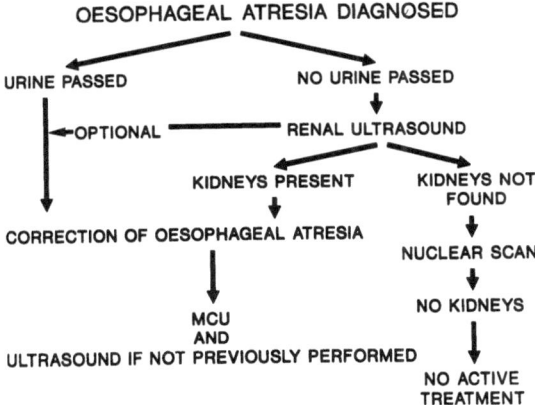

Figure 16.2 Algorithm for the investigation of the urinary tract in infants with oesophageal atresia. Renal ultrasound can be performed routinely prior to surgery in all patients.

scan will confirm the absence of functioning renal tissue. Bilateral renal agenesis, which occurs in almost 1% of oesophageal atresia patients, is a contra-indication to surgical repair of the oesophagus (see Chapter 20). Many patients with bilateral renal agenesis do not have features suggestive of Potters syndrome in the presence of oesophageal atresia.

References

Atwell, J. D. and Beard, R. C. (1974) Upper urinary tract anomalies associated with esophageal atresia and tracheoesophageal fistula. *J. Pediatr. Surg.*, **9**, 825–31.

Barnes, J. C. and Smith, W. L. (1978) The VATER association. *Radiology*, **126**, 445–9.

Bishop, P. J., Klein, M. D., Philippart, A. I., Hixson, D. S. and Hertzler, J. H. (1985) Transpleural repair of esophageal atresia without a primary gastrostomy: 240 patients treated between 1951 and 1983. *J. Pediatr. Surg.*, **20**, 823–8.

Holder, T. M., Cloud, D. T., Lewis, J. E. and Pilling, G. P. (1964) Esophageal atresia and tracheo-esophageal fistula: a survey of its members by the Surgical Section of the American Academy of Pediatrics. *Pediatrics*, **34**, 542–9.

Louhimo, L. and Lindahl, H. (1983) Esophageal atresia: primary results of 500 consecutively treated patients. *J. Pediatr. Surg.*, **18**, 217–29.

Phelan, E. and Chetcuti, P. (1991) Renal anomalies in the long-term follow-up of oesophageal atresia. *Pediatr. Radiol.*, (in press).

Romsdahl, M. M., Hunter, J. A. and Grove, W. J. (1966) Tracheo-esophageal fistula and esophageal atresia: surgical management and results at a university hospital. *J. Thorac. Cardiovasc. Surg.*, **52**, 571–8.

Smellie, J. and Normand, C. (1979) Reflux nephropathy in childhood. in *Reflux Nephropathy* (eds C. J. Hodson and P. Kincaid-Smith), Masson et cie, New York.

Waterston, D. J., Bonham-Carter, R. E. and Aberdeen, E. (1962) Oesophageal atresia: tracheo-oesophageal fistula. A study of survival in 218 patients. *Lancet*, i, 819–22.

Weigel, W. and Kaufman, H. J. (1976) The frequency and types of other congenital anomalies in association with tracheo-oesophageal malformations. *J. Clin. Pediatr.*, **15**, 891–94.

17 *Orthopaedic abnormalities*

D. R. V. DICKENS

When oesophageal atresia first became amenable to operative management, it seemed unlikely that the babies would require orthopaedic
treatment; but in the event, the orthopaedic surgeon has become a very
important member of the team involved in the management of oesophageal atresia and tracheo-oesophageal fistula, particularly in relation to
scoliosis and radial aplasia.

Although the treatment of orthopaedic anomalies does not take precedence over the treatment of the oesophageal atresia itself, the orthopaedic surgeon is involved early in the treatment of some of the
anomalies such as congenital dislocation of the hip and talipes equinovarus. Other anomalies, like scoliosis from hemivertebrae, are progressive through childhood, while chest wall deformity secondary to thoracotomy appears later in life.

The range of orthopaedic anomalies which occur in association with
oesophageal atresia is extensive (Table 17.1), but spinal problems are by
far the most numerous and demanding of the surgeon.

17.1 Spinal abnormalities

Spinal anomalies were present in 17% of the 387 patients in whom the
radiological and clinical records allowed adequate evaluation; other
series have reported an incidence varying from 2% to 75% (Holder *et al.*,
1964; Louhimo and Lindahl, 1983; Stevenson, 1972; Weigel and Kaufman, 1976). Vertebral anomalies were uncommon in patients with an
'H'-fistula, but occurred frequently in patients with oesophageal atresia
who also had renal and anorectal anomalies.

Spinal and rib anomalies may co-exist, but this is not invariable (Table
17.2). The type and distribution of congenital vertebral anomalies is
shown in Table 17.3.

Table 17.1   Orthopaedic anomalies in oesophageal atresia (387 patients)

Structural vertebral abnormalities		59
Scoliosis		48
Rib abnormalities		94
Radial abnormalities		13
Absent radius	11	
Hypoplasia radius	2	
Absent thumb (part of radial club hand)		13
Isolated thumb abnormalities		15
Absent first metacarpal	3	
Hypoplasia thumb	6	
Accessory thumb	3	
Trigger thumb	3	
Congenital dislocation of hip		6
Congenital talipes equinovarus		8
Others: Arthrogryposis, short femur, curly toes, poly-dactyly, adductor contracture of hip		

Table 17.2   Vertebral and rib anomalies

Total number of patients evaluated for spinal and rib anomalies	387
Spinal abnormalities:	66
Structural abnormality of spine	59
Scoliosis with 'normal spine' (idiopathic scoliosis)	7
Rib abnormalities:	94
with normal spine	68
with abnormal spine	26

17.1.1 SCOLIOSIS

In 1987 we reviewed 302 survivors following repair of oesophageal atresia and tracheo-oesophageal fistula for evidence of chest wall deformity (Figure 17.1) and scoliosis. Seventeen patients with tracheo-oesophageal fistula without atresia, in whom the fistula had been divided through a cervical approach, were excluded from further consideration because it was thought unlikely that, in the absence of congenital vertebral anomalies, the cervical approach could have contributed to subsequent scoliosis or anterior chest wall deformity. The incidence of scoliosis and vertebral anomalies in the remaining patients

Table 17.3 The type and level of congenital vertebral anomalies in patients with oesophageal atresia

	Formation defects	Segmentation defects	Mixed defects	Total
Cervical	0	3	0	3
Cervicothoracic	2	3	3	8
Upper thoracic	8	2	4	14
Lower thoracic	8	0	6	14
Thoracolumbar	1	3	2	6
Lumbar	1	2	1	4
Lumbosacral	6	3	0	9
Sacral	8	0	0	8
Coccygeal	1	0	0	1

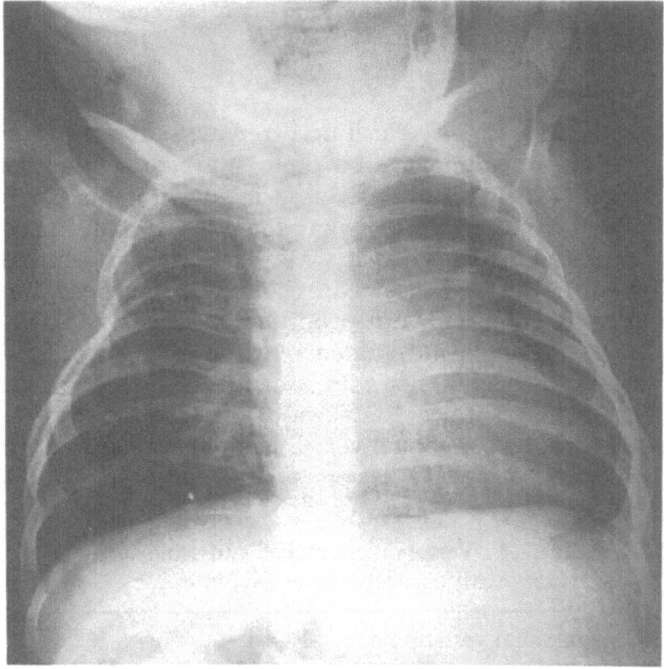

Figure 17.1 Radiograph documenting chest wall deformity following thoracotomy for oesophageal atresia.

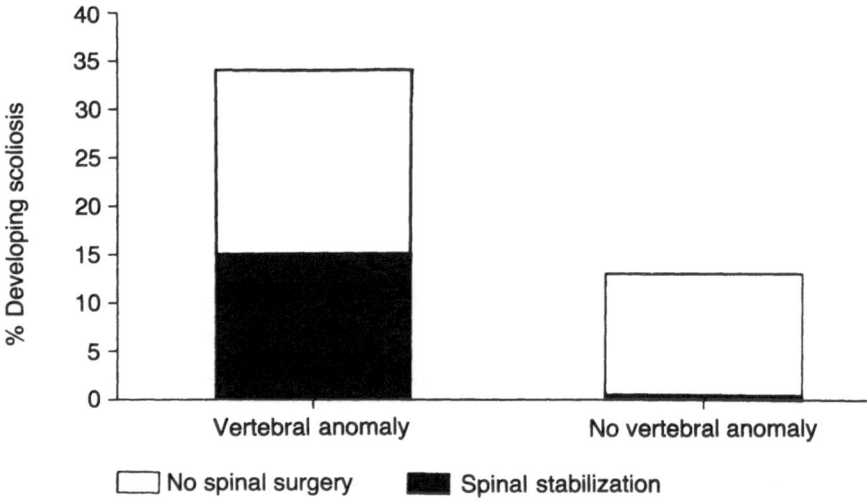

Figure 17.2 Scoliosis is more common and more severe when there is a coexisting congenital vertebral anomaly.

is summarized in Table 17.4. Scoliosis occurred more frequently and was more severe in those patients with a pre-existing congenital vertebral anomaly (Figure 17.2); and scoliosis associated with mixed vertebral anomalies in the lower thoracic spine had the worst prognosis (Chetcuti *et al.*, 1989). The severity of scoliosis was assessed by measurement of the Cobb angle, i.e. the angle created by joining a line from the top of the vertebra most tilted into the upper portion of the curve to a line from the bottom of the vertebra most tilted into the lowest portion of the curve. Whereas 15% of patients with a congenital vertebral anomaly subsequently required surgical stabilization of their spine, less than 0.5% of those without a congenital vertebral anomaly required surgery.

Table 17.4 Vertebral anomalies and scoliosis in survivors with oesophageal atresia ($n = 285$)

Congenital vertebral anomaly	53
No congenital vertebral anomaly	232
Scoliosis	48
with congenital vertebral anomaly	18
without vertebral anomaly	30

Of the 30 patients presenting with scoliosis in the absence of a vertebral anomaly:

— 10 were minimal clinically so that no further radiological assessment was made
— 17 had a Cobb angle of 15–20°
— 2 had a Cobb angle of 20–25°
— 1 had a Cobb angle greater than 40°.

Thoracic curves were convex to the right in ten, and to the left in 20. There were no significant sex differences between the left- and right-sided curves. The effect on respiratory function is detailed in Chapter 25.

It is our experience that rib resection (rather than an intercostal approach) and multiple thoracotomies increased the likelihood of the subsequent development of scoliosis and chest wall deformity (see Chapter 25).

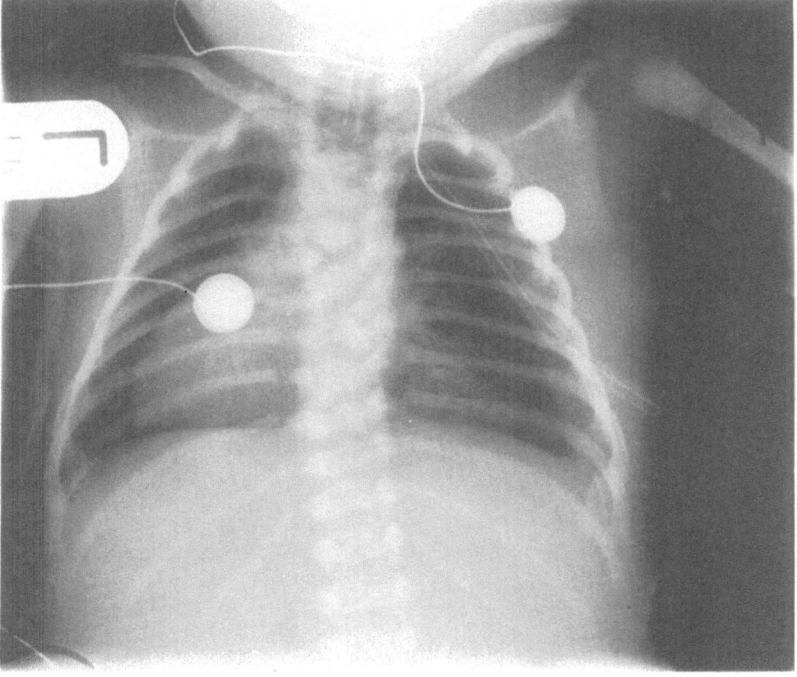

Figure 17.3 Spinal anomalies in oesophageal atresia are common. In this infant there are hemivertebrae of T5 – T7. The lesion is balanced with no deformity.

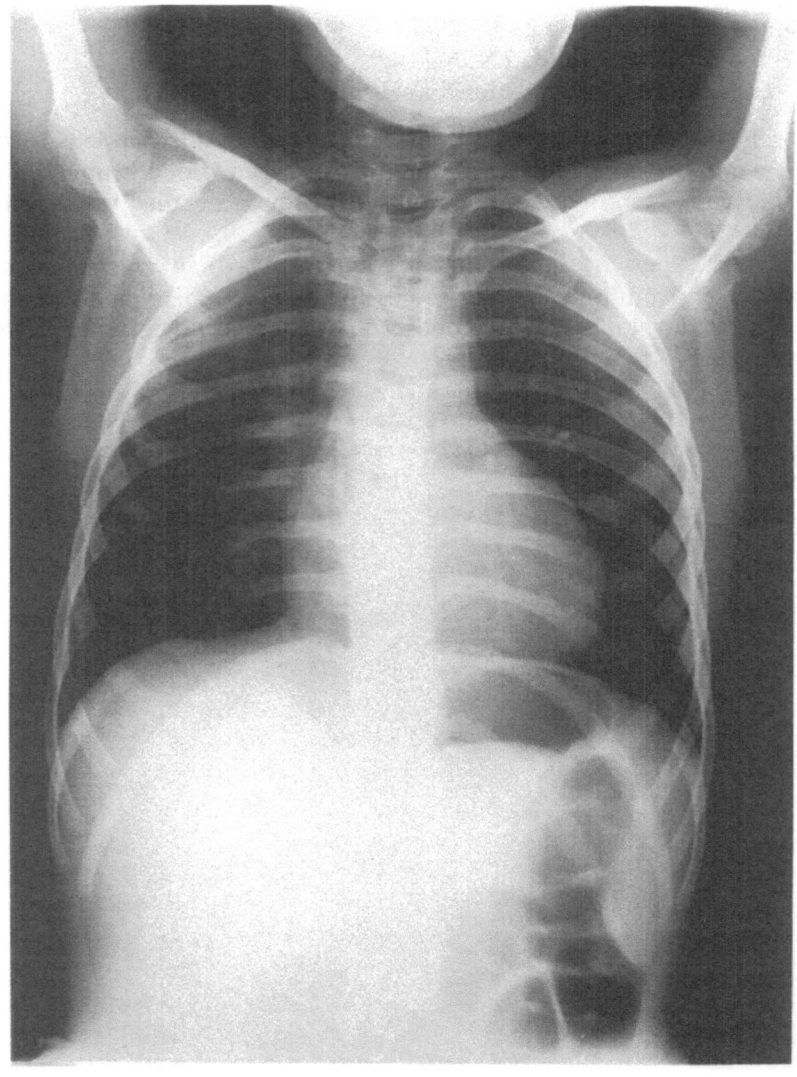

Figure 17.4 Oesophageal atresia infant with block vertebrae T2/3, representing failure of segmentation.

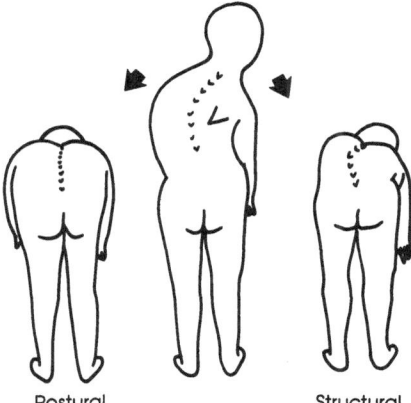

Postural   Structural

Figure 17.5 The clinical assessment of scoliosis. The forward bend test can be done during school screening and will detect structural scoliosis. (Reproduced with kind permission from Hutson and Beasley, 1988.)

Diagnosis of scoliosis

In view of the high incidence of spinal anomalies (Figures 17.3 and 17.4), it is recommended that all patients with oesophageal atresia should have a full spinal X-ray, AP and lateral during their first admission. The children should be followed until skeletal maturity, with annual review to assess the spine. The forward bend test done for school screening should be adequate for the clinical detection of scoliosis (Figure 17.5). If asymmetry is detected, full length PA and lateral films should be obtained to determine the presence and severity of the curve. If curves are detected, they must be kept under observation until skeletal maturity. Patients with congenital curves are more likely to have significant urinary tract abnormalities and it must be confirmed that their urinary tract was fully investigated during infancy. If scoliosis surgery is contemplated, the patient must be investigated to exclude cord tethering and diastematomyelia by myelography, CT scan or magnetic resonance imaging (MRI), or a combination of these. Respiratory function tests should also be performed preoperatively, as patients with scoliosis have an appreciable reduction in lung volume (Chetcuti *et al.*, 1989).

Prognosis

In the absence of a congenital vertebral anomaly, scoliosis tends to be minor and does not progress. On the other hand, scoliosis in the presence of a congenital vertebral anomaly is often progressive and may become severe (Figure 17.6).

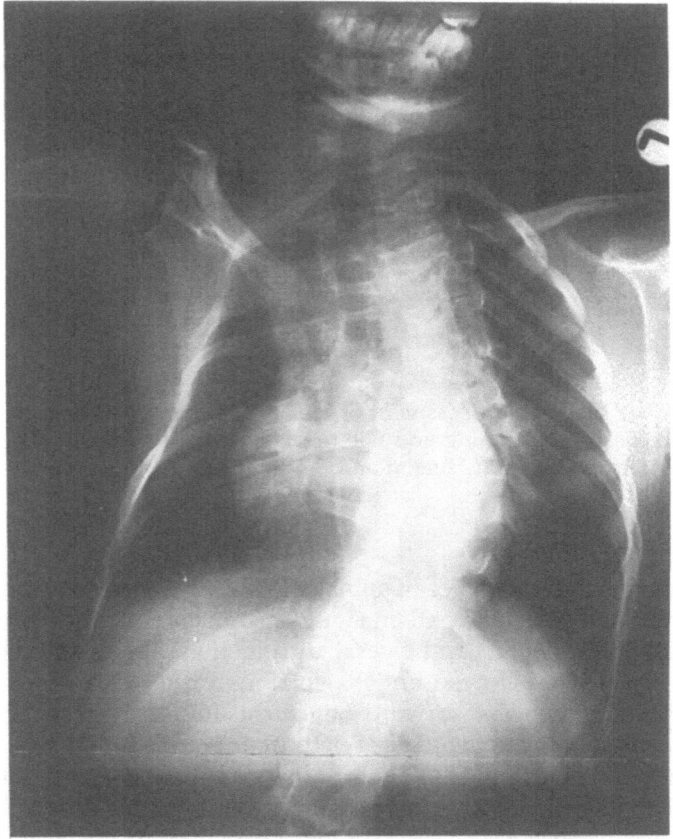

Figure 17.6   Scoliosis in the presence of a congenital vertebral anomaly can be progressive and may become severe. The child has multiple vertebral anomalies associated with scoliosis and fused ribs.

Treatment

Progressive curves are kept under close observation. If they increase above 20°, bracing is indicated, especially in those with normal vertebral anatomy. Bracing for congenital curves has not been found to be successful.

Curve progression above 40° in the growing child can be managed operatively in most cases. The optimum time for stabilization and fusion is close to skeletal maturity, and preferably over the age of ten years. If progression is due to failure of segmentation, e.g. unilateral unsegmented bar, early fusion over a short segment is indicated. Severe and

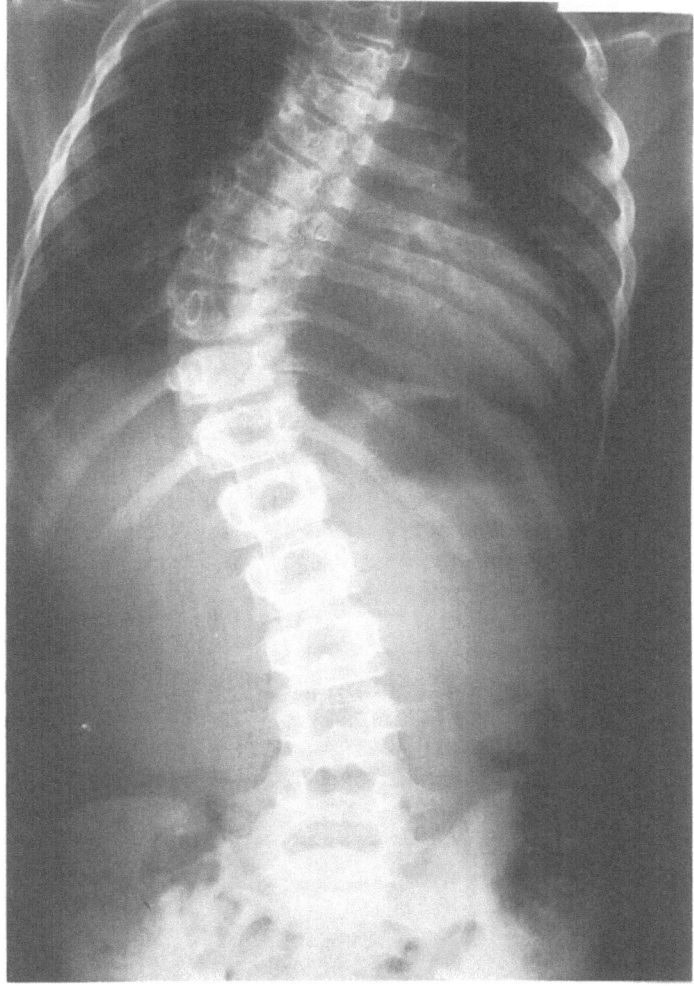

Figure 17.7 Spinal deformity with no obvious vertebral anomaly, before surgery.

progressive scoliosis in a child under the age of ten is difficult to treat: one option is non-fusion rodding combined with bracing and with repeated rod adjustment. This may prevent further progression of the curve until the child is at an age suitable for spinal fusion. In the past, most spinal fusions have employed Harrington instrumentation (Figures 17.7 and 17.8). In recent times, the Cotrel-Dubousset instrumentation is preferred where feasible.

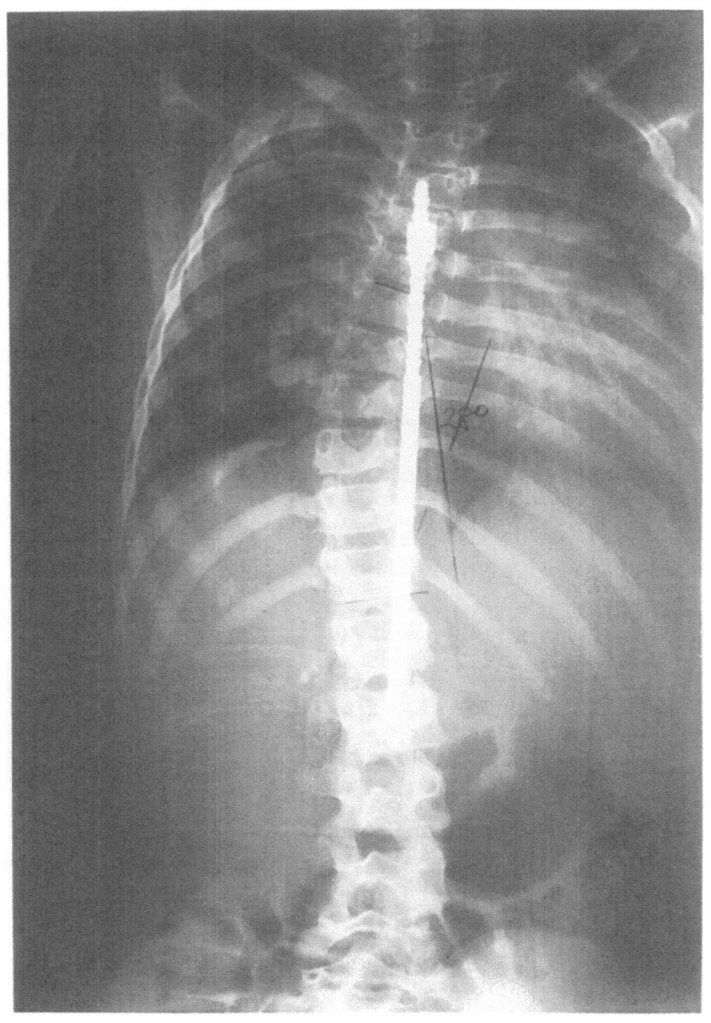

Figure 17.8 Same case as in Figure 17.6, following Harrington fusion.

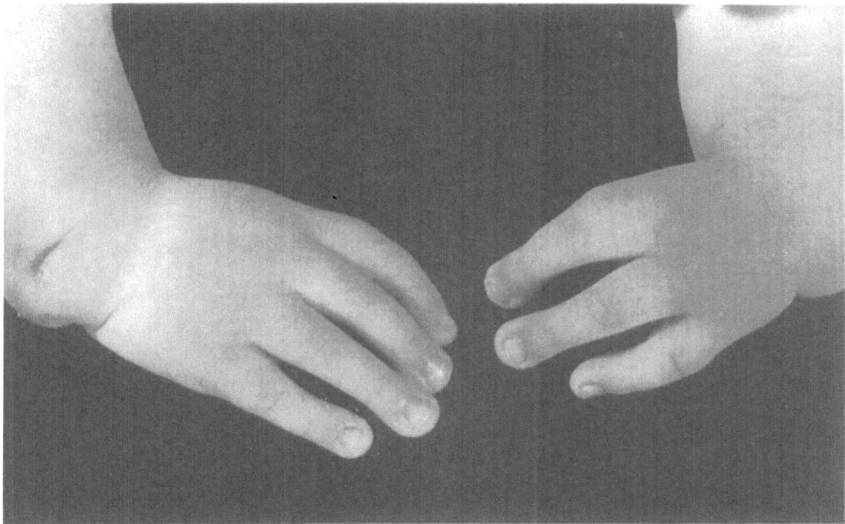

Figure 17.9 Bilateral radial club hand.

17.2 Limb abnormalities

17.2.1 RADIAL CLUB HAND AND THUMB ABNORMALITIES

Radial club hand was seen in 13 patients (Figure 17.9). In 11 of these there was complete absence of radius; two patients had radial hypoplasia. All cases were associated with aplasia or absence of the thumb. The thumb anomalies noted in the presence of a normal forearm included absence of the first ray (three patients); vestigial thumbs (six patients); accessory thumbs (three patients); and trigger thumb (three patients).

Diagnosis

The diagnosis of radial club hand and thumb anomalies is apparent on clinical inspection at birth. Plain radiological investigation will indicate the extent of bony deficiency and give an indication as to the potential for reconstruction (Figures 17.10 and 17.11).

Management

The usual management of the radial club hand has been by centralization, usually with excision of the central carpus and implantation of the ulna into the space. In more recent times, we have employed a soft tissue procedure, associated with ulnar shortening, on occasions placing

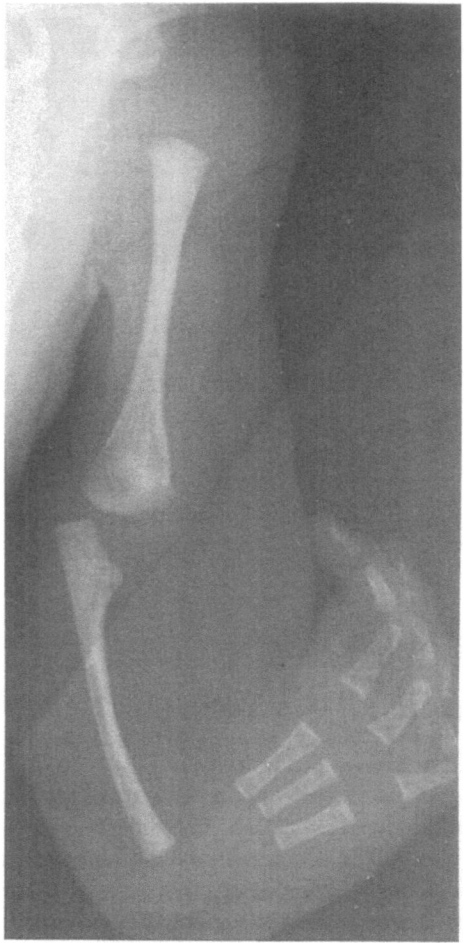

Figure 17.10   Radiograph of left hand and arm. Same patient as Figure 17.9.

the wrist simply on the end of the ulna and producing muscle balance. This procedure is usually carried out at the age of 6–12 months. After the carpus, wrist and digits have been aligned with the ulna, an intramedullary wire is passed through the third ray and down the ulna, and retained for three months. Following removal of that wire, splintage is continued for a further three months. Whether pollicization is indicated depends on the presence or absence of a contralateral thumb, the quality of sensation, and the stability of the situation. Pollicization, if performed, is usually attempted at 1–2 years of age.

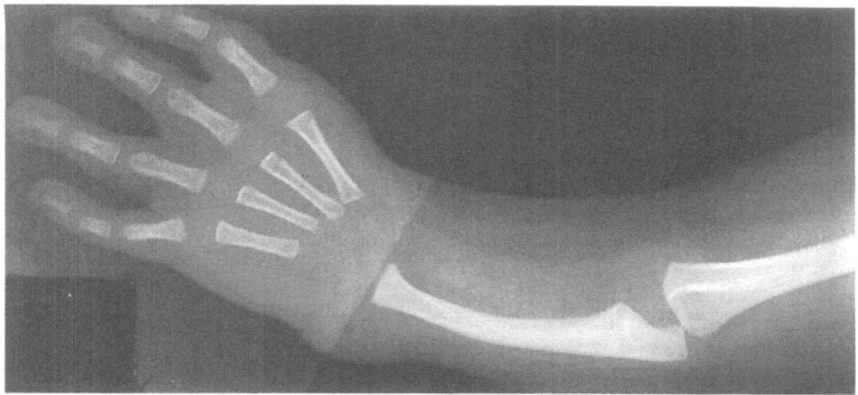

Figure 17.11 Radiograph of right hand and arm. Same patient as Figures 17.9 and 17.10. Note the radial aplasia and absence of thumb.

17.3 Congenital dislocation of the hip

Congenital dislocation of the hip occurred in six patients. On each occasion it was treated along conventional lines. Currently, this involves a harness initially.

17.4 Congenital talipes equinovarus

Congenital talipes equinovarus also occurs more often than one would expect (Table 17.1). It is treated with serial plasters and if this fails after 2–3 months, with soft tissue release forthwith.

References

Bishop, P. J., Klein, M. D., Philippart, A. I., Hixson, D. S. and Hertzler, J. H. (1985) Transpleural repair of esophageal atresia without a primary gastrostomy: 240 patients treated between 1951 and 1983. *J. Pediatr. Surg.*, **20**, 823–8.

Bond-Taylor, W., Starer, F. and Atwell, J. D. (1973) Vertebral anomalies associated with esophageal atresia and tracheo-esophageal fistula with reference to the initial operative mortality. *J. Pediatr. Surg.*, **8**, 9–13.

Chetcuti, P., Dickens, D. R. V. and Phelan, P. D. (1989) Spinal deformity in patients born with oesophageal atresia and tracheo-oesophageal fistula. *Arch. Dis. Child.*, **64**, 1427–30.

Cobb, J. R. (1948) Outline for the study of scoliosis. in *Instructional Course*

Lectures, The American Academy of Orthopaedic Surgeons, J. W. Edwards, Ann Arbor, MI, pp. 261–75.

Cotrel, Y. (1986) *New Instrumentation for Surgery of the Spine*. Freiund Publishing House Ltd.

Dickens, D. R. V. and Myers, N. A. (1987) Oesophageal atresia and vertebral anomalies. *Pediatr. Surg. Int.*, **2**, 278–81.

Holder, T. M., Cloud, D. T., Lewis, J. E. and Pilling, G. P. (1964) Esophageal atresia and tracheo-esophageal fistula: a survey of its members, by the Surgical Section of the American Academy of Pediatrics. *Pediatrics*, **34**, 542–9.

Hutson, J. M. and Beasley, S. W. (1988) *The Surgical Examination of Children*. Heinemann Medical Publishers, Oxford.

Louhimo, L. and Lindahl, H. (1983) Esophageal atresia: primary results of 500 consecutively treated patients. *J. Pediatr. Surg.*, **18**, 217–29.

Stevenson, R. E. (1972) Extra vertebrae associated with esophageal atresia and tracheoesophageal fistulae. *J. Pediatr.*, **81**, 1123–9.

Weigel, W. and Kaufman, H. J. (1976) The frequency and types of other congenital anomalies in association with tracheo-oesophageal malformations. *J. Chir. Pediatr.*, **15**, 891.

PART SIX
Care of the Child and Family

18   *Nursing care*

H. M. TELFER and G. E. McDONNELL

Nursing care plays an important part in the management of infants with oesophageal atresia. From the first sign that all is not well shortly after delivery until discharge from hospital these infants need knowledgeable and skilful nursing care. The nurse may be the first person to notice excessive drooling or respiratory distress in a newborn infant, prompting introduction of an oesophageal tube to confirm the diagnosis. Later, the specialist neonatal nurse must be constantly alert for early signs of change in condition, which may occur rapidly. Finally, the nurse plays a supportive role in the convalescence and long-term follow-up of the patient.

18.1   At birth

The immediate nursing priority in treating infants with oesophageal atresia is the prevention of aspiration into the respiratory tract. Aspiration results from:

1. Secretions accumulating in the blind upper oesophageal pouch spilling over into the trachea;
2. Reflux of gastric contents up the distal oesophagus and through the fistula (Filston and Izart, 1985).

18.1.1   MANAGEMENT OF SECRETIONS

The blind upper pouch should be suctioned every 10 to 15 minutes, or more frequently if required (Figure 18.1). This necessitates constant attention and meticulous care by the attending nurse for whom it is a prime responsibility. When the baby is asleep or settled, suction may be required less frequently. The initial suction determines how far subse-

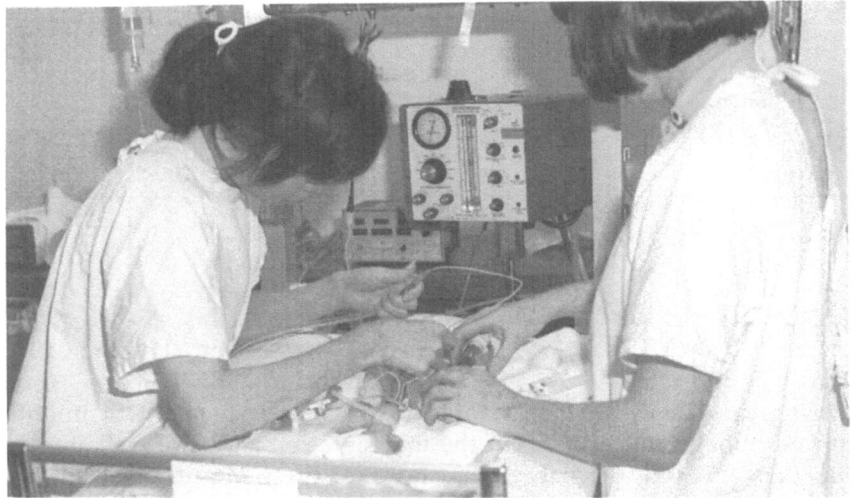

Figure 18.1 The blind upper oesophageal segment is suctioned frequently to prevent the accumulation of saliva and to reduce the likelihood of aspiration.

quent catheters need be inserted and this measurement can be displayed on the baby's cot. The upper pouch should be kept empty in a manner which avoids trauma to the mucosa: a size 8–10 French gauge suction catheter should be introduced gently through the mouth until the resistance of the blind oesophageal pouch is felt; the catheter is then withdrawn slightly before suction is applied to avoid direct trauma or perforation of the fundus of the pouch. A suction pressure of 200 cm H_2O is adequate and the catheter should be rotated between the thumb and forefinger as it is slowly withdrawn.

18.1.2 PREVENTION OF ASPIRATION OF THE GASTRIC CONTENTS

Ideally, the infant should be nursed in the prone position or on the right side, with the head slightly elevated. In practice, however, the demands of access often result in the infant being nursed supine, particularly if he or she is premature and requires intensive monitoring and resuscitation (Figure 18.2). The infant should be handled as little as possible and allowed to settle. One reason for this is that when the infant becomes agitated and cries, abdominal distension may develop when air is pushed down the distal fistula into the stomach. Gastric

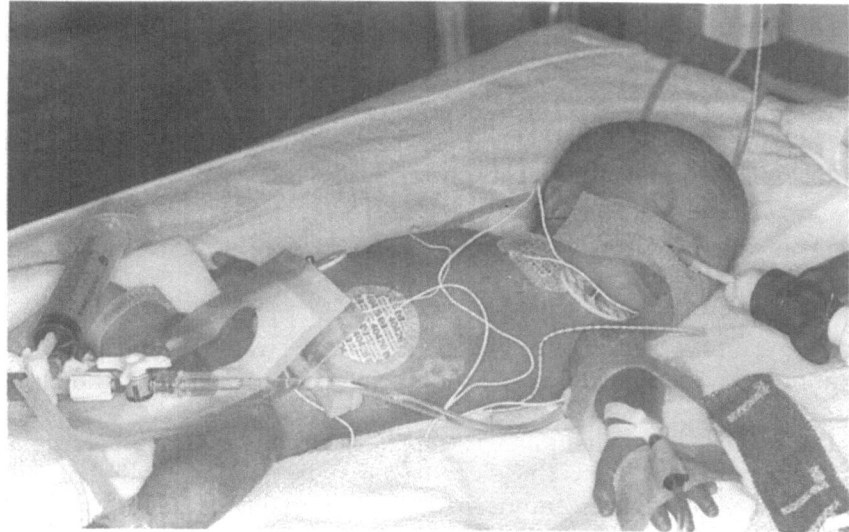

Figure 18.2 The requirements of resuscitation and monitoring may determine the position in which the infant is nursed. Most infants with oesophageal atresia do not require endotracheal intubation preoperatively.

distension increases the risk of reflux of gastric contents and elevation of the diaphragm interferes with the mechanics of ventilation. A dummy teat may be useful to help comfort the infant but oral feeds must not be given.

18.1.3 GENERAL BABY CARE

The maintenance of an optimal thermal environment is one of the most important aspects of neonatal care. The infant is nursed in an incubator or a radiant heater cot and the temperature controlled. The latter has the advantage of allowing easy access (Figure 18.1). The heart rate, respiratory rate and breathing patterns must be recorded and any changes in these observations, particularly the onset of apnoea or respiratory distress, may indicate that the upper pouch is full of secretions and suction is required (Gauntlett *et al.*, 1986). Monitor leads should be placed in the appropriate position to detect apnoea before the onset of bradycardia. These babies cannot be fed orally; therefore, blood glucose levels need to be measured to detect hypoglycaemia.

18.1.4   PLANNING TRANSFER

The nurse may be involved in the organization of transfer of the baby
to the tertiary institution. In Victoria, the Newborn Emergency Transport Service is used to transfer these infants (Chapter 7). A specialized
nurse will be part of the transporting team.

18.2   On admission to the tertiary centre

All the nursing procedures commenced at the referring hospital are
continued, with meticulous attention being paid to suction of the blind
upper pouch.

The specialist neonatal nurse is trained to be constantly alert for signs
of changes in condition. These changes may be subtle initially and not
always easy to interpret, emphasizing the importance of skilful specialist
nursing staff. One responsibility of the nurse is to ensure monitoring is
not disrupted during preoperative investigative procedures.

18.3   The postoperative period

18.3.1   MANAGEMENT OF SECRETIONS

Upper oesophageal and pharyngeal secretions may require suction
occasionally in the early postoperative period, as oedema around the
anastomotic site may impair swallowing. As the oedema subsides, the
need for suction lessens. Suction of the upper oesophagus must be
performed with care to avoid damage to the anastomosis. The length of
the suction catheter to be inserted is determined at operation and this
measurement is clearly displayed in a convenient position. The distance
is marked on a tape measure attached to the head of the cot (Figure
18.3). The suction catheter is not introduced beyond this length, preventing trauma to the anastomosis by the catheter.

18.3.2   PAIN RELIEF

The problem of pain relief in infants remains a difficult area to
manage. Intercostal nerve blocks and intrapleural local anaesthetics at
surgery have not been widely employed in neonatal surgery until
recently and last only four to six hours after completion of the operation.
Nursing assessment of pain postoperatively in infants is difficult and
must take into account the baby's immature central nervous system.

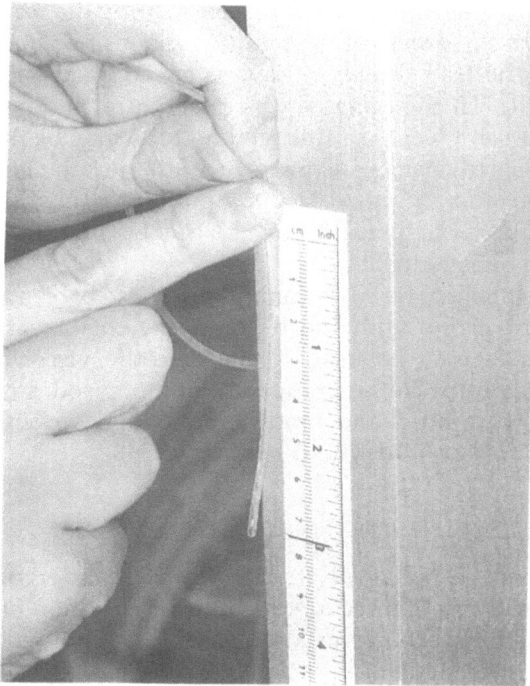

Figure 18.3 The distance the suction catheter can be introduced from the gums is clearly marked on a measure attached to the head of the cot.

Signs of pain include restlessness, haemodynamic instability, and changes in the state of alertness (D'Apolito, 1984). Intravenous morphine infusions have been used effectively in infants receiving ventilatory assistance, but their use outside intensive care units is not encouraged (Beasley and Tibballs, 1987). The pharmacokinetics of narcotics in infants is poorly documented and there is a risk of respiratory depression and overdose. If used in intensive care units, narcotic antagonists (e.g. Narcan) must be available to counteract overdose effects, such as hypoventilation and hypotension.

Gentle handling will reduce postoperative pain and discomfort. A soft towelling roll tucked behind the infant's back with the wound uppermost may be helpful. In subsequent days, the prone position appears to assist in keeping the baby settled.

18.3.3 FLUID BALANCE AND NUTRITION

Fluid and electrolyte balance is maintained and total blood glucose monitored; and the urine is tested for reducing substances twice a day.

After 3–5 days, oral feeds are introduced. During the first feed the nurse must be alert for signs of respiratory distress which may indicate inhalation of the feed. Breast feeding is encouraged and established as early as practical. If the infant is very premature, and oral feeds are not possible for several weeks, a fine feeding tube may be inserted through the anastomosis to enable gavage feeds until the baby is mature enough to suck. Care must be taken to avoid accidental dislodgement of the tube, although it can usually be replaced by the surgeon with little danger to the anastomosis.

Gastro-oesophageal reflux is common in these babies and it is helpful to nurse them prone with the head of the cot elevated after feeds. Thickened feeds may be used to increase the viscosity of milk and further reduce reflux. In the premature infant episodes of reflux may be associated with apnoea and bradycardia, often without coughing or visible milk in the oropharynx (Rushton, 1988).

18.3.4 PREVENTION OF INFECTION

The infant with oesophageal atresia who has undergone major thoracic surgery is at risk of infection due to the disruption of skin integrity, immature defence mechanisms and possible contamination of the lungs by aspiration. The signs of infection are often non-specific and include irregular respiration, apnoeic spells, lethargy, poor feeding and temperature instability. Early recognition of these signs will enable prompt investigation and treatment. Prophylactic antibiotics during surgery may have contributed to the current low rate of sepsis after thoracotomy.

18.3.5 PROLONGED HOSPITALIZATION

Most infants progress well without complications and are ready for discharge about 7–10 days after surgery. However, a small group of patients develop complications, or have an anatomical variant which necessitates a prolonged hospital stay. Infants with oesophageal atresia in the absence of a fistula have special nursing needs. The early management of these patients involves creation of a gastrostomy and suction of the blind upper pouch until oesophageal anastomosis is performed at 2–3 months. The goals of nursing management for these patients with long-gap oesophageal atresia are summarized in Table 18.1.

Management of upper pouch secretions

Frequent intermittent suction is performed to ensure the upper pouch does not fill with secretions. Vigilant nursing is required to identify

Table 18.1 Nursing goals in long-gap oesophageal atresia

1. Prevention of aspiration: keep the upper pouch free of secretions to prevent pulmonary complications
2. Provision of optimal nutrition, including care of the gastrostomy
3. Provision of an environment which facilitates normal growth and development and encourages the parents to be involved in the daily care of their infant
4. Preparation for discharge from hospital

signs that indicate that the infant needs further suctioning: an increase in respiratory effort, nasal flaring, restlessness and circumoral cyanosis. Usually this requirement becomes less frequent as the baby grows, becomes more settled, and gets used to being suctioned. A timer clock to remind staff when suctioning is due is useful. Previously we used a Replogle tube, consisting of a double lumen tube with an intake air line, inserted into the upper pouch and connected to continuous suction. Many problems were encountered with this method, including trauma to the mucosa, and intermittent suctioning is now favoured.

Nutrition

Optimal nutrition should be provided by enteral gastrostomy feeds. The promotion of rapid weight gain and oesophageal growth is important; therefore, if the mother's breast milk is not available, a high caloric artificial feed should be used. During gastrostomy feeds the infants are encouraged to suck on a dummy teat which has been dipped in the milk. This allows the satisfaction of hunger to be associated with the sensation of stomach filling and enables the infant to learn to suck. Salt supplements are added to the gastrostomy feed to replace the accumulative loss from saliva. Replacement of sodium chloride due to this loss has a positive effect on weight gain. As the baby grows, the gap between the ends of the oesophagus decreases and facilitates delayed primary repair (Puri *et al.*, 1981).

Care of the gastrostomy

Once a gastrostomy is performed, great care must be taken to prevent inadvertent dislodgement of the tube before there has been sufficient time for the track to become established. Premature dislodgement can be lethal if the tube is replaced intraperitoneally rather than in the stomach.

Care of the gastrostomy site postoperatively should be performed using aseptic technique for the first week to prevent infection and to promote a healthy, well-healed stoma. The site should be cleaned with isotonic saline daily. If there is discharge, a small gauze dressing can be wrapped around the tube. When the dressings are changed the gastrostomy tube is withdrawn until the resistance of the abdominal wall is felt; this brings the stomach wall against the abdominal wall. The tube is held at right angles to the abdomen before it is secured with tape, preventing leakage from around the stoma. Once the stoma is well healed and skin intact, gastrostomy care involves a clean technique. Parents are taught to wash around the site with soap and water during the normal bathing procedure and to secure the tube with tape. There is no need to use a dressing and it is normal to have a small amount of discharge from around the tube.

Complications of gastrostomy include infection, excoriation of the skin due to gastric acid leakage and accidental dislodgement of the tube. If the tube does fall out inadvertently, it is essential that it is replaced promptly before the stoma closes. Replacement is by simple reinsertion using a metal introducer to direct the tube. The gastrostomy tube itself may deteriorate and break, in which case it should be removed and replaced.

Parents' involvement in care and feeding

Parents are encouraged to be involved in their baby's care. The treatment of long-gap oesophageal atresia can extend over many months, during a critical time in the child's development. Nurses must consider the physical restrictions placed on the baby, as well as the normal social and emotional opportunities which are compromised. It is essential to provide an environment which allows parents to establish a close bond with their infant. A trusting relationship between parents and staff helps parents relate to their infant comfortably, to ask questions and to participate in the care of their infant. This creates a foundation which can be built upon for ongoing teaching prior to discharge.

The concept of Primary Nursing allows the co-ordination of nursing activities and enables liaison with other professionals. Other responsibilities include planning the nursing care and teaching the parents how to care for their infant. It is important that the parents' readiness to learn is assessed. It is often best to begin with small nurturing tasks, such as nappy changes, then move to other parentcraft skills as confidence increases. Activities involving parents should respect their other commitments so that the family unit is not placed under additional stress. It takes time to teach parents the techniques of suctioning the blind upper pouch, gastrostomy feeds and care of the gastrostomy site, but once learned, allows them greater responsibility in their baby's care.

A delayed primary oesophageal anastomosis is performed at about 8–10 weeks of age when the oesophageal segments have grown sufficiently. Postoperatively, the initial oral feedings may be difficult; the infants appear to have problems co-ordinating sucking, swallowing and breathing. Careful administration of the first feed by a skilled nurse, elevating the head of the infant and using a slow teat, will prevent coughing or choking initiated by rapid delivery of milk.

Oral feeding may take many weeks to establish in an older infant. When he tires he should not be forced to continue; instead, the feed should be completed via the gastrostomy. The attitude to feeding must be one of extreme patience and gentleness and should not be a rigid routine to achieve specified quantities each feed (Shannon, 1979). An infant will benefit most in this transitional period if his responses and quirks are documented in the nursing care plan and all feeds given in a similar way. The baby may become confused if a variety of approaches to feeding are attempted. The mother can be especially effective in establishing oral feeds if she is helped to feel at ease whilst feeding. Our experience has demonstrated that these infants often adapt better to breastfeeding than to bottle feeding.

Nurses need to be watchful during feeds for signs of complications. For example, anastomotic strictures may become symptomatic in the early postoperative period as disinterest in feeding, persistent coughing and small vomits with mucus.

The characteristic brassy cough of tracheomalacia is common but unless associated with respiratory complications, requires no precautions (Chapter 22).

18.3.6 DISCHARGE PLANNING

Discharge planning begins early in hospitalization with the development of parenting skills (Table 18.2). Shortly before discharge, there needs to be a time when the mother, and possibly the father, 'live in'

Table 18.2 Discharge planning checklist

---

1. Parenting skills satisfactory:
    oral feeds
    recognize different crying needs
    minimize gastro-oesophageal reflux
    gastrostomy care
2. Advise on action to be taken if:
    gastrostomy tube comes out or breaks
    food stuck in oesophagus
    oesophageal stricture develops
3. Names and telephone numbers of resource hospital personnel given to parents
4. Notify Maternal and Child Health nurse (or equivalent) of discharge

---

and take responsibility for their baby's care, where resources are at hand if required.

Gastrostomy tube feedings may still need to be used until oral feeds are well established. The parents need to know the techniques of gastrostomy care and what to do if the tube falls out or breaks. Written instructions will reinforce what has been learned and practised.

Prior to discharge, the Maternal and Child Health nurse is notified, so that she can establish home support and help the parents develop their normal parenting role. Parents should be given the names and telphone numbers of resource hospital personnel who may be contacted if concerns arise.

References

Beasley, S. W. and Tibballs, J. (1987) Efficacy and safety of continuous morphine infusion for postoperative analgesia in the paediatric surgical ward. *Aust. NZ J. Surg.*, **57**, 233–7.

d'Apolito, K. (1984) The neonate's response to pain. *Am. J. Mat. Child Nursing*, **9**, 256–7.

Filston, H. C. and Izart, R. J. (1985) *Congenital Abnormalities that Present with Respiratory Distress in the Surgical Neonate.* Appleton-Century-Crofts, Norwalk, Connecticut, pp. 104–5.

Gauntlett, I., Hochman, M. and Duncan, A. W. (1986) Tracheal compression by the upper pouch in oesophageal atresia without tracheo-oesophageal fistula. *Pediatr. Surg. Int.*, **1**, 243–5.

Puri, P., Blake, N., O'Donnell, B. and Guiney, E. J. (1981) Delayed primary anastomosis following spontaneous growth of esophageal segments in esophageal atesia. *J. Pediatr. Surg.*, **16**, 180–3.

Rushton, C. H. (1988) The surgical neonate: principles of nursing management. *Pediatr. Nursing*, **14**, 143–6.

Shannon, R. M. (1979) in *Comprehensive Paediatric Nursing* (eds G. M. Scipien, M. U. Barnard, M. A. Chard, J. Howe and P. J. Phillips), McGraw Hill, New York, p. 762.

19 *Support of the family*

H. SPEIRS and J. H. GRAHAM

The family of a patient born with oesophageal atresia requires psychosocial support from the moment the diagnosis is first suspected. In the future this may commence before birth if an antenatal diagnosis has been made. More often the need commences when the diagnosis is made shortly after the birth. Initially, psychosocial support is given to the parents but later help may also be required by other members of the extended family. Many medical and paramedical disciplines are involved in the care of babies with oesophageal atresia and their families, and each has specific responsibilities which may continue well into childhood. Central to ongoing care is the involvement of the surgeon who operates on the baby; he has a responsibility to communicate with the parents before surgery, and after the baby is discharged from hospital he must co-ordinate follow-up and ensure that the parents have ready access to him and the other support facilities as required.

19.1 Response of parents to an infant born with oesophageal atresia

The events occurring after the birth are contrary to the parents' expectations which have evolved during pregnancy. The anticipated postnatal experiences of joy, celebration and loving, as family members share in welcoming the newest member, are compromised and may be disrupted further if the infant is premature or has major coexisting abnormalities. The response of the parents to the unexpected trauma is dependent on factors internal and external to the family (Table 19.1). These factors determine the capacity of the family to cope with and adapt to their newfound situation.

19.1.1 ADAPTATION TO PARENTHOOD

Pregnancy and parenthood create stresses from adaptation to changing roles, relationships, responsibilities and life-styles. Continuity is

Table 19.1   Factors determining parents' response to birth of an infant with oesophageal atresia

— Individual personality traits
— The stability of marital and family relationships and social supports
— The religious, social and cultural values and experiences of the family
— Past life experiences, crises and losses
— Progress before and during pregnancy; e.g. previous infertility, pregnancy loss, problems during pregnancy or an unplanned pregnancy
— Coexisting social crises, e.g. financial stresses, social isolation, single parenthood

Table 19.2   Summary of factors which influence successful adaptation to the crisis situation (Speirs and Darling (1985))

Recognition of crisis behaviour patterns
Response to stresses specific to the birth of a baby with oesophageal atresia
Issues relating to environmental stresses
Tasks of the family to assist adaptation
Tasks of health care professionals to promote family well-being
Issues relating to siblings and extended family
Specific experiences – chronic hospitalization, disability, ethical issues, neonatal death

disrupted and the individual may lose his or her sense of control and equilibrium. Normally, this is within the context of a maturation process or transition from one developmental stage to another (Hobbs, 1984) but when a family experiences the birth of an infant requiring specialized neonatal care, this developmental crisis is compounded. Depending on how the situation is handled the outcome may vary from a healthy positive adaptation to the crisis, to breakdown in individual or family function. A number of considerations influence the success of this adaptation (Table 19.2) and an understanding of these is important in the overall management of the family.

Crisis behavioural patterns

The parent of an infant with oesophageal atresia is vulnerable and feels a sense of helplessness, uncertainty, powerlessness, and disorganization. Acute anxiety may be expressed in helpless dependent behaviour, open hostility or anger (Turnquist *et al.*, 1988). Responses are not related to the actual complexity or prognosis of the oesophageal atresia but rather to the individual's perception of the situation. Commonly parents express feelings of being submerged or 'being hit by a tidal wave'. If they have not previously faced a major crisis in their lifetime they may feel frightened (Truswell *et al.*, 1988). They have concern for the safety and survival of the newborn infant, and may feel some relief when the infant is transferred to a specialized unit for surgery. Alternatively there is a sense of helplessness and despair as the mother and child are separated (Speirs and Darling, 1985). Contact between the mother and infant before transfer is vital (Davis and Hawkins, 1985); personal contact may be reinforced by the provision of 'polaroid photos'.

Issues specific to the birth

At birth the parental hopes and expectations of the pregnancy are shattered. There is a sense of shock and disbelief and an overwhelming sense of sadness, loss and grief. The sense of loss is multifactorial (Table 19.3). The image of a new mother feeding, cuddling and bathing her new baby is blurred as mother and baby are separated. The feelings of failure and inadequacy are reinforced as she waits 'empty-handed' in a maternity ward among healthy mothers and babies. Awareness of her role in protecting and nurturing the infant can affect her self-esteem.

Separation of mother from her infant who requires specialized care impedes bonding as does the response of the mother to the birth of an 'imperfect child'. The factors determining this emotional response are summarized in Table 19.4. Parents ask 'Why me?' 'What is it that I have done or not done?' There is a searching back through the pregnancy seeking an explanation to make sense of the confusion they are experiencing. A sense of guilt is common (Koop *et al.*, 1975) and may be overwhelming.

There is also a marked change in the role of the father. The father tends to have a passive role within the 'normal' maternity situation, but now becomes an active participant. He is the link between mother and child whilst he struggles to cope with his own response to the situation.

Table 19.3 The types of loss experienced following the birth of an infant with oesophageal atresia

1. Loss of expectations of the pregnancy
2. Loss of 'healthy normal' baby
3. Losses associated with anticipated parenting roles, relationships and experiences
4. Losses associated with separation of mother and child
5. The threat of actual loss as parents fear the infant may die, i.e. the experience of anticipatory grief.

Table 19.4   Factors influencing the reaction of the parent to an imperfect infant

---

Is the anomaly visible?
Is the anomaly correctable?
Is the condition life-threatening?
Are there future medical needs?
The future in terms of normal development?
Is the condition hereditary?
Reaction of family members to the abnormality
Cultural values and perceptions of the abnormality
Availability and perceived quality of health care (Frietag-Koontz, 1988)
The parents' perception of 'why' the anomaly is present
When and how parents are told of the anomaly
Intelligence and background of parents
Comprehension of the nature of the treatment required to correct the anomaly

---

Few men are equipped to step easily into this role and there may be a conflict between the roles of husband and father, particularly when the mother and child are in different hospitals.

The information parents most want to hear is that the child will survive with a good quality of life. Information must be realistic, honest and expressed in a manner which is interpretable by the parents. A primary 'block' in registering what they are told is common during stress. For this reason the same information must be provided on several occasions, preferably by the same person with more than one staff member present at the interviews.

The parents' response to the uncertainties of ongoing treatment may generate profound stress and anger, which is sometimes directed at the medical profession. This may be exacerbated by societal expectations that the medical world can cure all. For some who have a child with a complex anomaly, e.g. chromosomal aberration, the sense of responsibility, guilt or failure may be almost unbearable and a parent may become totally immobilized or withdrawn.

Environmental aspects

Parents and families have to grapple not only with the crisis of the birth of an infant requiring specialized care but also with the stress related to the unfamiliar surroundings of the sophisticated neonatal intensive care unit (Sands, 1983). For many families, travelling to an inner city tertiary institution can be difficult and stressful. They should be told how to find the hospital and its neonatal unit. In the Intensive Care Unit there is a lack of privacy and a multiplicity of new people which can be unsettling at the least, and occasionally overwhelming. For many days there may be enforced inactivity, of waiting and watching, either in a waiting area or by the baby's bedside. The frustration of this, often under-estimated by staff, is commonly the trigger for expressions of anger. The technology around the infant is noisy and bewildering: a multitude of tubes, tapes, infusions, pumps, monitors and respirators, each with its own alarm system. Often the parents' perception of the baby's appearance is at variance with the medical opinion as to the infant's condition.

Parents are often hesitant to touch their baby for fear of either causing it distress or interfering with the apparatus or routines of its specialized care; this heightens their sense of helplessness and loss of control (Carter *et al.*, 1985). Without psychosocial support for parents the environment in the Intensive Care Unit is not likely to be conducive to parenting or interacting with the baby. Parents are commonly left with a sense of 'I have had a baby but it is no longer mine' and may become passive participants in care.

Other family members

Members of the extended family are important in providing support to the parents. They may also require support, as the whole family may be coping poorly. Grandparents in particular tend to be vulnerable as they observe their own child suffering. Furthermore, grandparents, attempting to support the family, may constitute a source of conflict as they grapple with their own sense of helplessness.

Many families have other siblings who are confronted with their own sense of disaster. Their responses are dependent on their age and conceptual development. Even with a normal birth siblings can feel displaced and rejected. These feelings may be exaggerated and the stability of family relationships put in jeopardy. It is worthwhile taking time to address the responses of the siblings with the family (Troy *et al.*, 1988). Although children are more adaptable than adults they still need an explanation appropriate to their life experiences and conceptual development. Siblings can be incorporated into the situation by visiting, bringing toys, letters or drawings of their choice for the baby. Children are perceived to be a distraction in the neonatal unit but this need not be so (Schwab, 1983).

Additional family stresses

Prolonged hospitalization may create additional burdens on the family (Table 19.5). Sensitivity to the subtleties of the family dynamics assist in their recognition, many of which can be alleviated.

Table 19.5   Additional family stresses

Excess time and costs involved with travelling

The shrinking of one's world between home and hospital

Financial stresses which may relate to 'hidden costs', e.g. travel, phone or to work absences

Coping with family and friends who either no longer ask about the baby, or alternatively ask why the baby isn't home yet

Stresses on child/family relationships increasing as each member struggles with the uncertainty and disruption to family life

Uncertainty in regard to the length of hospitalization, future treatments and the degree of disability the child may develop

---

19.2   Support of the family

All staff caring for the infant with oesophageal atresia play a role in meeting the psychosocial needs of the family. The key to success is the early identification of specific problems and good communication at all times.

19.2.1   AFTER ANTENATAL DIAGNOSIS

Although a definite diagnosis of oesophageal atresia is rarely made in the fetus, it is likely that in the future more cases will be diagnosed *in utero*. When an antenatal diagnosis is made consultation with a paediatric surgeon is obligatory so that he can meet the parents-to-be to explain what the condition means and outline the measures needed to treat it. The approach should be one of 'guarded optimism' taking into account that co-existent anomalies may have been identified. The paediatric surgeon may be asked by the obstetrician for advice on the appropriate mode and place of delivery. Ideally the baby should be born in a tertiary institution accustomed to the care of babies with neonatal problems. The method of birth will not be influenced by the diagnosis of oesophageal atresia. Adaption and planning can also be enhanced by non-medical sources e.g. social workers.

19.2.2   WHEN A DEFINITIVE DIAGNOSIS HAS BEEN MADE

Care of the family commences as soon as the diagnosis of oesophageal atresia has been made. The parents' expectation of the delivery of a normal healthy infant has not been fulfilled, and almost immediately their infant is transferred to another hospital. A simple explanation of the problem and likely outcome needs to be given to both parents. This is the first and most important statement to be made to the parents since they will often only 'hear' and remember the first statement made. The father, if at all possible, should accompany the infant to the paediatric centre. Here he will meet the surgeon and nursing staff involved in the care of his baby. Later, he will be able to take the information back to the mother. However, she also needs direct communication from the surgeon. Nursing staff often need to reinforce what has been said, and give further explanation.

19.2.3 THE FIRST ADMISSION

There must be good communication between staff members and this will facilitate communication with the family. The surgeon is the 'team leader' and as well as co-ordinating and directing treatment should be in a position to give the family as much support as required. In so doing he must recognize the role played by his medical colleagues, e.g. neonatologists and intensivists, and paramedical staff, e.g. nursing and social workers. At various times there will be a need for the parents to speak with or be counselled by another specialist, e.g. cardiologist, cardiac surgeon, thoracic physician, orthopaedic surgeon, urologist, gastroenterologist or geneticist. The surgeon is responsible for ensuring that there is adequate and appropriate consultation and communication.

When the mother visits for the first time, which may also be the first time she meets the surgeon, an effort must be made to arrange an interview to acquaint her with details of her child's treatment and progress.

Staff need to be conscious of the vulnerability of parents and of the fluctuations in their responses from day to day. An awareness of their coping behaviours and defence mechanisms is helpful. Withdrawal is common and may reflect difficulty in expressing emotions publicly and the myth that 'if I don't get involved, my distress will be less'. Selective listening may reflect the parents' struggle to make sense of the emotio-

Table 19.6 How to help the parents cope

---

1. Minimize the stress of separation of parents from child
2. Re-establish parents' relationship with their baby
3. Help them understand the nature of the anomaly, and the prognosis
4. Provide easy access for information
5. Increase the individual's sense of control by enabling participation in processes, decisions and care
6. Recognize early where additional support is required.

Table 19.7 Parental tasks

Learn to cope with temporary 'loss' of baby
Face the reality of the infant's condition
Understand oesophageal atresia and its implications
Deal with and express feelings
Learn the 'system'; become familiar with the hospital setting
Develop parent/infant relationships
Recognize and deal with co-existing stress
Plan for the future

(Speirs, Siegel, Nobel and Hamilton)

nal turmoil and the anxiety which they are experiencing. Staff must be careful not to engage in reinforcing negative behaviour but give parents the time and space they require. The attitude of staff may influence parental responses and behaviour, helping them to adapt to their new situation (Table 19.6). This adaptation requires that the parents accomplish a number of tasks (Table 19.7). They must have access to key personnel to help them understand their child's progress and provide them with additional support as required. Expression of feelings tends to be open and spontaneous when communication and interaction with staff is healthy and parents feel 'safe'.

Parents should be encouraged to touch, talk to, photograph and share experiences with their baby. They must be allowed to undertake simple parenting tasks, even at a stage when the infant is acutely ill.

In summary, the primary objectives of staff in supporting the family are to help parents feel at ease and to allow them contact with their baby (Siegel, 1982).

19.2.4 THE ROLE OF THE SOCIAL WORKER

Whereas the roles of the surgeon and the nursing staff are relatively easy to define, the part played by the social worker will vary from baby to baby and family to family. Nevertheless, the medical social worker is an integral part of the team and it behoves the medical staff to keep her informed of all developments. She should be involved as early as possible, preferably preoperatively, and the involvement continues throughout the period of hospital admission and following discharge from hospital.

It is important to minimize the adverse impact of the child's condition on family relationships and lifestyle. A balance between the specific needs of the child and the needs of the family as a whole has to be maintained. This requires an understanding of family dynamics and the family's ability to cope with stressful situations. The social worker may initiate specific interventions and problem-solving strategies to regain the sense of control and harmony within the family.

Just as the surgeon identifies, and adjusts his response to, the various clinical situations in the child, so too it is important for the social worker to recognize the range of abilities and methods which different individuals (even the several members of a family) will display in coping with the situation in which they find themselves. Parents should, therefore, be spared excessive and stereotyped advice which takes no account of the variations in relatives' responses.

Sensitivity of this nature is the hallmark of the good social worker.

19.2.5 PREPARING FOR DISCHARGE FROM HOSPITAL

Successful repair naturally leads to a state of euphoria in the parents. However, the joy of going home is often accompanied by a new sense of crisis as the parents finally take full responsibility for the care of their baby. Part of discharge planning involves the parents coming to 'live in' at the hospital to experience 24 hour care to gain confidence in their own parenting abilities.

Parents receive instructions on how best to care for their infant prior to discharge, and parents whose infant is in need of specialized care have liaison with and referral to community support services organized well in advance of discharge. They may also require practical and financial assistance.

Occasionally there are problems in obtaining practical community support for families with infants with 'special needs', e.g. gastrostomy feeds. Often these children are not catered for by existing services for the disabled. This may create immense stress on families when extended networks are unable to maintain adequate and functional support.

19.3 The role of independent parent support groups

In several regions parent support groups have been set up to provide long-term comfort, advice and assistance to the families of children with oesophageal atresia. Raising funds for research into oesophageal atresia and related disorders has been an important additional role of some of these groups.

19.3.1   OESOPHAGEAL ATRESIA RESEARCH AUXILIARY (AUSTRALIA)

Since 1922 the Royal Children's Hospital in Melbourne has encouraged the public development of voluntary support groups known as Auxiliaries. The aim of the original auxiliary was to 'interest the public in the hospital, to provide goods, and to raise money'. Whereas much of the work of the auxiliaries in the first 50 years or so was concerned with knitting, sewing and providing items such as bedding for the hospital, the groups that were formed in the 1970s and 1980s focused mainly on raising funds to enable the hospital to improve capital equipment and to finance research. More recently, additional auxiliaries have been established to provide parental support and promote research into specific medical conditions. The Oesophageal Atresia Research Auxiliary (OARA), set up in 1980, is an example of this latter type. The constitution of the Oesophageal Atresia Research Auxiliary lists three objectives (Table 19.8).

An annual donation of $5000 from the Windermere Foundation, an administrator of charitable donations, has provided OARA with a solid financial backing and enabled it to fund a number of studies into oesophageal atresia-related problems, including evaluation of the association of dysfunction of the oesophagus with lung disease following the repair of oesophageal atresia (Le Soeuf *et al.*, 1987) and a long-term

Table 19.8   The main objectives of the Oesophageal Atresia Research Auxiliary

Objective 1:

To raise funds to be useful for research and especially for the employment of qualified persons appointed or nominated by the Royal Children's Hospital Research Foundation to perform research in the field of oesophageal atresia or related conditions.

Objective 2:

To raise funds for family counselling to be set up in accordance with those measures generally suggested by medical persons associated with the Royal Children's Hospital.

Objective 3:

To offer comfort, advice and assistance on a personal level, in consultation with Royal Children's Hospital Social Work Department, wherever necessary or possible, to families directly involved in oesophageal atresia or related conditions.

follow-up study of survivors of repair of oesophageal atresia (Chetcuti *et al.*, 1988). The OARA has actively promoted research into these and other problems of oesophageal atresia and related conditions. This research has resulted in numerous contributions to the world literature and has modified aspects of the investigation and management of oesophageal atresia within the Royal Children's Hospital.

In co-operation with the Social Work Department of the Hospital, OARA has established a small fund which is used (at the discretion of the Social Work staff) to support families of new-born oesophageal atresia patients. This fund has helped to pay transport and accommodation costs when a welfare need was clearly evident.

Until recently most families of new patients have left the hospital unaware of the existence of the Auxiliary, and only discovered it at a much later date. Now, families are given a 'resource kit' on oesophageal atresia during the first admission. Only in this way can the support work of the Auxiliary be made effective.

19.3.2 TOF SUPPORT GROUP (UK)

In the United Kingdom, an organization known as TOFS (Tracheo-Oesophageal Fistula Support) functions as a registered charity 'to sup-

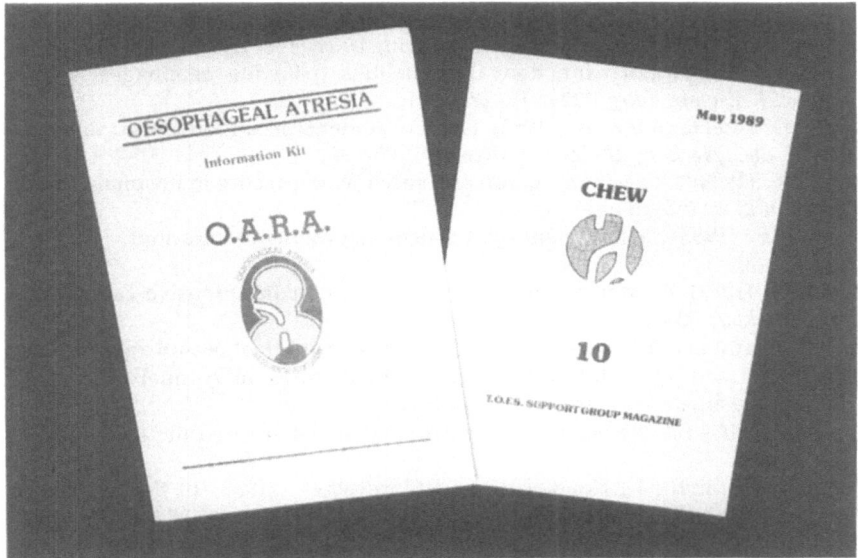

Figure 19.1 The OARA information kit given to parents during the first admission, and an issue of the TOFS Support Group newsletter, 'CHEW'.

port babies born unable to swallow'. This organization is an active, rapidly expanding one. Its current aim is to hold a regular national conference on oesophageal atresia. The first conference was held in 1987 and the second in 1989.

TOFS group sends out a regular newsletter, 'Chew', to its members (Figure 19.1). The contents provide news and useful information for the families of patients with repaired oesophageal atresia.

References

Carter, M., Miles, M., Buford, T. and Hassanein, R. (1985) Parental environmental stress in pediatric intensive care units. *Dimens. Crit. Care Nurs.*, **4**, 180–8.

Chetcuti, P., Myers, N. A., Phelan, P. D. and Beasley, S. W. (1988) Adults who survived repair of congenital oesophageal atresia and tracheo-oesophageal fistula. *Br. Med. J.*, **297**, 344–6.

Davis, D. and Hawkins, J. (1985) High risk maternal and neo-natal transport: psychosocial implications. *Dimens. Crit. Care Nurs.*, **4**, 368–79.

Frietag-Koontz, M. (1988) Parental grief in diagnosis of severe neurological impairment. *J. Perinat. Neonat. Nurs.*, **2**, 45–55.

Hobbs, M. (1984) Crisis intervention in theory and practice. *Br. J. Med. Psychol.*, **57**, 23–34.

Koop, C. E., Schnaufer, L., Thompson, G., Haecker, T. and Dalrymple, D. (1975) The social, psychological and economic problems of the patient's family after successful repair of oesophageal atresia. *Z. Kinderchir.*, **17**, 125.

Le Soeuf, P. N., Myers, N. A. and Landau, L. I. (1987) Etiological factors in long-term respiratory function abnormalities following esophageal atresia repair. *J. Pediatr. Surg.*, **22**, 918–22.

Noble, D. and Hamilton, A. (1981) Families under stress. Perinatal social work. *Health Soc. Work*, **6**, 28–35.

Sands, R. (1983) Crisis intervention and social work practice in hospitals. *Health Soc. Work*, **8**, 253–61.

Schwab, F. (1983) Sibling visiting in a neonatal intensive care unit. *Pediatrics*, **71**, 835–8.

Siegel, R. (1982) A family-centred program of neonatal intensive care. *Health Soc. Work*, **7**, 50–6.

Speirs, H. and Darling, Y. (1985) Psychological aspects of oesophageal atresia. Presented at Royal Children's Hospital, Melbourne, at Annual Meeting of Oesophageal Atresia Research Auxiliary.

Troy, N. (1988) Sibling visiting in the neonatal intensive care unit. *Am. J. Nurs.*, Jan, 68–70.

Truswell, S., Blyth, J., Kendall, S. and Shipway, P. (1988) In the eye of the storm: crisis intervention in hospitals. *Aust. Soc. Work*, **141**, 38–43.

Turnquist, D., Harvey, J. and Anderson, B. (1988) Attributions and adjustments to life-threatening illness. *Br. J. Clin. Psychol.*, **27**, 55–65.

20 Case selection

N. CAMPBELL

20.1 The problem

When oesophageal atresia is associated with other abnormalities that may result in death or poor quality of life, the question can be asked: 'Should the oesophageal atresia be repaired?'

Oesophageal atresia and its variations are almost always technically correctable, but the outcome in terms of survival and quality of life may be determined by factors other than the oesophageal atresia. This means that clinicians involved in the care of babies with oesophageal atresia may be faced with the question of whether they should proceed with surgery or not. Implicit in this question is knowledge that without surgery death will follow, and the belief that the interests of some babies may be best served by allowing them to die. More than half the babies with oesophageal atresia have associated malformations (Chapter 14). They may also be very premature or suffer from other serious conditions, such as birth asphyxia and perinatal infections. Associated malformations may be single, multiple or part of a recognized syndrome, or the VATER and CHARGE associations. Associated chromosome abnormalities include Trisomy 18 and Trisomy 21. The premature baby less than 32 weeks' gestation is at risk of hyaline membrane disease, perinatal infection and intracerebral haemorrhage. Fetuses with oesophageal atresia are as much at risk of perinatal asphyxia as other fetuses: modern techniques can result in short-term survival of these babies, even with severe established brain damage. Finally, babies in whom the diagnosis of oesophageal atresia is delayed can develop serious lung disease from aspiration of milk feeds or gastric and pharyngeal secretions.

20.2 Ethical background

Oesophageal atresia associated with incurable or other serious conditions is one of a number of clinical situations in which there might be

Table 20.1 The selective non-treatment debate

1. Under what circumstances may treatment be withheld or withdrawn?
2. Who should make the decision?
3. What criteria should be applied?
4. What kinds of treatment may be withdrawn?
5. When curative treatment has been withdrawn, what palliative care is acceptable?
6. What should be the aims of public policy?

justification for withholding treatment. Almost everyone involved in the debate – doctors, nurses, bio-ethicists, parents and lawyers – agrees that withholding treatment is appropriate in at least some circumstances. For example, most would accept that withholding mechanical ventilation from babies with anencephaly, and surgery from babies with oesophageal atresia and bilateral renal agenesis, is appropriate, but beyond this there is little consensus. The major questions in the selective non-treatment debate (Table 20.1) are discussed below:

1. Under what circumstances may treatment be withheld or withdrawn? Should it be only when early death is inevitable, or may it include cases where survival is likely, but the resulting quality of life will be poor?
2. Who should make the decision: doctors, parents, ethics committees, or courts of law?

    Doctors have technical medical knowledge and experience of long-term outcome; but are not trained in moral issues. In our pluralistic society, the moral views of parents are at least as valuable as those of others, they are able to see best the interests of their baby and family, and it is they who will have to cope with the consequences of the decision. However, they will be in emotional turmoil, and the best interests of their baby may conflict with their own.

    Hospital ethics committees can ensure that all appropriate expertise is brought to bear, that there are no communication blocks between doctors, nurses and parents, and that emotions do not cloud the issues; but they are not responsible for the outcome, and tend to see their role as upholding principles rather than seeking out the best possible solution for the individual.

    Involvement of the law courts may allow resolution of legal questions which are central to decision-making, and protect individual rights; but their processes tend to be slow, law reform lags behind public opinion, and law courts are too inflexible to decide issues which often have no satisfactory legal solution.

3. What criteria should be applied? Should they relate to the baby's best interests, and nothing else, or to the interests of the family as well? The impact of a seriously handicapped baby on the family members is considerable and continues for a long period. Should babies have the same rights as everyone else, and their right to life prevail over all else, or should the rights and interests of siblings and parents be given equal or greater weight? Can the rights and interests of babies and the rest of their families ever really be viewed separately?

   When the economic costs of caring for impaired survivors are counted in millions of dollars, should this be taken into account when community resources are finite?

4. What kinds of treatment may be withdrawn? Is it reasonable to withdraw complex life-support systems and major surgery, or ordinary care such as antibiotics, fluids and nutrition? Should feeds be withheld if they merely prolong a life of poor quality?

5. When curative treatment has been withdrawn, what palliative care is acceptable? Should analgesics or sedatives be given, even though they may depress respiration, reduce the desire to feed, and shorten life? Is there indeed a place for active termination of a baby's life when pain or other distress is unremitting?

6. What should be the aims of public policy? Should governments aim to be involved in selective non-treatment decisions, to ensure that individual rights and the law are upheld, and the public interest protected? Should they legislate to establish guidelines or laws, and maintain surveillance of institutions caring for sick babies? Or should governments leave selective non-treatment issues to families and doctors acting in good faith?

20.3 Quality of life

Although a few feel that treatment may be withdrawn only when death is imminent and inevitable, there is a larger body of opinion which believes that the quality of life of the baby is a further factor which should be considered. Some believe that the implications of the baby's survival for the quality of life of the family – parents, and present and future siblings – may also justify consideration.

20.3.1 QUALITY OF LIFE OF THE BABY

A number of factors influence a baby's quality of life (Table 20.2).

Table 20.2   Factors influencing the quality of life of the baby

1. Intellectual handicap
2. Physical handicap
3. Other factors:
    Ongoing pain or other distress
    Permanent physical ill-health: a shortened life-span: an increased risk of
    acquired diseases such as infections, malignancies
    Physical disfigurement
    Urinary or faecal incontinence
    Sexual problems
    Psychological and emotional disturbance

Mental handicap

Most clinicians would accept that if severe intellectual handicap is
certain, it may be appropriate that treatment be withheld. Examples
include the baby with Trisomy 18, or hydranencephaly. It is assumed
that such babies are incapable of awareness of self and the world, and
thus unable to give or experience love or other human pleasures. If it is
held that the most important consideration is the capacity to achieve at
least limited independence, selective non-treatment may be entertained
in infants with milder degrees of mental defect, as occurs in such
conditions as Down's syndrome, and the CHARGE association.

Parents' subjective views vary widely. Some accept a child with severe
intellectual disability as long as there is a possibility of at least some
interaction. Others view mild handicap, as in Down's syndrome, as an
unmitigated disaster.

Physical status

It is accepted by many that gross physical handicap, such as that
caused by high neural tube defects, is sufficient reason to withhold
treatment. While there is an almost infinite variety of combinations of
physical handicaps, they should be considered in terms of their functional results. Will the child be able to sit, stand or walk, with or without
special aids? Will some degree of independence be possible? If there are
associated problems such as visual handicap, colostomy, incontinence
or missing limbs, will the special skills required to cope with them be
attainable?

Combinations of factors

A number of other factors which may affect quality of life are listed in
Table 20.2. In conjunction with intellectual and physical handicaps, they

have a compounding rather than an additive effect on the quality of life. Physical handicaps, which might not seriously affect the life of a child of normal intellect, may result in far poorer function when combined with severe intellectual disability.

20.3.2   QUALITY OF LIFE OF THE FAMILY

The survival of a seriously handicapped child imposes physical, financial and emotional burdens on the rest of the family. Added to the parents' grief and guilt, these burdens may cause marital breakdown and major behavioural problems in siblings. The mother is often left to care for the family unaided. Given finite family resources, the rights and needs of normal siblings must be balanced against the increased needs of the handicapped child.

20.3.3   QUANTIFYING QUALITY OF LIFE

Attempts have been made to make the assessment of the effects of handicap or chronic illness on the quality of life less subjective. Scoring systems for various handicaps, illness and other impediments to normal life, together with formulae for giving weightings to various combinations, have been devised (Kind *et al.*, 1982). Although they can help to clarify issues in resource allocation, they are of little help in individual cases.

20.4   An approach to selective non-treatment

The guidelines employed in selective non-treatment issues at the Royal Children's Hospital are described below:

1. Withdrawal of curative treatment should be considered when there is little hope of survival or when quality of life will be unacceptably poor;
2. In these cases, the consultants should inform the parents about all relevant aspects of diagnosis and prognosis, but need not remain neutral. In most cases they should indicate clearly what they believe could be the best decision.
3. The final decision on whether or not to treat an infant who is not expected to survive, or who is likely to have a very poor quality of life, belongs to the parents.

    If parents want treatment to continue despite medical advice to the contrary, treatment must be continued in good faith. If parents want treatment withdrawn, contrary to medical advice, resolution in favour of continuing can almost always be achieved with frank, respectful discussions, avoiding confrontation. Resort to the law is seldom, if ever, necessary. Hospital ethics committees have no place in prospective decision-making for individual babies.

4. The baby's best interests are the most important consideration; but other factors including the effect of the baby's continuing defects on the rest of the family may have some influence on decisions.

5. When it is agreed by all that it is correct to withdraw curative treatment, no treatment likely to prolong life unnecessarily should be continued. This includes oxygen, antibiotics, intravenous therapy, and feeding by any artificial means.

6. When curative treatment is withdrawn, the baby should be made comfortable, and the emotional needs of the family and staff attended to. The use of analgesics and sedatives to make the infant comfortable may incidentally shorten the baby's life. Nursing staff are actively involved in decision-making and in some cases, may initiate the discussion among clinical staff.

20.4.1   SELECTIVE NON-TREATMENT IN BABIES WITH OESOPHAGEAL ATRESIA

In 44 cases there was a deliberate decision made not to treat the infant on account of associated anomalies (Table 20.3). In patients with oesophageal atresia and distal tracheo-oesophageal fistula, definitive operative treatment was withheld in 6.5% up until 1972 and in 13% from 1973 (Figure 20.1), in part reflecting the increased number of patients admitted with major chromosomal defects and other lesions associated with a poor prognosis. In order to clarify the ethical issues involved, it is useful to classify babies with oesophageal atresia and associated life-threatening or handicapping conditions as shown in Table 20.4.

Babies for whom early death is inevitable

It does not benefit the baby to repair the oesophageal atresia when there is bilateral renal agenesis. Ethical decision-making is thus straightforward; no quality-of-life issues are involved. Neither morality nor the law would require treatment which is futile, not offering any hope of benefit to the patient. Only two of the 15 babies with renal agenesis or gross dysplasia and hypoplastic lungs had typical 'Potter's Syndrome'; the remaining 13 babies had combinations of imperforate anus, cardiac malformations, sacral and vertebral anomalies, radial aplasia or dysplasia, duodenal atresia and genital anomalies. In recent years, these babies

Table 20.3 The Royal Children's Hospital oesophageal atresia series: babies in whom surgery was decided against because of associated anomalies ($n = 44$)*

Patients	
Renal agenesis or gross dysplasia with pulmonary hypoplasia ± multiple other major anomalies	15
Trisomy 18	11
'Inoperable' cardiac malformations ± other major anomalies	6
Gross Central Nervous System malformations	3
Trisomy 21	3
CHARGE association	3
Unknown	3

*There were additional patients who arrived moribund or in whom the diagnosis of oesophageal atresia was made at post mortem.

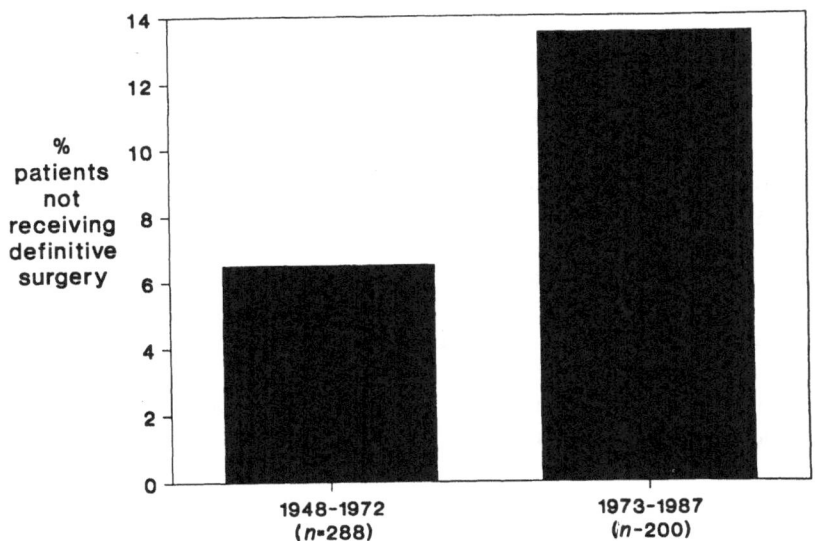

Figure 20.1 Patients with oesophageal atresia and distal tracheo-oesophageal fistula in whom definitive operative treatment was withheld.

Table 20.4   Situations in which withholding surgery might be considered

---

A.   Babies in whom early death is inevitable
1.   Renal agenesis with pulmonary hypoplasia
2.   Inoperable cardiac malformations

B.   Babies who may survive but with severe intellectual handicap
1.   Trisomy 18
2.   Major structural brain abnormalities
3.   Acquired severe brain injury
(a) Severe birth asphyxia
(b) Very low birthweight babies with intracerebral haemorrhage

C.   Babies with less intellectual handicap with or without physical handicaps
1.   Down's syndrome
3.   CHARGE association

D.   Babies with normal intellectual prognosis but severe physical handicaps

---

have been successfully resuscitated at birth, transferred to the surgical unit and investigated. The families have been advised of the futility of active treatment and most have agreed to treatment withdrawal. All active measures have been stopped and replaced with palliative care.

The oligohydramnios of fetal renal dysplasia can be balanced *in utero* by the polyhydramnios of oesophageal atresia, so that the fetal lungs grow relatively normally and the baby may have surprisingly little evidence of pulmonary hypoplasia and intrauterine compression. One baby who had absent kidneys on ultrasound confirmed at post-mortem, had no respiratory distress and appeared to pass small amounts of 'urine' per urethra. For this reason alone, it is appropriate to perform renal ultrasonography on all babies with oesophageal atresia prior to surgery.

The six babies who had oesophageal surgery withheld because of associated cardiac lesions considered inoperable were all born before 1980. Recent progress in cardiac surgery and intensive care means that most complex cardiac malformations can be treated successfully – by stages, if necessary – with eventual cardiac transplantation as an option if staged surgical procedures fail. Objective counselling of parents, with realistic detailing of the problems involved and the chances of success, is mandatory if such a course is to be offered. The few arguably inoperable conditions (hypoplastic left heart syndrome, some complex cyanotic lesions involving a single ventricle or inadequate pulmonary arteries and some cases of idiopathic hypertrophic cardiomyopathy) are very uncommon in association with oesophageal atresia. Close consultation between neonatologist, cardiologist and cardiac surgeon is needed to decide whether to proceed, and the timing of the diagnostic and surgical procedures.

Babies in whom severe developmental handicap is certain

In these babies there is usually a shortened life-span as well. Since active treatment enables survival for some time, decisions to withhold oesophageal repair or other life-saving measures involve judgements about the quality of life the baby will have with survival.

Babies with Trisomy 18 are severely mentally defective. Without active treatment of associated malformations, 50% are dead within a month, and less than 10% survive to one year. Trisomy 18 has been the commonest reason for withholding treatment in the last decade. In the last five years, all cases were actively resuscitated at their hospital of birth and transferred on ventilators. Clinical recognition was usually easy, and the diagnosis confirmed by bone marrow chromosome analysis within hours. Once the diagnosis was made, mechanical ventilation was ceased and most died within minutes – although four recent infants have lived longer than 48 hours, and one for six days.

Major structural brain abnormalities include anencephaly, hydranencephaly and gross hydrocephalus (Figure 20.2); in each of these conditions, gross mental deficiency is the rule. Anencephalic babies seldom survive beyond a few minutes or hours, but since the severity of the lesion is variable, and they are seldom given active support, the potential for survival of some with less complete lesions, is unknown. Survival beyond a year of life has been reported, as has one case with anencephaly and oesophageal atresia.

The developmental prognosis for hydrocephalus and other structural brain lesions is variable and may be difficult to predict but with a combination of microcephaly, large encephalocele, dilated ventricular system and absent corpus callosum (holoprosencephaly) severe mental deficiency can be expected.

The acquired severe brain lesions that might influence decisions in babies with oesophageal atresia are severe birth asphyxia and large intracerebral haemorrhage (Grade IV) in the very low birthweight baby (birthweight < 1500 g).

Babies with lesser intellectual handicap with or without physical handicap

Decisions in this group are based on quality-of-life judgements, and attitudes vary widely. In general, those who consider quality-of-life judgements relevant in decision-making believe mental handicaps have a greater negative effect on quality-of-life than physical handicaps. This

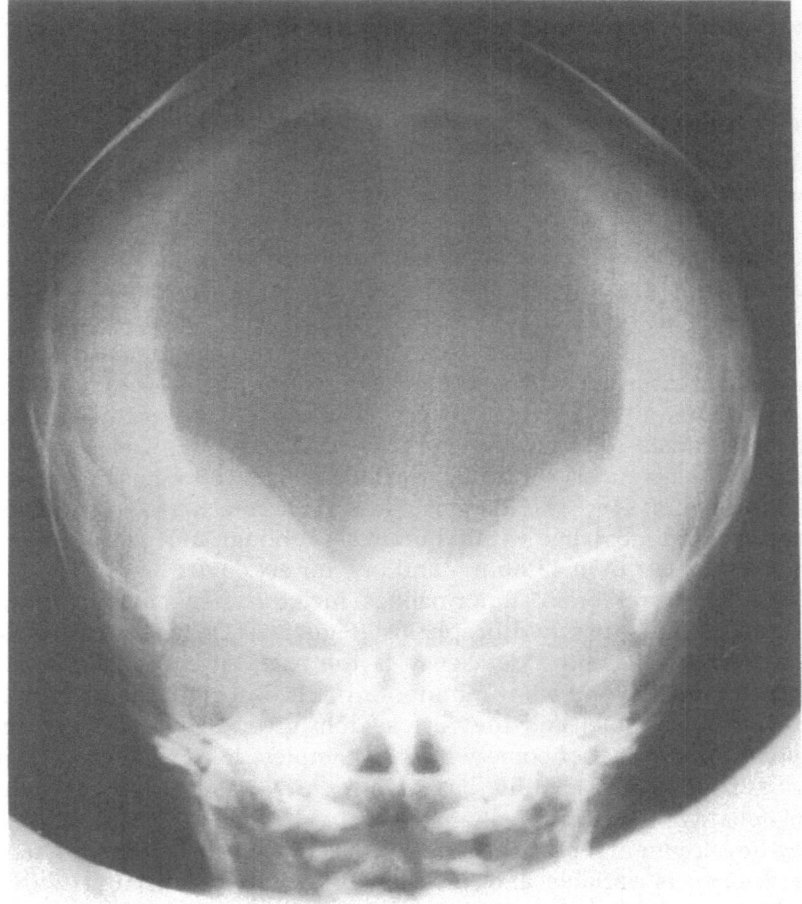

Figure 20.2 Gross hydrocephalus.

is especially so for those who believe it is appropriate to consider the quality of life of the family as well as the baby.

The management of the baby with Down's syndrome and oesophageal atresia has created much controversy, since medical, legal and parental attitudes vary so much. To some parents survival of a child with Down's syndrome is seen as disastrous; to others, whilst a cause for sadness, it is not seen as justifying withdrawal of treatment. In recent cases in which the courts have become involved, both in Britain and the United States, decisions have favoured surgery. Medical opinion remains divided, and many still maintain that quality of life in

Down's syndrome children and their families is sufficiently poor that parents should be allowed a choice.

In ten babies with Down's syndrome, three had surgery withheld (Table 20.3). Our current policy is to advocate surgery unless the parents are adamantly against it.

The early literature on CHARGE association indicated that over 90% of survivors were mentally retarded, many seriously. Our more recent experience and that of others (Oley *et al.*, 1988) of children with CHARGE association has been better, with about one-third of survivors mentally normal, or nearly so.

Surgery was withheld in three of the five patients with CHARGE association and oesophageal atresia. Of the two survivors, one is dull-normal, the other seriously retarded. Our current approach is to advocate surgery but not to proceed if parents are strongly against it.

Babies with normal intellectual prognosis but probable severe physical handicaps

Those who believe it is reasonable to withhold treatment on quality-of-life judgements are usually influenced more by intellectual handicaps than by physical handicaps. Most would not consider withholding surgery because of severe physical handicaps alone. Nevertheless it is routine practice in many centres to withhold surgery from babies with high neural tube defects on the basis of severe physical handicaps alone, significant intellectual handicaps being uncommon.

If surgery is withheld from a baby with oesophageal atresia and severe physical handicaps, death is inevitable. We believe that babies with malformations which will result in severe permanent disabilities are not always best served by life-preserving surgery.

20.5 The withdrawal of treatment

Once the decision is made not to operate on a baby with oesophageal atresia, death is inevitable. The aims of care change from the preservation of the baby's life to the reduction of suffering, and the support of family and staff through the emotional distress of withdrawal and death.

The baby with unrepaired oesophageal atresia may suffer from:

1. Accumulation of secretions in the blind upper pouch causing distressing choking episodes. Aspiration pneumonia, dyspnoea and hypoxia may ensue.
2. Hunger, since the baby cannot be fed.

3. Distress resulting from associated abnormalities or their management, e.g. mechanical ventilation, endotracheal tube care, or, in the baby with anorectal or genitourinary anomalies, pain from bowel obstruction or urinary tract obstruction. Measures which prolong life prolong these distresses, and are therefore against the baby's interests.

Most measures aimed at relieving distress will hasten the baby's death. Although this is in the baby's interest, it has ethical and legal implications and may be emotionally distressing to parents and staff. Nevertheless, it is our belief that all care likely to prolong life should be withdrawn, except pharyngeal suction.

Parents should be given an outline of what is involved in withdrawal and palliative care, and options for their involvement. When parents have been fully informed, and centrally involved in the decision-making process, many of them see it as natural that they will also participate fully in palliative care. However, some do not, and initially wish to withdraw from the situation, feeling overwhelmed. It is best to advise with sensitivity, that whilst it is natural not to be able 'to cope', it is also 'natural' to see their child through his final illness. Of parents whose babies have had treatment withdrawn in our Unit (not just those with oesophageal atresia), 94% chose to maintain the closest involvement with their babies until their death. No parents thus involved have subsequently expressed regret: all have been positive that seeing their baby through his or her death was the most appropriate thing to do.

20.5.1 BABIES ON VENTILATORS

Ventilation is ceased and the baby extubated. Since the resulting hypoxia may be distressing, the baby is given 0.1–0.2 mg/kg of morphine intravenously beforehand. Babies with severe brain abnormalities, such as Trisomy 18, may be considered unaware and do not need analgesia or sedation but if uncertainty exists, morphine administration should be used for these babies as well.

Parents are given options for their involvement before respiratory support is withdrawn. Would they like to hold their baby for a period whilst still alive before extubation, and be with him for extubation and thereafter? Would they like to hold their baby before extubation, but then leave? Would they like to be given their baby after extubation? Or would they prefer not to be present at all? Would they like their baby to be brought to them elsewhere, in a quiet place, after extubation? What other family members or friends would they like with them during treatment withdrawal?

The great majority opt for the first alternative. They must be prepared in advance for the colour changes, gasping and other agonal events, or they will find them distressing and more difficult to cope with.

Following extubation, oxygen-dependent babies usually die within minutes. After death, parents usually appreciate the removal of all intravascular catheters and other equipment. They usually wish to remain with the baby for an hour or more; some require several hours, and wish to bath the baby and perform other rites. Any sense of hurry should be avoided. The parents should be given long periods to be alone with their dead baby.

Occasionally babies with oesophageal atresia have lived for many hours – one for four days – following extubation. Parents should be prepared in advance for this possibility, otherwise they may find it emotionally intolerable.

20.5.2 BABIES IN OXYGEN

The administration of oxygen into an incubator or head box is much less invasive than mechanical ventilation, and therefore less distressing to the dying baby, but it will prolong the dying process. Whether oxygen should be withdrawn is decided with the parents. If it is withdrawn, morphine is given intravenously beforehand, and repeated as required. Oxygen can be given temporarily via a nasal cannula to make it easier for the parents to nurse their baby before the oxygen is finally withdrawn. Parents are given the same options for their involvement in the withdrawal process as with withdrawal of mechanical ventilation. If it is decided not to withdraw oxygen, subsequent management is along the lines outlined below.

20.5.3 OTHER SITUATIONS

Babies who remain in oxygen, or who need neither oxygen nor mechanical ventilation prior to withdrawing treatment, will live longer once treatment is withdrawn than those described above. Antibiotics and intravenous fluids are withdrawn and parenteral analgesia (morphine) is given. Because of the blind upper pouch, numerous choking episodes will usually occur, during which the baby is very distressed, but does not die. Repeated suctioning of the upper airway will relieve these episodes and minimize aspiration. It will thus prolong the baby's survival, and for this reason might not be considered to be in the baby's interests. However, staff and parents find it impossible not to intervene during these distressing episodes. Thus repeated suctioning of the airway is usually necessary and appropriate, even though all other life-prolonging treatment has been withdrawn.

As the baby becomes dehydrated from withdrawal of parenteral fluids, salivary and other secretions reduce and choking episodes cease. Dehydration also has a beneficial effect on dyspnoea and other symptoms resulting from heart failure or lung disease. These benefits are not seen when hydration is maintained with intravenous fluids. The longest survival in our institution of a baby with unrepaired oesophageal atresia has been six days after cessation of active measures.

Parents can be encouraged to live in the hospital with the baby and other family members during the dying process. Given the requirements of frequent airway suctioning, it is not usually appropriate for the baby to go home. Furthermore, most parents are not emotionally ready to take dying babies home until several days of treatment withdrawal have elapsed. Parents choose to maintain very close involvement with their dying baby, either by living in the hospital or by paying prolonged daily visits. The great majority express a strong desire to be with the baby at the time of death, and are distressed and disappointed if the baby dies in their absence.

Parents require much support, re-explanation of their baby's condition and reassurance as the baby dies. Palliative care requires much more of the surgeon's and physician's time than active management. Nursing staff and junior medical staff also need much support, and opportunities for discussion of the issues and the process. They bear the immediate stress with the parents at the cot side. At least daily discussions between medical and nursing staff of the baby's and family's progress are essential. Conscientious objection to being involved in withdrawal of treatment and palliative care (which seldom occurs in our experience) must be respected.

20.5.4 AUTOPSY

Autopsy should be performed in all babies dying following withdrawal of treatment. It seems to help many parents to have objective confirmation after death of conditions which may have seemed abstract or unreal in the discussions during the baby's life. In some cases autopsy is essential for genetic counselling. It is best to discuss autopsy well before death, as part of the discussions about treatment withdrawal. Parents are less likely to be disturbed by the idea, and more likely to agree, than if autopsy is first brought up after death.

20.5.5 GRIEF COUNSELLING

An experienced social worker is invaluable in providing assistance and support to parents during withdrawal discussions and implementation. Grief counselling should start when the decision to withdraw treatment is made. Most families benefit from continuation of counselling in the days and months after death. Some families will benefit from referral to a parent support group. It is best to advise the family of such groups and let them decide for themselves if they wish to make contact. A few families benefit from continuation of counselling for years after the baby's death.

Genetic counselling is best done about three months after the baby's death.

References

Kind, P., Rosser, R. and Williams, A. (1982) Valuation of quality of life: some psychometric evidence. in *The Value of Life and Safety* (ed. M. W. Jones-Lee), Elsevier/North Holland, Amsterdam.

Oley, C. A., Baraitser, M. and Grant, D. B. (1988) A re-appraisal of the CHARGE association. *J. Med. Genet.*, **25**, 147–56.

PART SEVEN
The Problems

21 Oesophageal complications

A. W. AULDIST and S. W. BEASLEY

Mortality in oesophageal atresia has declined to the point now where death is expected only in those who have severe associated anomalies (Chapter 24). Consequently, reduction of morbidity and improvement in the quality of life have become the principal aims of therapy. Much of the morbidity of oesophageal atresia relates to complications of the oesophageal anastomosis, such as anastomotic leak, stricture formation and recurrent tracheo-oesophageal fistula (Figure 21.1); these complications of repaired oesophageal atresia are discussed in this chapter.

21.1 Anastomotic leak

The problem of leakage from the oesophageal anastomosis has posed a major challenge to surgeons ever since the first repair of oesophageal atresia; and over the years the fear of leakage (and its consequences) has been responsible for several changes in surgical technique. These include the type of anastomosis employed, the extra-pleural approach and the use of staged procedures. In relation to the type of anastomosis, the classic two-layered Haight telescoping anatomosis was developed in an attempt to lessen the risk of leakage but it was found to produce a high stricture rate (Coran, 1989; Myers *et al.*, 1990). More recently, recognition that the one-layered, end-to-end anastomosis has a relatively low leakage and stricture rate has made it the anastomosis of choice.

21.1.1 DEFINITION OF ANASTOMOTIC LEAK

Leakage from the anastomosis may vary enormously in significance, from a minor leak on contrast radiology in a well infant, to complete anastomotic disruption with mediastinitis, empyema, pneumothorax and septicaemia. Assessment of anastomotic leak must take into consideration its severity and sequelae. For descriptive purposes, we have

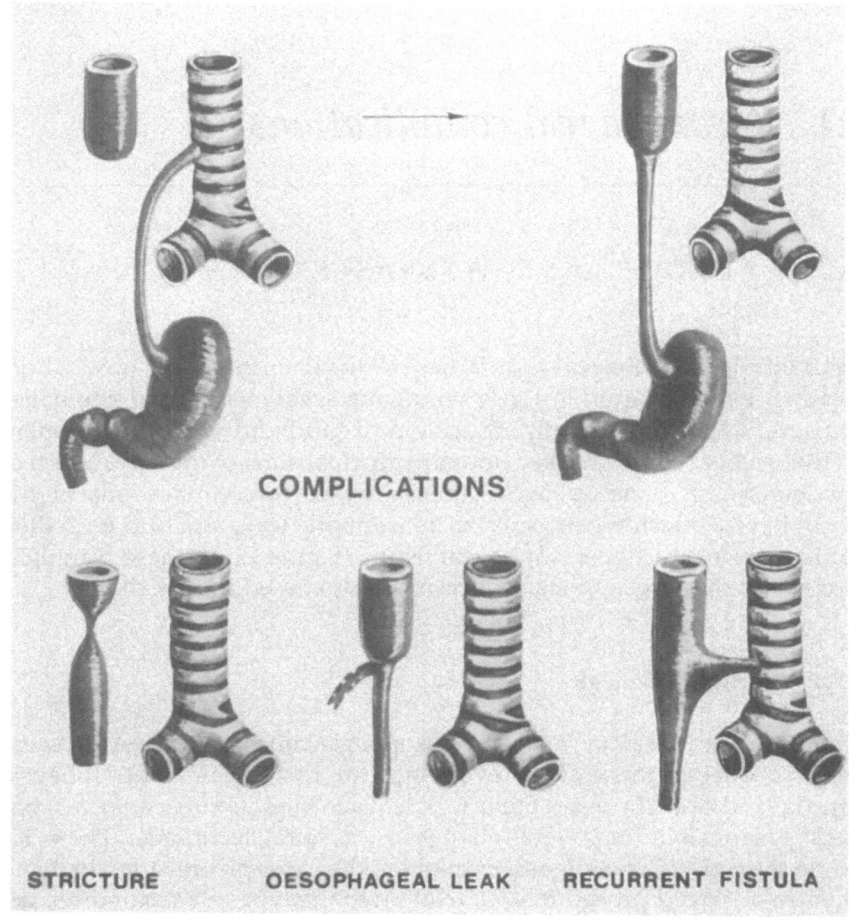

COMPLICATIONS

STRICTURE   OESOPHAGEAL LEAK   RECURRENT FISTULA

Figure 21.1 The oesophageal complications of repaired oesophageal fistula.

found it useful to define leak as follows:

1. *Incidental*: Small radiological leak, no clinical symptoms.
2. *Minor leakage*: Saliva in chest drain, but clinically well.
3. *Major leakage*:
   (a) mediastinitis or abscess
   (b) pneumothorax, empyema
   (c) radiologically confirmed major oesophageal disruption

21.1.2 INCIDENCE

The incidence of leakage has decreased over the decades as recognition of the predisposing factors has led to modification of surgical

Table 21.1 Severity of leak after primary anastomosis in 200 consecutive patients with oesophageasl atresia and distal fistula

	Number	%
No leak	158	79.0
Radiological leak, infant asymptomatic	17	8.5
Minor leak:		
Saliva in chest drain < 1 week	14	7.0
Saliva in chest drain > 1 week	5	2.5
Major leak:		
Empyema/mediastinitis	4	2.0
Lung abscess	2	1.0

technique. In a series of 224 patients described by Coran (1989) the overall incidence of leak was 8.5%. Spitz (1988) reported 34 leaks in a total of 199 patients (17%). The majority were minor but in seven cases the leak was major and included complete disruption in six. At the Royal Children's Hospital since 1970, major anastomotic leak has been an uncommon problem occurring in only 3% of 200 consecutive primary anastomoses (Table 21.1).

21.1.3 CONTRIBUTING FACTORS

Early leakage is likely to occur if the anastomosis is constructed poorly and the sutures are not placed or tied correctly. Excessive tension and ischaemia of the oesophageal ends may be additional factors which contribute to leakage (Table 21.2). The likelihood of leakage due to these latter factors may be diminished if the oesophagus is mobilized carefully (McKinnon and Kosloske, 1990). The extent of oesophageal dissection undertaken is a balance between that dissection required to gain length to avoid excessive tension at the anastomosis and injury to the blood supply of both oesophageal ends which may occur when the oesophagus is mobilized extensively or myotomies are performed. Spitz *et al.*

Table 21.2 Factors which may contribute to leakage from the oesophageal anastomosis

Incorrectly placed sutures
Insecure sutures
Excessive tension at anastomosis
Ischaemia of oesophageal ends
Infection

(1987) found a statistically significant increase in the rate of anastomotic leak when braided silk was used, compared with polyglycolic acid and prolene. There was no significant difference in leak rate between patients with or without reflux (Spitz, 1988). In 27 of his 199 patients the anastomosis was difficult and under maximum tension: in these a high leakage rate might have been expected but there were only two leaks, both of which were minor.

At the Royal Children's Hospital the incidence of anastomotic leak in oesophageal atresia with distal tracheo-oesophageal fistula since 1970 was related to gestation and length of gap as shown in Figures 21.2 and 21.3. In this series, leak was more common when the gap between the oesophageal ends was more than 4 cm, but even in this group the leakage rate in the last decade has been lower than in previous years. It is possible that a period of paralysis and assisted ventilation postoperatively may help prevent leakage in some patients (Spitz *et al.*, 1987), but our decline in leakage rate has occurred irrespective of assisted ventilation. Anastomotic leak was more common after an end-to-side anastomosis (25%) than an end-to-end anastomosis (12%) (Figure 21.4). This compared with an incidence of 17% (8/47) in patients with a one-layered anastomosis and 6.2% (11/177) in patients with a Haight anastomosis in the series described by Coran (1989).

Although most of our postoperative leaks occurred in intubated patients, these often involved anastomoses constructed under greater

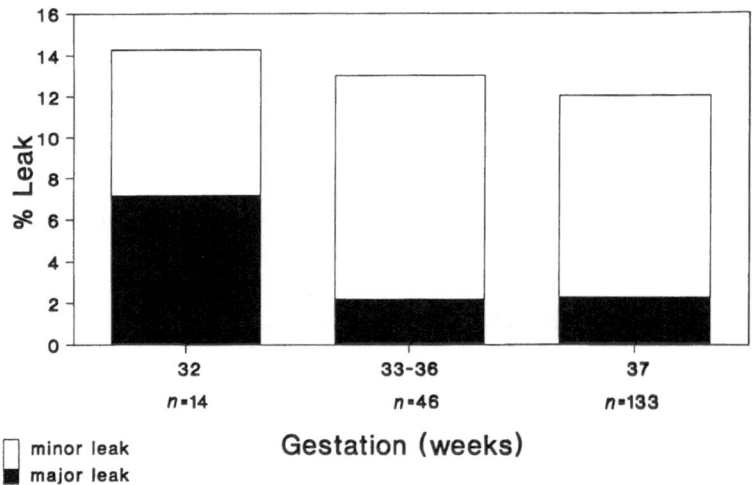

Figure 21.2   The relationship of anastomotic leakage to gestation in oesophageal atresia and distal tracheo-oesophageal fistula between 1970 and 1984.

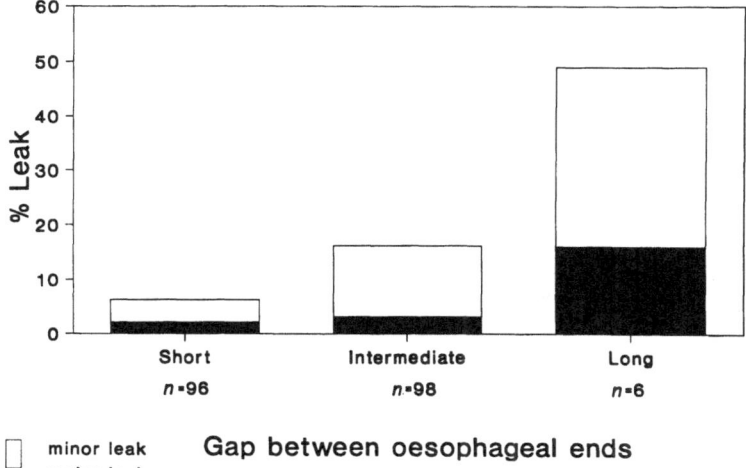

minor leak
major leak

Gap between oesophageal ends

Figure 21.3 Relationship between length of gap between oesophageal segments and anastomotic leak in oesophageal atresia and distal tracheo-oesophageal fistula (200 consecutive patients). Short gap = < 2 cm; intermediate gap = 2–4 cm; long gap = > 4 cm.

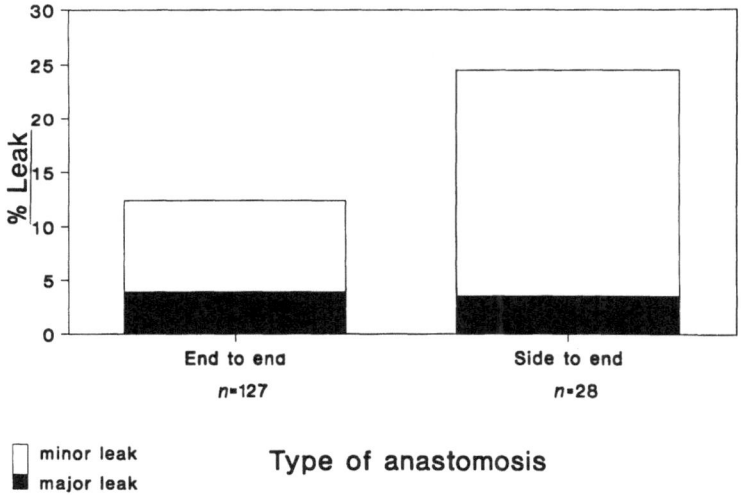

minor leak
major leak

Type of anastomosis

Figure 21.4 Incidence of leak according to the type of anastomosis. Not included in this figure are five anastomoses in conjunction with circular myotomies (three leaked) and nine Haight anastomoses (one leaked).

Table 21.3 Relationship of endotracheal intubation to the development of an anastomotic leak in oesophageal atresia and distal tracheo-oesophageal fistula (*n* = 200)

Intubation	No intubation		Intubation	
	No.	%	No.	%
Preoperative period				
No. of patients	168		32	
Leak	21	12.5	4	12.5
(minor)	17		2	
(major)	4		2	
Postoperative period				
No. of patients	92		108	
Leak	7	7.6	17	16.0
(minor)	6		12	
(major)	1		5	

tension or following extensive mobilization of the oesophagus (Table 21.3). Nevertheless, our data are unable to demonstrate a beneficial effect of paralysis and assisted ventilation on leakage rate.

The relationship of leak to subsequent stricture formation and recurrent tracheo-oesophageal fistula is shown in Table 21.4, and the effect of gastrostomy in Figure 21.5.

Table 21.4 Relationship of leak to stricture and recurrent fistula in 200 patients

	Stricture		Recurrent fistula	
	Nil	Present	Nil	Present
Number of patients reviewed	179	21	192	8
Number of patients with leak	21	4	23	2
% leak	11.7	19.1	12	25
P value	0.5		0.3	

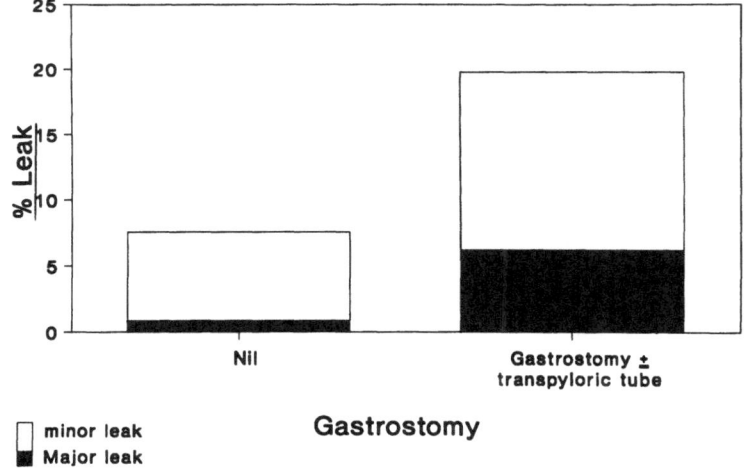

Figure 21.5 Effect of gastrostomy on the incidence of anastomotic leak in oesophageal atresia and distal tracheo-oesophageal fistula in 200 consecutive patients between 1970 and 1984.

21.1.4 DIAGNOSIS

The easiest way to diagnose a leak is to observe saliva in the chest tube. If the presence of saliva in the chest tube is not certain the baby can be given methylene blue to swallow; if a leak is present it will appear in the chest tube. In 8.5% an asymptomatic leak was demonstrated on barium swallow in patients in whom no saliva had drained from the chest tube (Table 21.1). In patients in whom a chest tube is not used the development of a pneumothorax or pyrexia is suggestive of a leak. A persistent leak should be studied by barium swallow to assess the extent of anastomotic disruption (Figure 21.6). The volume of the leak can be compared with the total fluid intake and is one factor in deciding management. The presence of systemic features (pyrexia, septicaemia) will also influence treatment.

21.1.5 TREATMENT

Most leaks can be successfully managed conservatively. Safe total parenteral nutrition enables oral feeds to be stopped. Antibiotics are commenced and the leak will usually close spontaneously. Radical intervention, such as cervical oesophagostomy, is necessary rarely and should be reserved for the patient in whom supportive therapy has been unsuccessful. A long-standing leak may require gastrostomy to allow

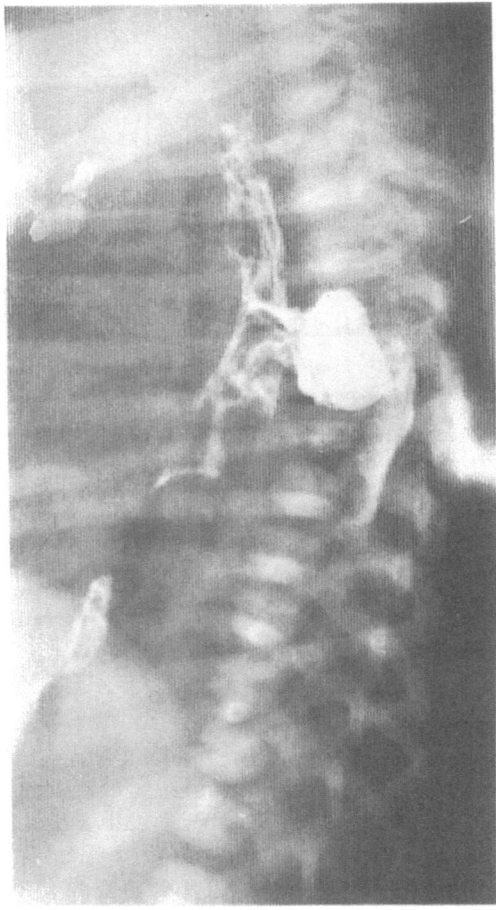

Figure 21.6   A barium swallow demonstrates the extent of anastomotic disruption.

continuation of enteral feeds. In this situation gastrostomy combined with a transpyloric tube or an antireflux procedure may be beneficial so that reflux from the stomach does not perpetuate the leak. Complete disruption of the anastomosis is now rare, but has been an indication for cervical oesophagostomy and subsequent oesophageal replacement in less than 2% of those with a distal fistula.

21.1.6   PREVENTION

Careful handling of the oesophagus, minimal mobilization of the oesophagus and the use of an end-to-end one-layered anastomosis with interrupted polyglycolic acid sutures may contribute to a low leakage rate. Postoperative paralysis and assisted ventilation of patients with a long gap or tension on the anastomosis may be helpful (Spitz *et al.*, 1987).

21.2 Recurrent tracheo-oesophageal fistula

A recurrent tracheo-oesophageal fistula is a severe and potentially dangerous complication of oesophageal atresia. In the early years patients with this complication often died, but with improvements in supportive care it is possible to treat these patients successfully.

21.2.1 INCIDENCE

The incidence of recurrent fistula ranges from 3 to 14% (Table 21.5).

Table 21.5 Overall incidence of recurrent tracheo-oesophageal fistula (Rec-.TOF)

Author	(years)	No. of patients	No. Rec.TOF	%
Leendertse-Verloop *et al.*	(1975–84)	77	8	10
Hicks *et al.*	(1967–79)	82	4	5
Bishop *et al.*	(1974–83)	60	4	7
Beardmore	(1962–77)	52	7	14
Touloukian	(1968–79)	38	3	8
Ein *et al.*	(1965–82)	250	23	9
Ghandour *et al.*	(1975–85)	242	20	8
RCH, Melbourne	(1948–88)	498	15	3

21.2.2 CONTRIBUTING FACTORS

At Great Ormond Street the development of a recurrent fistula was related to the use of silk suture material but not to tension on the anastomosis (Spitz *et al.*, 1987). Two patients developed recurrent fistulae after ligation and division of the oesophagus without anastomosis, as part of a staged procedure. In Toronto, a higher incidence of recurrent fistula after end-to-side anastomosis has been reported (Ein *et al.*, 1983). This observation has resulted in the end-to-side anastomosis being abandoned in most centres. Tension on the anastomosis was not found to be a significant aetiological factor in Toronto, and it is interesting that

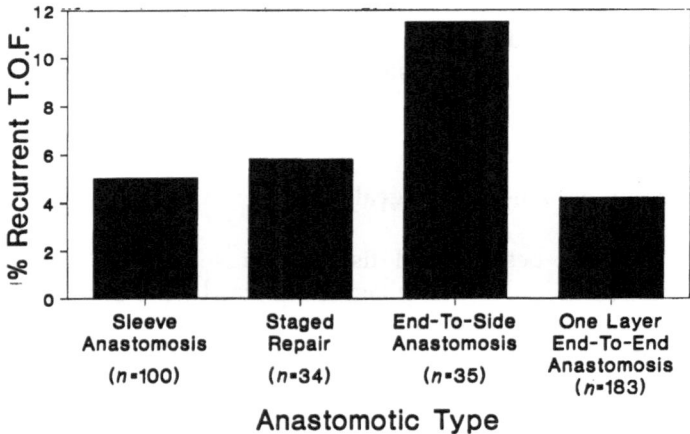

Figure 21.7   Relationship of recurrent tracheo-oesophageal fistula to the type of anastomosis.

eight of their 23 recurrent fistulae had neither anastomotic leak nor stricture.

In Melbourne, the primary end-to-end anastomosis with one layer of interrupted sutures had the lowest rate of recurrent fistula (Figure 21.7) and the end-to-side anastomosis the highest.

21.2.3   SECOND RECURRENCE OF FISTULAE

Second recurrence of tracheo-oesophageal fistulae has been reported. At Great Ormond Street there were four patients of the original 23 with a recurrent fistula who developed a second recurrence, and two of 20 recurrent fistulae in Toronto. There were two second recurrences in the Melbourne series.

21.2.4   PATHOGENESIS

It is likely that some recurrent fistulae are caused by an anastomotic leak resulting in infection in the area of the repair (Figure 21.8), particularly when the anastomosis is in direct contact with the site of tracheal closure. However, it is difficult to explain how such a local infection could cause a recurrent fistula when there is no clinical or radiological evidence of leak or stricture in the region of the anastomosis. Tension on the anastomosis and anastomotic leak in combination may enhance the chance of recurrent fistula.

Some fistulae present months or years after the primary operation, in the absence of any intervening symptoms. It may be that in some of

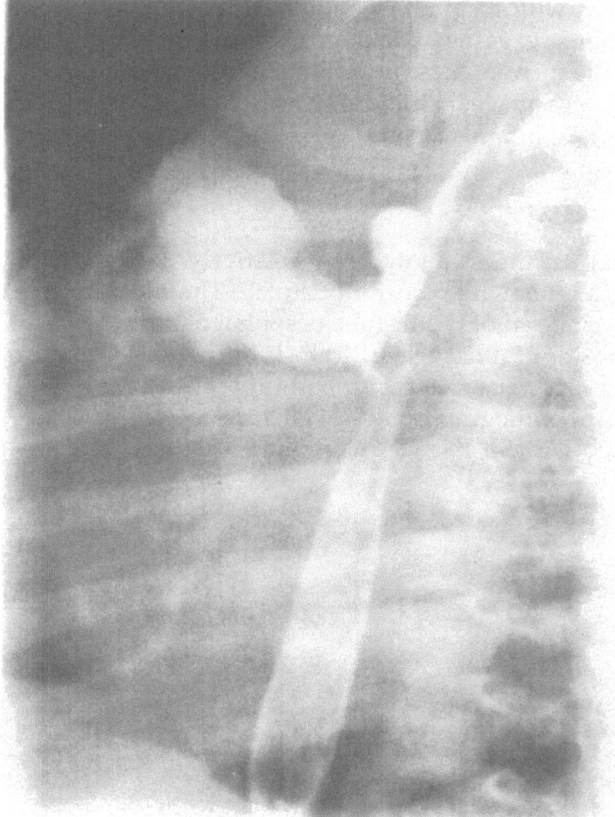

Figure 21.8 Major leakage from the oesophageal anastomosis causing local infection in the region of the repair is likely to have contributed to the development of a recurrent tracheo-oesophageal fistula in this patient.

these patients, use of a suture material such as silk creates a persistent granulomatous reaction.

Once established, a recurrent fistula allows saliva and food into the trachea. In patients with gastro-oesophageal reflux, acid may gain access to the respiratory tract as well. This causes inflammation in the tracheobronchial tree, atelectasis and repeated episodes of pneumonia.

21.2.5 CLINICAL PRESENTATION

Recurrent fistulae have been diagnosed as early as a few days after the primary operation, but some do not present for many years. A few patients are diagnosed at the time of routine barium swallow, but the majority present with respiratory and/or swallowing symptoms. These include coughing, gagging, choking, cyanosis, apnoea, dying spells, wheezing and recurrent chest infections; and may simulate the symptomatology of oesophageal stricture (Haight, 1969). The typical presentation is that of an infant who coughs and splutters with each feed.

21.2.6 DIAGNOSIS

A conventional barium swallow has a relatively poor yield of positive diagnoses in patients with recurrent fistulae. The most reliable method of diagnosis is cine-radiographic tube oesophagography with the patient in the prone position. A nasogastric tube is introduced into the oesophagus and the oesophagus filled with barium while the tube is gradually withdrawn. Cine-radiographs are taken in a lateral view during this procedure (Figure 21.9). Bronchoscopy has been advocated as another

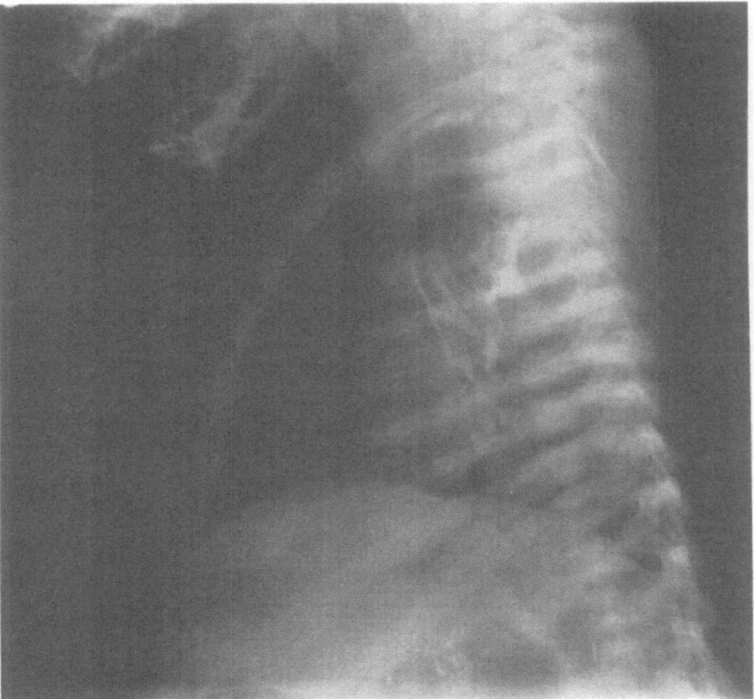

Figure 21.9 Radiograph taken during cineradiography demonstrates a recurrent tracheo-oesophageal fistula.

method of diagnosis (Gans and Berci, 1971; Benjamin, 1981; Randolph, 1986). The recurrent fistula usually arises from the pouch of the original fistula and enters the oesophagus at or just below the anastomotic repair site (Benjamin, 1981). The advent of modern bronchoscopes may encourage bronchoscopy to be more widely used in this situation in the future.

21.2.7 TREATMENT

Despite isolated reports of spontaneous closure of recurrent fistulae, an indefinite waiting policy is not appropriate. Even in those in whom the symptoms subside for a time, it is unlikely that spontaneous closure will occur. In Toronto no operation for recurrent fistula was done within five weeks of the first, and at Great Ormond Street the recommendation is that the surgeon waits at least eight weeks from the original procedure (Spitz, 1988). Early operation is made difficult by inflammation between the oesophagus and trachea and the chance of causing damage to the original anastomosis is high. In Melbourne, the policy is to wait at least four weeks from the first operation, and of even more importance, is the requirement that the patient is in optimal respiratory and general condition. The advent of reliable intravenous nutrition means that gastrostomy is no longer necessary and feeding the patient via a nasogastric tube is discouraged because reflux may aggravate the respiratory problem if gastric contents are aspirated. The operative approach is through the original right fourth interspace and access is transpleural. Some surgeons have found that the passage of a fine ureteric catheter through the fistula will facilitate its localization during the operative repair (Spitz *et al.*, 1987). Stay sutures are placed on the fistula when it is identified. It is preferable to avoid using tapes around the oesophagus because of the increased dissection required. The fistula is divided and each end closed with 5/0 interrupted polyglycolic acid sutures. Mediastinal tissue can be placed between the ends of the divided fistula. The postoperative management is the same as after a primary operation, although some surgeons delay instituting oral feeds for a longer period.

There are now several reports of endoscopic obliteration of recurrent tracheo-oesophageal fistulae. Rangecroft *et al.* (1984) described endoscopic diathermy obliteration of the fistula whereas others have used tissue adhesives (Gdanietz and Krause, 1975; Pampino, 1979; Waag *et al.*, 1979) or a combination of a tissue adhesive and sclerosing agent (Izzidien Al-Samarrai *et al.*, 1987). The use of these techniques may have special application in regions where additional surgery has an unacceptably high morbidity or where parents are reluctant to allow their child to undergo surgery (Izzidien Al-Samarrai *et al.*, 1987).

A transtracheal approach to the fistula (Martin *et al.*, 1986) and the use of a vascularized pedicle of pericardium to separate the trachea and oesophagus during repair of recurrent tracheo-oesophageal fistula (Botham and Coran, 1986) have been described.

21.2.8   PREVENTION

A variety of recommendations have been recorded to avoid recurrent tracheo-oesophageal fistulae. These include division and careful closure of the original fistula with meticulous placement of interrupted polyglycolic acid sutures and placement of interposing pleura, pericardium or intercostal muscle between the divided fistula and the oesophageal anastomosis. We do not believe that interposition of tissue is feasible in the usual case; reliance on division of the fistula (rather than ligation alone) and meticulous anastomosis is all that should be necessary. It has been possible to avoid recurrent fistulae in our last 70 patients born with oesophageal atresia and distal fistula.

21.3   Anastomotic stricture

Anastomotic stricture is the most common reason for further surgery to the oesophagus after repair of oesophageal atresia.

Oesophageal stricture can be defined as a narrowing of the oesophagus which requires treatment. There is no universally agreed definition of stricture following oesophageal atresia surgery, and many definitions have been used. For example, Coran (1989) defined a stricture as a narrowing requiring more than two dilatations. For the purposes of this discussion a stricture is defined as any narrowing at the anastomosis requiring surgical treatment, including dilatation.

21.3.1   INCIDENCE

Direct comparisons of the incidence of stricture are difficult because different institutions have used a variety of definitions of stricture and applied them to different subgroups of patients. Oesophageal strictures requiring dilatation or other surgical treatment were present in about 30% of our survivors since 1979. This compares with an overall incidence of 19% in Coran's (1989) series of 224 patients and 74/199 (37%) reported by Spitz (1988) from London.

21.3.2 FACTORS INFLUENCING STRICTURE FORMATION

Careful handling of the oesophagus to avoid damage to the blood supply of the oesophageal ends and construction of the anastomosis under as little tension as possible would be expected to minimize the incidence of stricture formation (Table 21.6) but the effect of these and other factors which may influence stricture formation is difficult to quantify. Spitz *et al.* (1987) found an increased incidence of stricture when silk was used for the anastomosis, compared with either polyglycolic acid or polypropylene. Children with gastro-oesophageal reflux had a significant increase in stricture formation (Table 21.7). There was a higher incidence of stricture formation in patients who leaked from their anastomosis.

An oesophageal stricture may occur co-incidentally in association with a recurrent fistula, but there is no evidence of an increased incidence of stricture when a recurrent fistula develops.

Table 21.6 Factors which may contribute to stricture formation

Rough handling of oesophagus at time of repair
Ischaemia
Tension on anastomosis
Suture material, e.g. silk
Gastro-oesophageal reflux
Anastomotic dehiscence
Type of anastomosis, e.g. 2 layer

Table 21.7 Effect of gastro-oesophageal reflux (GOR) leak, and anastomotic type on stricture formation

	No. of patients	Stricture	No Stricture	% Stricture
GOR	61	39	22	64
No GOR	110	30	80	27
Leak	30	20	10	67
No leak	151	54	97	36
One-layer anastomosis	47	2	45	4
Haight anastomosis	177	41	136	23

*Data derived from Spitz *et al.* (1987) and Coran (1989).

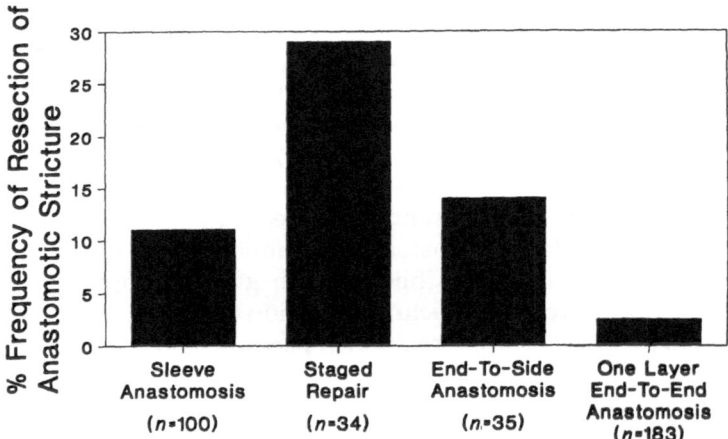

Figure 21.10   The frequency of resection of an anastomotic stricture according to the type of anastomosis constructed.

Coran (1989) found a greatly increased incidence of stricture with a two-layer (Haight) anastomosis, compared with the one-layer anastomosis. In our series, resection of an anastomotic stricture was required most commonly with staged repairs and least commonly with a primary one-layer end-to-end anastomosis (Figure 21.10).

21.3.3   CLINICAL PRESENTATION

Patients with a stricture have feeding difficulties and dysphagia as their major symptoms. The first symptom in babies is often 'slow feeding' and excessive regurgitation, with or without cyanotic episodes. Older patients often present with foreign body impaction of food in the oesophagus. Many patients complain of dysphagia with certain foods, e.g. sausages, and the food bolus may be regurgitated, or pass onwards with the help of swallowed fluid. In such a patient the possible diagnoses include stricture, oesophageal dysmotility or a combination of both.

21.3.4   DIAGNOSIS

Diagnosis of an oesophageal stricture is suspected from the history and confirmed either by endoscopy or barium swallow. Endoscopy is used as the first investigation when the child presents with foreign body impaction. The presence of a stricture should be noted at the time of removal of the foreign body, and provided that the foreign body has not been present for too long it is of value to dilate the stricture at the same time. In other patients, a barium swallow is the appropriate first investigation. The procedure has the advantage of demonstrating gastro-oesophageal reflux in patients where the stricture is not too tight to allow sufficient barium into the stomach. Other associations such as recurrent fistula may also be identified.

21.3.4 TREATMENT

In patients with mild narrowing of the oesophagus, one or two dilatations may be all that is required. In patients with associated gastro-oesophageal reflux, it will usually be necessary to perform an antireflux operation. Gastro-oesophageal reflux is documented in about 40% of patients after repair of oesophageal atresia and about half of these develop a significant anastomotic stricture. Although in the past such strictures were managed by dilatation alone, there is now widespread acceptance (Pieretti *et al.*, 1974) that the reflux should be treated surgically. When an anastomotic stricture is suspected, a barium swallow should be performed (Figures 21.11 and 21.12). Constant narrowing on X-ray is diagnostic, and should prompt the radiologist to look for evidence of gastro-oesophageal reflux. Once the contrast study has demonstrated the stricture, endoscopy is performed to complete its assessment, obtain a biopsy at the site of narrowing and dilate it. A Nissen fundoplication is required for those with a stricture and gastro-oesophageal reflux (Chapter 23). After a successful antireflux operation, the stricture will usually improve over several weeks but may require one or two further dilatations. In the unlikely event that the stricture fails to resolve or respond easily to dilatation after an antireflux operation, the stricture should be resected.

Method of dilatation

Many methods of dilatation have been used over the years. They include dilatation under a general anaesthetic using a Hurst mercury-filled bougie or with a more rigid gum elastic bougie; retrograde dilatation using Tucker bougies railroaded through the stricture on a string through a gastrostomy; and balloon dilatation under radiographic control (Ball *et al.*, 1984). This last method has certain theoretical advantages over other methods (McLean and Le Veen, 1989) and early experience suggests it may be very effective. The use of steroids injected into the stricture has been advocated but is unproven for resistant strictures. It may have a place as a 'final try' before proceeding to resection. A small number of strictures resistant to all forms of dilatation will need resection. In the early part of our series, this was relatively common (Myers *et*

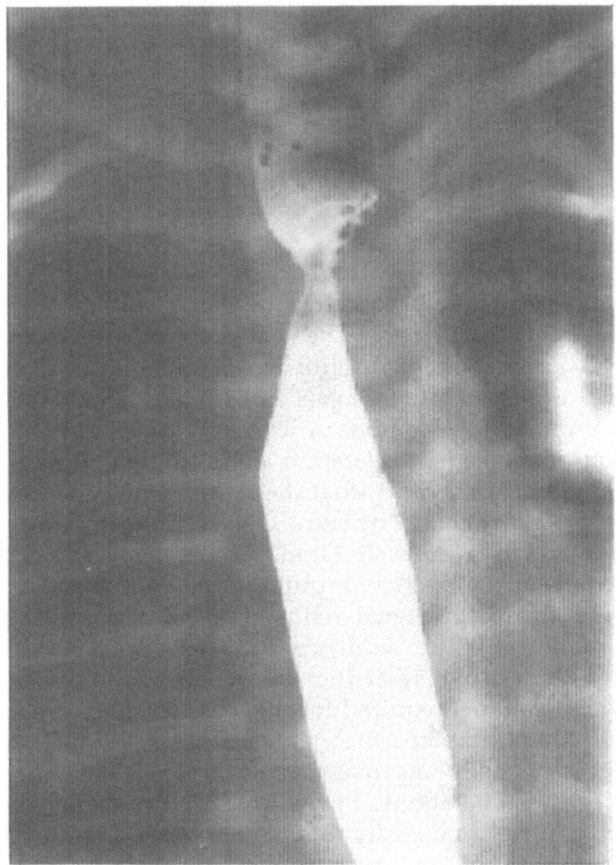

Figure 21.11 Barium swallow demonstrates an anastomotic stricture: constant narrowing of the oesophagus is diagnostic.

al., 1990) but since the introduction of the Nissen fundoplication has been most uncommon.

21.3.5 PREVENTION

A single-layered, end-to-end anastomosis using non-absorbable sutures, such as polyglycolic acid, gives a low incidence of stricture. The anastomosis should be constructed accurately with the least possible tension between the ends. Interference of the blood supply of the oesophagus should be kept to a minimum. If these guidelines are

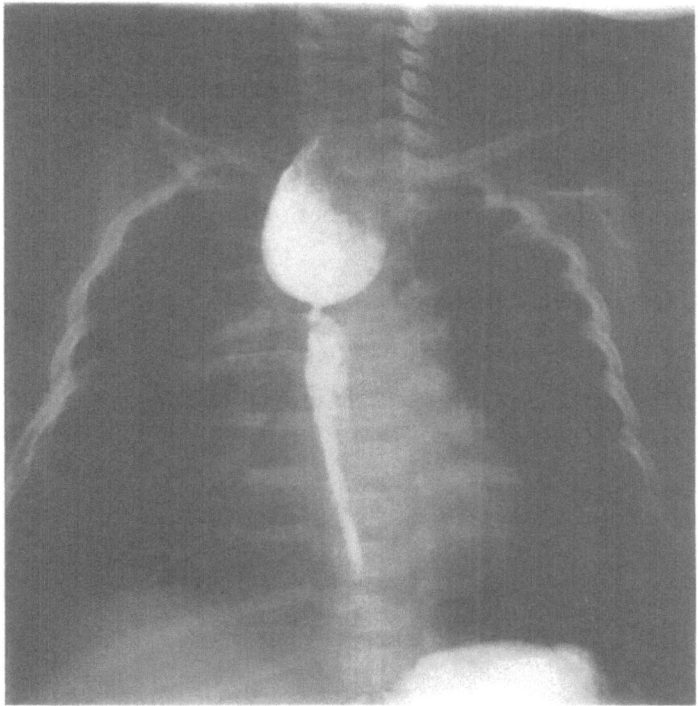

Figure 21.12 A severe anastomotic stricture which ultimately required resection. Note the distension of the proximal oesophagus.

followed, the incidence of stricture will be confined largely to those with significant gastro-oesophageal reflux for whom antireflux surgery as soon as the stricture becomes symptomatic is indicated.

21.4 Motility problems

Oesophageal motility is abnormal both before and after repair of oesophageal atresia (Chapter 5). It is probable that injury to vagal fibres from mobilization of the oesophagus worsens the oesophageal dysmotility; and thus should be kept to a minimum. Abnormal motility is responsible for minor dysphagia in most patients (Chapter 25). In some, solid food may obstruct the oesophagus at or around the site of the anastomosis without any evidence of an actual stricture on X-ray or at endoscopy. These patients seem to improve gradually with age, but in the meantime need to be taught to chew their food well and drink with their meals. The abnormal oesophageal motility may contribute to tracheal aspiration, as the oesophagus does not empty normally during the swallowing process. It may also account for the increased number of patients suffering complications of gastro-oesophageal reflux. The fact that the oesophagus does not empty normally allows fluid from the stomach to sit in the lower oesophagus for a longer period of time than in patients with normal muscular action.

21.5 Uncommon complications

21.5.1 OESOPHAGEAL DIVERTICULUM

A pseudodiverticulum can occur following leakage from the anasto-mosis but this usually heals satisfactorily without long-term mechanical

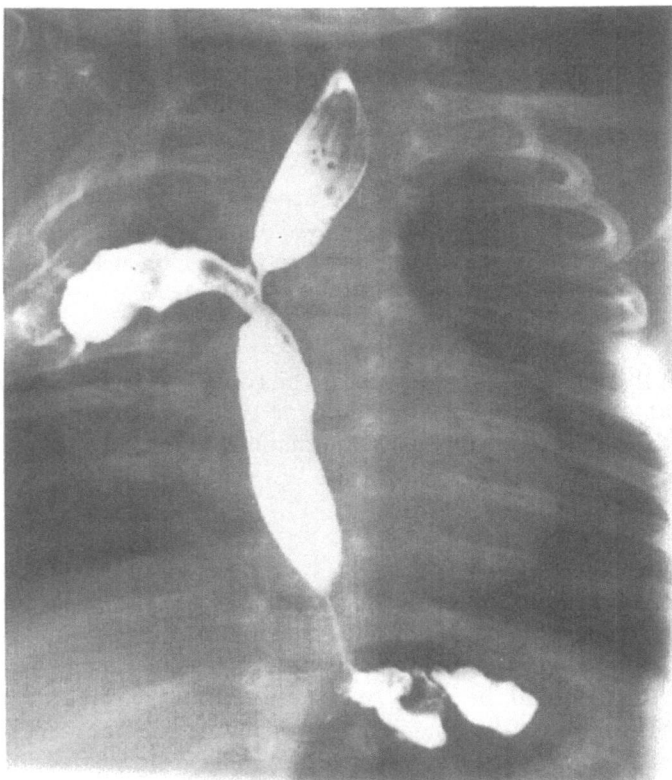

Figure 21.13   A pseudodiverticulum of the oesophagus may occur after leakage from the anastomosis.

complications (Figure 21.13). Ballooning at the site of a circular myotomy is common and a diverticulum may develop (Taylor and Myers, 1989).

21.5.2 SHELF AT SITE OF ANASTOMOSIS

This has occurred in a few patients and may, at least in some, be due to an asymmetric anastomosis (Figure 21.14). If the oesophagotomy in the upper oesophagus is made off-centre (i.e. not at the most dependent portion of the oesophagus) the final radiological appearance of the oesophagus may be unsatisfactory and the shelf may contribute to foreign body impaction. In most cases the narrowing is overcome by serial oesophageal dilatations (Figure 21.15).

21.5.3 RUPTURED STOMACH

This should be included as a direct complication of treatment of oesophageal atresia and usually occurs where high pressure ventilation

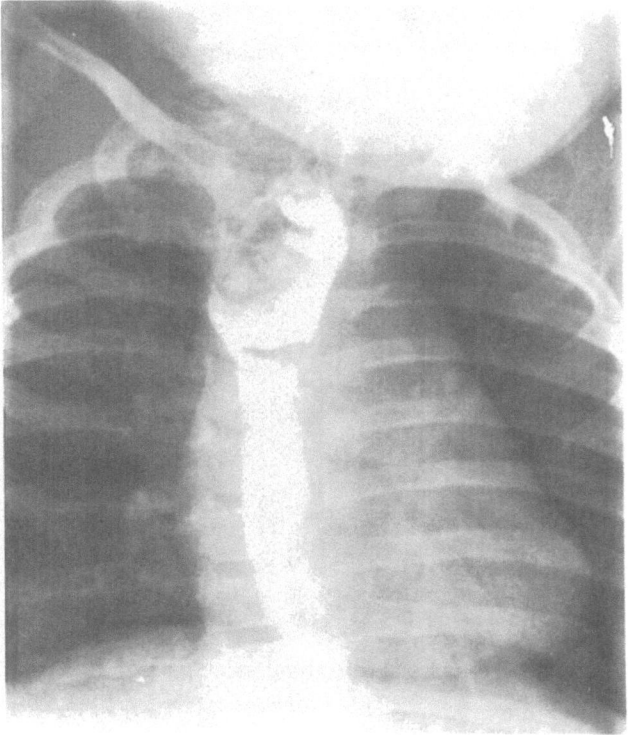

Figure 21.14 A shelf on one side of the anastomosis is probably due to an asymmetric anastomosis.

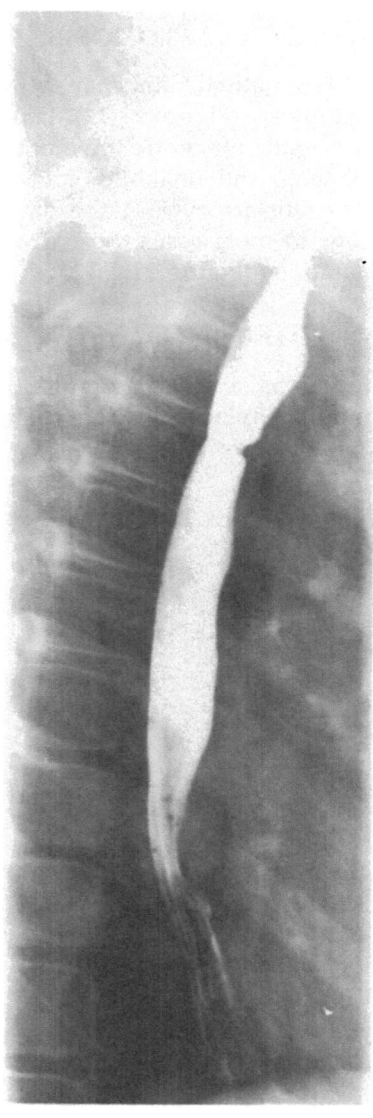

Figure 21.15 Response to serial dilatation: same patient as Figure 21.14.

is necessary in premature babies with oesophageal atresia and a distal fistula (Chapter 9). It highlights the importance of early division of the fistula, even in the presence of severe lung disease (Holmes *et al.*, 1987; Beasley *et al.*, 1989).

21.6 Complications specific to the less common variants

21.6.1 UPPER POUCH FISTULA

This group has a high incidence of complications because of its rarity and the great variation in the methods of treatment that have been used (Chapter 11). Complications that have occurred are listed in Table 11.2.

21.6.2 OESOPHAGEAL ATRESIA WITHOUT FISTULA

This anatomical group has a higher mortality and morbidity (Myers *et al.*, 1987). The increased incidence of leakage and stricture is related to the long gap between oesophageal segments and the mobilization and tension required to bridge the gap. Fistula formation between the oesophagus and the tracheobronchial tree is less common, mainly because the trachea has always been intact.

21.6.3 'H' FISTULA

The incidence of recurrent fistula is higher in this group than in patients with a distal fistula. The close proximity of the tracheal and oesophageal suture lines may be the most important contributing factor.

References

Ball, W. S., Strife, J. L., Rosenkrantz, J., Towin, R. B. and Noseworth, J. (1984) Oesophageal strictures in children: treatment by balloon dilatation. *Radiology*, **150**, 263–4.

Beardmore, H. E., Peitsch, J. B. and Stokes, K. B. (1978) Oesophageal atresia with tracheo-oesophageal fistula. *J. Pediatr. Surg.*, **13**, 677–81.

Beasley, S. W., Shann, F. A., Myers, N. A. and Auldist, A. W. (1989) Developments in the management of oesophageal atresia and tracheo-oesophageal fistulas. *Med. J. Aust.*, **150**, 501–3.

Benjamin, B. (1981) Endoscopy in oesophageal atresia and tracheo-oesophageal fistula. *Ann. Otol. Rhinol. Laryngol.*, **90**, 376–82.

Bishop, P. J., Klein, M. D., Philipart, A. I., Hixson, D. S. and Hertzler, J. H. (1985) Transpleural repair of oesophageal atresia without a primary gastrostomy: 240 patients treated between 1951 and 1983. *J. Pediatr. Surg.*, **20**, 823–4.

Botham, M. J. and Coran, A. G. (1986) The use of pericardium for the management of recurrent tracheo-oesophageal fistula. *J. Pediatr. Surg.*, **21**, 164–6.

Coran, A. G. (1989) Current management of oesophageal atresia and tracheo-oesophageal fistula. *Bull. Soc. Sci. Med. Grand-Duche Luxembourg*, **3**, 29–51.

Ein, S. H., Stringer, D. A., Stephens, C. A., Shandling, B., Simpson, J. and Filler, R. M. (1983) Recurrent tracheo-oesophageal fistulas: seventeen year review. *J. Pediatr. Surg.*, **18**, 436–41.

Gans, S. L., Berci, G. (1973) Inside Tracheo-esophageal fistula: New Endoscopic Approaches. *J. Pediatr. Surg.*, **8**, 205.

Gdanietz, K. and Krause, I. (1975) Plastic adhesives for closing esophago-tracheal fistula in children. *Z. Kinderchir.*, **17**, 137–8 (Suppl).

Ghandour, K. E., Spitz, L., Brereton, R. J. and Kiely, E. M. (1990) Recurrent tracheo-oesophageal fistula: experience with 24 patients. *Aust. Paediatr. J.*, (in press).

Haight, C. (1969) in *Pediatric Surgery*, vol. 1, 2nd edn (eds W. T. Mustard *et al.*), Year Book Medical Publishers, Chicago, Chapter 28.

Hicks, L. M. and Mansfield, B. P. (1981) Oesophageal atresia and tracheo-oesophageal fistula. Review of thirteen years' experience. *J. Thorac. Cardiovasc. Surg.*, **81**, 358–63.

Holmes, S. J. K., Kiely, E. M. and Spitz, L. (1987) Tracheo-oesophageal fistula and the respiratory distress syndrome. *Pediatr. Surg. Int.*, **2**, 16–18.

Izzidien al-Samarrai, A. Y., Jessen, K. and Haque, K. (1987) Endoscopic obliteration of a recurrent tracheo-oesophageal fistula *J. Pediatr. Surg.*, **22**, 993.

Leendertse-Verloop, K., Tibboel, D., Hazebroek F. W. J. and Molenaar, J. C. (1987) Post-operative morbidity in patients with oesophageal atresia. *Pediatr. Surg. Int.*, **2**, 2–5.

Manning, P. B., Morgan, R. A., Coran, A. G. *et al.* (1986) Fifty years' experience with oesophageal atresia and tracheo-oesophageal fistula. *Ann. Surg.*, **204**, 446–51.

Martin, L. W., Cox, J. A., Cotton, R. and Oldham, K. T. (1986) Transtracheal repair of recurrent tracheo-oesophageal fistula. *J. Pediatr. Surg.*, **21**, 402–3.

McKinnon, L. J. and Kosloske, A. M. (1990) Prediction and prevention of anastomotic complications of oesophageal atresia and tracheo-oesophageal fistula. *J. Pediatr. Surg.*, **25**, 778–8.

McLean, G. K. and Le Veen, R. F. (1989) Shear stress in the performance of oesophageal dilatation: comparison of balloon dilatation and bougienage. *Radiology*, **172**, 983–6.

Myers, N. A., Beasley, S. W., Auldist, A. W., Kent, M., Wright, V. and Chetcuti, P. (1987) Oesophageal atresia: anastomosis or replacement? *Pediatr. Surg. Int.*, **2**, 216–20.

Myers, N. A., Beasley, S. W. and Auldist, A. W. (1990) Secondary oesophageal surgery following repair of oesophageal atresia with distal tracheo-oesophageal fistula. *Pediatr. Surg. Int.*, **25**, 773–7.

Pampino, H. J. (1979) Endoscopic closure of tracheo-oesophageal fistula. *Z. Kinderchir.*, **27**, 90–3 (suppl.)

Pieretti, R., Shandling, B. and Stephens, C. A. (1974) Resistant esophageal stenosis associates with reflux after repair of esophageal atresia: a therapeutic approach. *J. Pediatr. Surg.*, **9**, 355–7.

Randolph, J. G. (1986) in *Pediatric Surgery*, vol. 1, 4th edn. (eds K. J. Welch, J. G. Randoph, M. M. Ravitch, J. A. O'Neill and M. I. Rowe), Year Book Medical Publishers, Chicago, pp. 688–9.

Rangecroft, L., Bush, G. H., Lister, J. *et al.* (1984) Endoscopic diathermy obliteration of recurrent TOF. *J. Pediatr. Surg.*, **19**, 41–3.

Spitz, L. (1988) Oesophageal atresia – Symposium. Presented at the International Congress of Paediatric Surgery, Melbourne, Australia, November.

Spitz, L., Kiely, E. and Brereton, R. J. (1987) Oesophageal atresia: five year experience with 148 cases. *J. Pediatr. Surg.*, **22**, 103–8.

Taylor, R. G. and Myers, N. A. (1989) Management of a post-Livaditis-procedure oesophageal diverticulum. *Pediatr. Surg. Int.*, **4**, 238–40.

Touloukian, R. J. (1981) Long-term results following repair of oesophageal atresia by end-to-side anastomosis and ligation of the tracheo-oesophageal fistula. *J. Pediatr. Surg.*, **16**, 983–8.

Waag, K. L., Joppich, I., Manegold, B. C. *et al.* (1979) Endoscopic closure of tracheo-oesophageal fistula. *Z. Kinderchir.*, **27**, 93–5.

22 Tracheomalacia

L. SPITZ and P. D. PHELAN

22.1 Definition

Tracheomalacia is a structural and functional weakness of the trachea which results in partial respiratory obstruction in infants and children with oesophageal atresia and tracheo-oesophageal fistula.

Some degree of tracheomalacia is almost inevitable in infants born with oesophageal atresia and tracheo-oesophageal fistula. The significance and management of tracheomalacia in these patients remain areas of considerable uncertainty and controversy. The Melbourne approach to the management of infants with symptoms normally attributed to tracheomalacia has tended to be more conservative than that adopted in other centres. For example, over the last eight years, surgical correction of tracheomalacia has been attempted in Melbourne in only three of our oesophageal atresia and tracheo-oesophageal fistula patients, compared with an operative rate of 11.8% at Great Ormond Street (Kiely *et al.*, 1987).

For as long as the exact mechanisms and natural history of the tracheal obstruction in tracheomalacia are not well understood, and the benefits of aortopexy are not predictable, variations in the management of the condition will continue.

22.2 Pathogenesis

22.2.1 PATHOLOGY

The term tracheomalacia is probably inaccurate in that there is no evidence that the tracheal cartilage is intrinsically soft. Wailoo and Emery (1979) have demonstrated an absolute deficiency in cartilage in many patients, the majority of whom also show an increase in the length of the transverse muscle in the posterior tracheal wall. The cartilage is shorter than normal so it fails to give adequate support to the tracheal wall. The combination of deficient cartilage (seen in 75% of cases) and elongated muscle (in 60%) contributes to a soft tracheal wall which usually has a perimeter greater than normal. It has been postulated that the structural defect in the wall of the trachea is due to the inclusion of oesophageal muscle and squamous epithelium in the membranous part (Emery and Haddadin, 1971). This feature was present in 80% of cases of oesophageal atresia compared with 2.5% of controls.

On the other hand, Davies and Cywes (1978) have proposed that the flaccid trachea results from external pressure from the dilated proximal blind oesophageal segment *in utero*. It is difficult to reconcile this mechanism with the known distribution of tracheomalacia which involves the lower half of the trachea in about 60%. The deficiency of cartilage is limited to the site of the fistula in 30%; and in a small number, the whole trachea is abnormal.

22.2.2 PATHOPHYSIOLOGY

The functional consequences depend on the extent of tracheal involvement. When the abnormality is limited to the intrathoracic trachea, as is the case in the majority of patients, the symptoms and signs are the consequence of expiratory obstruction. They will occur when expiration becomes active and positive intrathoracic pressure is generated. The more forced the expiration, the greater the degree of tracheal collapse. Expiration is likely to become active in the presence of lower respiratory infection and with inhalation of foreign material into the lower respiratory tract. Once expiration ceases to be forced, and the extent of positive intrathoracic pressure is reduced, normal respiration is regained. Thus, in the common form of tracheomalacia, the signs are those of intermittent expiratory obstruction with normal inspiration. Inspiration becomes difficult only if there is gross hyperinflation of the lung as is seen with prolonged expiratory difficulty.

In infants with tracheomalacia, there is frequently a history of feeding difficulty and vomiting. An oesophageal stricture at the site of anastomosis may predispose to inhalation of saliva and food into the lungs, and distension of the oesophagus proximal to the stricture can compress a soft trachea. If expiratory difficulty occurs, this will increase the positive intra-abdominal pressure and facilitate gastro-oesophageal reflux. Thus gastro-oesophageal reflux may both cause and result from the expiratory obstruction of tracheomalacia.

Where there is involvement of the whole trachea, inspiratory obstruction in the extrathoracic trachea and expiratory obstruction in the intrathoracic trachea occurs. This combination is likely to produce severe symptoms and may be incompatible with life.

22.3 Incidence

It is probable that the majority of infants with oesophageal atresia and tracheo-oesophageal fistula have some degree of tracheomalacia. The 'seal-bark' cough of oesophageal atresia (the so-called 'TOF cough') is probably the result of tracheomalacia. The soft segment of the trachea sets up expiratory vibrations during the process of coughing which result in its barking quality. Clinical experience suggests that most infants with repaired oesophageal atresia and tracheo-oesophageal fistula have this symptom. In about 5%, symptoms of airways obstruction are moderate to severe and probably due to severe tracheomalacia.

It is uncertain whether tracheomalacia is limited to patients with tracheo-oesophageal fistula and oesophageal atresia. Patients with pure oesophageal atresia do not seem to have airways obstruction as frequently, unless there has been a distended upper oesophageal pouch before surgical correction of the atresia. In this situation, the obstruction is usually inspiratory. Similarly, major postoperative airways problems are uncommon in patients with an isolated tracheo-oesophageal fistula.

22.4 Symptomatology

The infant may present with problems within days or weeks of the oesophageal repair, but generally, presentation is delayed until the infant is a few months of age.

The harsh barking cough – the so-called TOF cough – is the most characteristic symptom and sign of tracheomalacia, and may be the first sign of impending problems. Its persistence into late adolescence and even adult life suggests that the tracheal abnormality is to some extent permanent.

The infant may be reluctant to feed because of difficulty in breathing during feeding. Cyanotic attacks may occur during feeds, and in severe tracheomalacia, respiratory arrest or 'near-miss' sudden infant death may occur (*vide infra*).

Infants and young children with oesophageal atresia seem to develop wheeze with intercurrent respiratory infections more readily than do other children. It is now recognized that 20–25% of the childhood population will wheeze as a result of asthma. However, the incidence of wheeze seems higher in oesophageal atresia (Chetcuti and Phelan, 1990) and it is probably unwise to attribute wheeze in infants who have been born with this abnormality to asthma unless there is substantial other supporting evidence, such as a family history of asthma or other allergic disorders. Making the distinction is probably important, as the use of beta-2 adrenergic drugs which can reduce tracheal muscle tone may aggravate rather than relieve the airways obstruction.

The occasional patient who develops episodes of severe expiratory airways obstruction can present major management problems. The episodes seem to occur during intercurrent respiratory infections and in children with feeding difficulties. Parents may notice a cough and wheeze which progresses to complete airways obstruction and cyanosis. If the obstruction is sufficiently severe, there may be loss of consciousness. This may then be called 'a near-miss' sudden infant death syndrome. While these obstructive episodes can be extremely frightening to parents and other observers, the frequency with which they have a fatal outcome is unclear. If gross hyperinflation has not occurred, then once the infant has lost consciousness, forced expiration will probably cease and the return of normal respiration should occur. In our series over the last 20 years, no infant or young child with a history of repeated obstructive episodes has died as a result of definite respiratory obstruction. However, there have been two incompletely explained deaths: one three-month-old infant without previous symptoms was found dead in its cot; and a nine-month-old infant developed severe respiratory distress soon after feeding and died before medical attention could be obtained. In this second case, there had been one previous similar, but less severe, episode. Autopsy failed to identify the cause of death, although tracheal obstruction from ingested food held up at a minor oesophageal stricture was suggested as a possible cause.

It is recognized that there is a complex interrelationship between feeding difficulties and the symptoms of severe tracheomalacia. Inhalation of a small amount of food into the lower respiratory tract may initiate forced expiratory effort. Regurgitation of stomach contents into the oesophagus may further obstruct the trachea, and if these reach the pharynx, they may be inhaled compromising respiration further.

22.5 Diagnosis

Attempts should be made to determine the presence and extent of tracheomalacia in infants and young children who have had one or more episodes of serious airways obstruction. Detailed investigation is not warranted if the only symptom present is a 'TOF cough'.

A lateral X-ray of the thoracic inlet will show a narrow slit-like appearance in the lower trachea, but in isolation this is of limited value. The two investigations most likely to produce useful information are bronchoscopy and cinetracheobronchography, and when required are complementary.

Bronchoscopy must be performed with the patient breathing spontaneously. If the patient is paralysed, there will be no active expiration and so it is impossible to assess the extent of tracheomalacia. When the patient is breathing spontaneously, a bronchoscope partly obstructs expiration and makes it active. The affected part of the trachea reveals a widened posterior wall with the anterior–posterior diameter of the trachea narrowed considerably. The trachea does not have its normal 'D' shape. Often the collapsing lumen is narrowed to a transverse slit which closes completely during expiration, and is most severe in the region of the previously closed tracheo-oesophageal fistula.

A cinetracheobronchogram with contrast, performed on a spontaneously ventilating patient, allows the extent of the expiratory tracheal collapse to be determined accurately. The degree of tracheal collapse is usually not possible to quantify at bronchoscopy. Both anterior–posterior and lateral projections are required, as it is with the latter that the degree of tracheal narrowing is most evident (Figures 22.1 and 22.2).

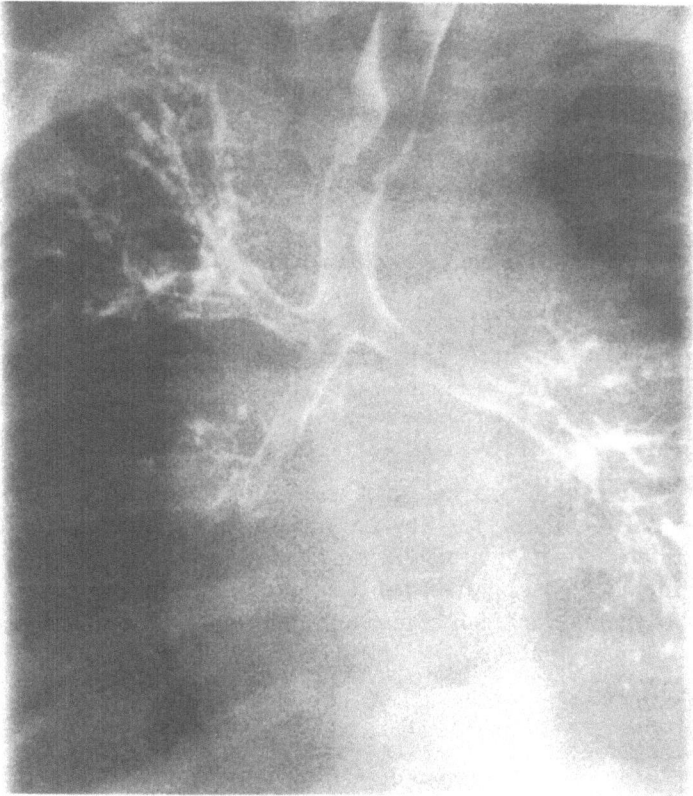

Figure 22.1 Cinetracheobronchography: AP view in infant with tracheomalacia.

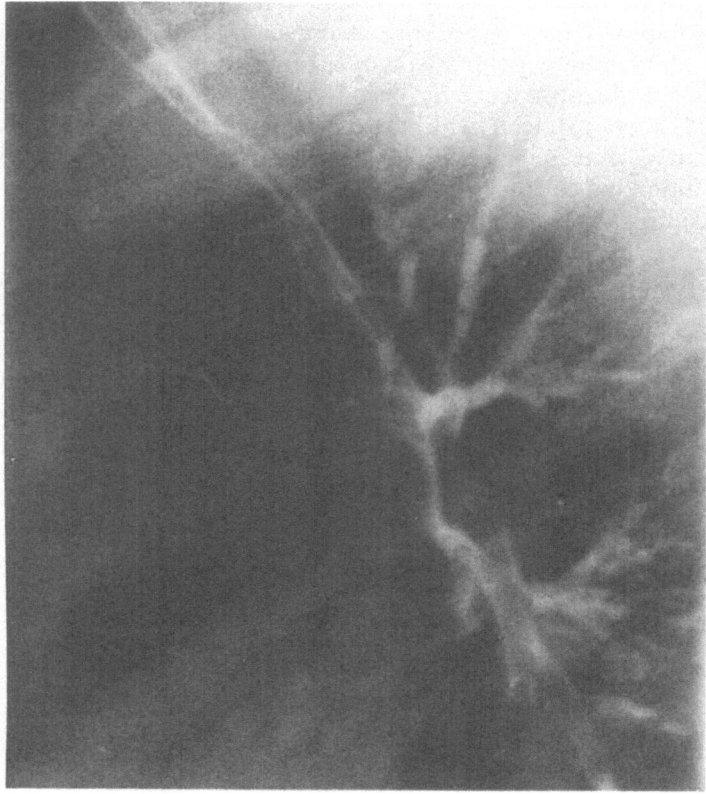

Figure 22.2   Cinetracheobronchography: the degree of tracheal narrowing in tracheomalacia is most evident in the lateral projection (same patient as in Figure 22.1).

Dynamic studies of the trachea, by Cine CT (Kimura *et al.*, 1990) provide an additional technique for the diagnosis of tracheomalacia and may demonstrate tracheal collapse during expiration.

Assessment of oesophageal function radiologically by barium swallow, and of the gastro-oesophageal sphincter by pH monitoring, will be indicated in many patients.

22.6   Management

The management of tracheomalacia remains controversial. However, it is agreed that where the symptoms are mild no active intervention is necessary. There is a tendency for improvement with time.

It is the child with recurrent cyanotic episodes due to expiratory obstruction who presents the difficult problem. Reintroduction of the procedure first used by Gross and Neuhauser (1948) to relieve compression on the trachea by an anomalous innominate artery, has encouraged a number of groups to recommend aortopexy as an effective procedure for the relief of tracheomalacia (Benjamin *et al.*, 1976; Kiely *et al.*, 1987).

The approach to the management of these infants at the Royal Children's Hospital, Melbourne, has been conservative and in the few patients in whom aortopexy has been performed, there has been little apparent benefit to the patients. Other centres (Filler *et al.*, 1976; Rode *et al.*, 1985; Spitz, 1986) have employed aortopexy more widely in tracheomalacia and seem pleased with the results. For example, at the Hospital for Sick Children, Great Ormond Street, London, over an eight-year period, 1980–87, 41 of 257 infants (16.2%) developed significant tracheomalacia, for which aortopexy was performed in 30 (11.8%).

The difference in the philosophy of the two centres is highlighted by the approach to the infant with gastro-oesophageal reflux. In Melbourne, great attention is paid to careful feeding of infants with moderate to severe tracheomalacia, with small amounts of soft foods until late in their first year. Any oesophageal stricture is dilated. If there is associated gastro-oesophageal reflux, this is managed by posturing and thickened feeds in the first instance, and by Nissen fundoplication if there are persistent respiratory symptoms or an oesophageal stricture develops. In London, the belief that the respiratory obstruction which occurs as a result of tracheomalacia may induce or aggravate associated gastro-oesophageal reflux, has encouraged the recommendation that the tracheomalacia be attended to first, in the expectation that the reflux will either resolve, or become less of a problem.

If the problem occurs in the early postoperative weeks, prolonged nasotracheal intubation with positive end expiratory pressure has been used. This seems to protect against the tracheal collapse. The natural history of tracheomalacia symptoms is that they seem to decrease with time. The first 6–12 months are usually the most worrying period, although we have had patients in their second year who have developed severe airways obstruction following the impaction of a bolus of food.

The association of tracheomalacia with a recurrent tracheo-oesophageal fistula is considered particularly hazardous. If an aortopexy is performed as the initial procedure, the aperture of a recurrent fistula may be widened and expose the infant to the risk of massive aspiration during feeding or vomiting. In this situation, repair of the recurrent fistula should take precedence, or both complications should be dealt with under the same anaesthetic.

At present we recommend conservative management in the first instance for a baby with severe tracheomalacia. If gastro-oesophageal reflux is a major problem, then a Nissen fundoplication may be indicated. Aortopexy should only be undertaken if life-threatening episodes continue despite these simpler measures. External splinting operations have not been shown to be effective.

22.7   Aortopexy

22.7.1   SURGICAL APPROACH

Aortopexy can be performed through an anterolateral thoracotomy (Schwartz and Filler, 1980; Kiely, 1988) or via a median sternotomy (Cohen, 1981): the former approach is described below.

Under general endotracheal anaesthesia, the infant is positioned supine on the operating table with a rolled towel beneath the shoulders and the left arm abducted (Kiely, 1988). A left transverse incision is made over the third rib, extending from the lateral border of the sternum medially to the mid-axillary line laterally (Figure 22.3). The pectoral muscles are divided with diathermy in the line of the incision, exposing the anterior half of the left third rib with its costal cartilage. Entry into the pleural cavity is gained through the second intercostal space.

The thoracotomy is held open by means of an infant-sized Finochietto retractor. The left lung is retracted laterally. The phrenic nerve, coursing along the surface of the pleura covering the posterior aspect of the superior mediastinum, is identified and carefully preserved. The left lobe of the thymus is mobilized by a combination of sharp and blunt dissection, coagulating small venules as they are encountered. The left lobe separates readily from the right, and at the

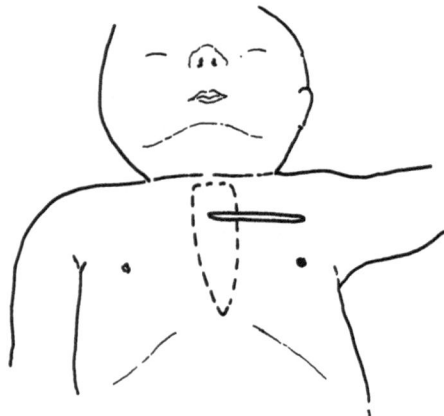

Figure 22.3   Incision for aortopexy.

isthmus where the main venous drainage is encountered, the vessel is coagulated and divided.

22.7.2 TECHNIQUE OF AORTOPEXY

The fascia covering the ascending arch of the aorta is opened to expose the adventitial surface. During this manoeuvre, the reflection of the pericardium on to the ascending aorta is deliberately opened. The surgeon has the choice of either suturing the exposed aorta directly to the posterior surface of the sternum using three interrupted sutures of 4/0 polypropylene, or of suturing a dacron patch on to the anterior surface of the aorta with continuous 5/0 polypropylene sutures and placing three 3/0 polypropylene sutures through the patch and, in turn, through the body of the sternum to be tied on to the anterior surface (Spitz, 1986). This manoeuvre has the effect of drawing the ascending arch of the aorta well forward. The fibrous connections between the posterior surface of the aorta and the anterior wall of the trachea then hold open the lumen of the trachea.

The wound is closed in layers with or without an intercostal drain.

22.7.3 POSTOPERATIVE MANAGEMENT

The intercostal drain is placed on an underwater seal and an early chest X-ray is taken to exclude a pneumothorax. Recovery from surgery is usually rapid and improvement in respiratory status occurs immediately. Oral feeding is commenced on the same day.

22.7.4 COMPLICATIONS

There are few complications from the procedure. Wound infection is rare, but the long-term cosmetic effect of the scar may not be ideal. At the Hospital for Sick Children, Great Ormond Street, recurrence of symptoms due to failure of the procedure has been unusual, and when it occurs may be due to a longer length of tracheomalacia, particularly where the proximal trachea is involved. In such cases, a repeat procedure may be required, which will involve either splitting of the manubrium sterni, or performing the tracheopexy via a cervical collar incision.

22.8 Conclusion

The term 'tracheomalacia' is a misnomer if it is taken to mean soft tracheal cartilage. Absolute deficiency of cartilage and elongation of the transverse muscle in the posterior tracheal wall are common accompaniments of oesophageal atresia with tracheo-oesophageal fistula and result in a soft tracheal wall. The common symptom is the so-called 'TOF cough' but occasional infants develop severe expiratory airways obstruction. If there is involvement of the whole trachea, then there may be an inspiratory component to the obstruction as well. Management is difficult, but most infants will respond to careful attention to feeding and occasionally surgical control of gastro-oesophageal reflux. Where these measures have not proved successful, aortopexy should be considered. While aortopexy seems effective in the hands of some groups, our experience with it has not been particularly encouraging.

References

Benjamin, B., Cohen, D. and Glasson, M. (1976) Tracheomalacia in association with congenital tracheo-oesophageal fistula. *Surgery*, **79**, 504–8.

Chetcuti, P. and Phelan, P. D. (1990) Lung function abnormalities in repaired oesophageal atresia and tracheo-oesophageal fistula. (in press).

Cohen, D. (1981) Tracheopexy – aortotracheal suspension for severe tracheomalacia. *Aust. Paediatr. J.*, **17**, 117–21.

Davies, M. R. Q. and Cywes, S. (1978) The flaccid trachea and tracheo-oesophageal congenital anomalies. *J. Pediatr. Surg.*, **13**, 363–7.

Emery, J. L. and Haddadin, A. J. (1971) Squamous epithelium in respiratory tract of children with tracheo-oesophageal fistula. *Arch. Dis. Child.*, **46**, 236–42.

Filler, R. M., Rossello, P. J. and Lebowitz, R. L. (1976) Life-threatening anoxic spells caused by tracheal compression after repair of oesophageal atresia: correction by surgery. *J. Pediatr. Surg.*, **11**, 739–48.

Gross, R. E. and Neuhauser, E. B. D. (1948) Compression of the trachea by an anomalous innominate artery: an operation for its relief. *Am. J. Dis. Child.*, **75**, 570–4.

Kiely, E. M. (1988) Aortopexy. in *Rob and Smith's Operative Surgery* (eds L. Spitz and H. H. Nixon) 4th edn, Butterworths, London, pp. 126–9.

Kiely, E. M., Spitz, L. and Brereton, R. J. (1987) Management of tracheomalacia by aortopexy. *Pediatr. Surg. Int.*, **2**, 13–15.

Kimura, K., Soper, R. T., Kao SCS *et al.* (1990) Aortosternopexy for tracheomalacia following repair of esophageal atresia: evaluation by cine-CT and technical refinement. *J. Pediatr. Surg.*, **25**, 769–72.

Rode, H., Millar, A. W. J., Vega, M. and Cywes, S. (1985) Oesophageal atresia – severe tracheomalacia and its correction by aortopexy. *Z. Kinderchir.*, **40**, 282–6.

Schwartz, M. Z. and Filler, R. M. (1980) Tracheal compression as a cause of apnoea following repair of tracheo-oesophageal fistula: treatment by aortopexy. *J. Pediatr. Surg.*, **15**, 842–8.

Spitz, L. (1986) Dacron patch aortopexy. *Progr. Pediatr. Surg.*, **19**, 117–19.

Wailoo, M. P. and Emery, J. L. (1979) The trachea in children with tracheo-oesophageal fistula. *Histopathology*, **3**, 329–38.

23 *Gastro-oesophageal reflux*

D. G. JOHNSON and S. W. BEASLEY

Gastro-oesophageal reflux is one of the most significant ongoing problems following successful repair of oesophageal atresia, with or without tracheo-oesophageal fistula. Normal babies often have gastro-oesophageal reflux (GOR) but in the presence of repaired oesophageal atresia, reflux is more common and its effect on an oesophagus which is already abnormal is to cause considerable additional morbidity.

23.1 Pathophysiology

A patient with corrected oesophageal atresia has an oesophagus in which there has been alteration of several of the factors which normally prevent gastro-oesophageal reflux (Table 23.1).

Table 23.1 Possible factors contributing to poor oesophageal motility and gastro-oesophageal reflux after repair of oesophageal atresia

1. Inherent oesophageal dysmotility in oesophageal atresia
2. Injury to branches of vagus nerve during surgical procedures
3. Upwards displacement and tension of lower oesophageal segment
   Reduction in length of intra-abdominal oesophagus
   Alteration of angle of HIS
4. Use of gastrostomy

23.1.1 DISORDERED PERISTALSIS

Studies of oesophageal function before repair of oesophageal atresia are rare, but the limited data available suggest oesophageal motility is probably abnormal in all patients (Chapter 5). On oesophageal manometry, the dysmotility is manifest as tertiary or unco-ordinated and

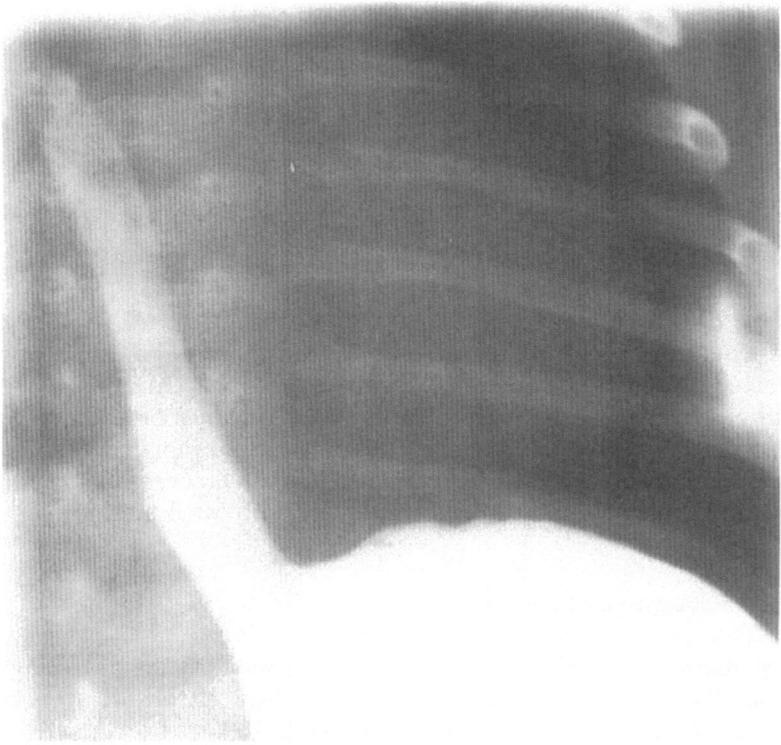

Figure 23.1   Poor oesophageal clearance and ineffective emptying of gastric content which has refluxed into the oesophagus is common in infants with repaired oesophageal atresia. This radiograph shows free reflux into the lower oesophagus.

non-propulsive peristalsis. The severity of the abnormality is variable, but a totally normal motility study in an infant following oesophageal atresia repair is rarely, if ever, obtained. The early postoperative barium study may show a to-and-fro movement of oesophageal content ('Yo-Yo peristalsis') and functionally the effect is poor oesophageal clearance; and when reflux occurs, there is ineffective emptying of gastric content from the oesophagus (Figure 23.1). Extensive surgical mobilization of the oesophagus may injure vagal fibres and interfere with oesophageal innervation, worsening the peristaltic abnormality. Normal function of the gastro-oesophageal junction is dependent on an effective oesophageal pump to propel food through the oesophagus into the stomach (Holder, 1988).

23.1.2 SHORT OR ABSENT INTRA-ABDOMINAL SEGMENT

O'Sullivan *et al.* (1982) have shown a clear relationship between the length of the intra-abdominal segment of oesophagus and the pressure needed to overcome the lower oesophageal sphincter pressure (LOSP) to cause reflux. It is likely that the length of the intra-abdominal oesophagus is the most important of all the mechanical factors which prevent reflux.

Following repair of oesophageal atresia, an intra-abdominal segment of oesophagus can rarely be demonstrated radiographically, although current techniques are not really adequate to identify or measure the length of oesophagus below the diaphragm. However, it is clear that the oesophagus is entirely above the diaphragm when a hiatal hernia is demonstrated. Endoscopy of symptomatic patients suggests that the junction of gastric and oesophageal mucosa is at or just above the point of diaphragmatic closure in most, reflecting little or no effective intra-abdominal segment. The reason for this anatomy in oesophageal atresia patients is not clear, but in some it may be related to surgical mobilization of the lower oesophageal segment to overcome a gap before oesophageal anastomosis, thereby drawing the lower oesophagus upwards towards the diaphragm, and reducing the length of intra-abdominal oesophagus. Displacement and alteration of the gastro-oesophageal junction may also make the angle of insertion less acute and further contribute to reflux. Asymptomatic patients are not endoscoped routinely, so we cannot be sure of the extent to which reduction of the intra-abdominal segment occurs after oesophageal repair.

23.2 Incidence

Leendertse-Verloop *et al.* (1987) from Rotterdam found in a study of the postoperative course of 77 oesophageal atresia patients with end-to-end anastomoses that gastro-oesophageal reflux had a major effect on morbid-operatively in 42 (54%), spontaneously in 30 and on provocation in 12. They found that gastro-oesophageal reflux had a major effect on morbidity, and played an important part in the occurrence of anastomotic strictures, anastomotic leaks and oesophagitis. Nissen fundoplication was performed in eight of these patients.

In another follow-up study of 25 patients between three and 83 months post-repair involving a detailed history, barium oesophago-gram, extended oesophageal pH monitoring and a gastro-oesophageal scintiscan, two-thirds of the patients had significant reflux on long-term

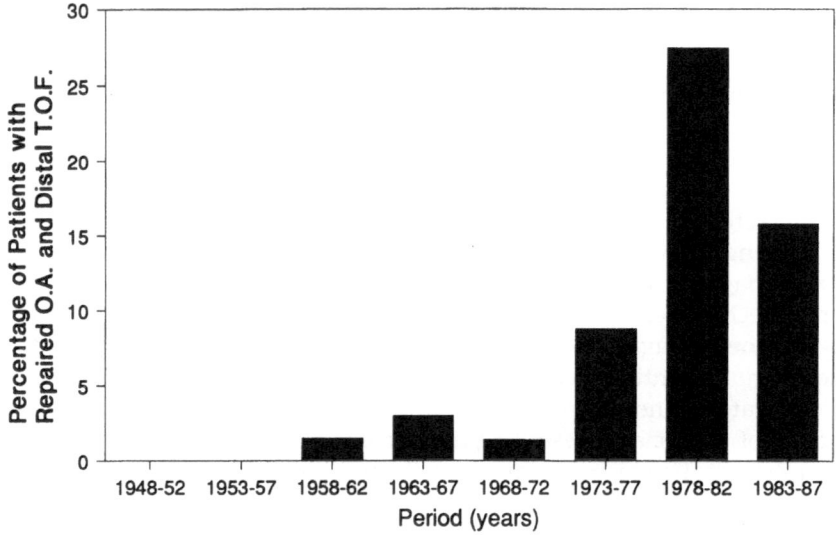

Figure 23.2　Number of patients with repaired oesophageal atresia (OA) undergoing Nissen fundoplication.

follow-up, 68% by pH monitoring and 64% by scintiscan (Jolley *et al.*, 1980). Symptomatic children were more likely to have major degrees of gastro-oesophageal reflux and slow gastric emptying than those without symptoms. The ultimate duration, long-term effects and significance of asymptomatic reflux were not determined, but three of the ten symptomatic patients required surgical control of the reflux.

In a subsequent study of 254 oesophageal atresia infants managed from 1972 to 1988, abnormal gastro-oesophageal reflux was demonstrated by barium oesophagography in virtually all the patients immediately postoperatively, as well as at six months follow-up. Disordered, poorly co-ordinated peristalsis was seen in most, but only a minority had significant symptoms or complications of reflux for which an anti-reflux operation was required in 30 (12%). With increasing awareness of the problem the percentage is likely to be higher in the future. Certainly, at the Royal Children's Hospital, the number of fundoplications being performed in children with repaired oesophageal atresia has increased in recent years (Figure 23.2), reflecting increased familiarity with the association between reflux and anastomotic and respiratory complications.

23.3 Symptoms and complications

Reflux symptoms can be grouped conveniently into three main categories.

Vomiting

Abnormal frequency or volume of vomiting may vary in significance from being an inconvenient nuisance to being a major problem causing retardation of growth and development and chronic malnutrition. While failure to thrive is sometimes an indication for fundoplication in children without oesophageal atresia, it is comparatively rarely so in children with oesophageal atresia.

Respiratory symptoms

Stridor, obstructive apnoea, recurrent pneumonia, and reactive airway disease can all be caused by reflux of gastric contents into the airway. Documentation of direct airway contamination is difficult and antireflux surgery to control these symptoms – which may have other causes – requires careful screening and preoperative evaluation. Reflux can cause respiratory disease, but respiratory disease by virtue of increased respiratory effort and increased negative intrapleural pressures can also cause reflux. Tracheomalacia often coexists with oesophageal atresia and contributes to the respiratory symptoms. Reflux in these patients may be exacerbated by the increased respiratory effort required to overcome the partial collapse of the tracheal lumen during expiration (Chapter 22). It may be difficult to decide whether initial surgical treatment is better directed towards correction of the reflux or the tracheomalacia.

Peptic oesophagitis

Irritability, pain on swallowing, refusal of feeds and blood-flecked vomitus are common manifestations of oesophagitis in children, and may be seen in infants as well as in older children. Oesophageal stricture with longitudinal shortening and circular contraction of the oesophagus may take years to develop, but significant reflux strictures in infants 3–9 months of age is also seen. Persistent reflux of acid to the level of oesophageal anastomosis following oesophageal atresia repair may cause continuing inflammation and stenosis at the anastomosis. In fact, most reflux strictures in patients occur at the anastomosis and respond to management only after elimination of the reflux (Pieretti *et al.*, 1974; Schwagten *et al.*, 1988; Hill, 1989).

23.4   Medical management

Medical management for symptomatic reflux following repair of oesophageal atresia is essentially the same as that for reflux from any cause. In treating reflux in infants and children it is hoped that anatomic growth and functional development will eventually favour the acquisition of competence of the lower oesophageal sphincter. Medical treatment aims to prevent complications of gastro-oesophageal reflux until spontaneous resolution of reflux has occurred. Upright or prone positioning, elevation of the head of the bed or cot, alteration of the physical characteristics of feeds, acid buffering, surface coating agents and drug manipulation of lower oesophageal sphincter pressure and gastric emptying, can all be utilized with effectiveness (Table 23.2).

Positioning is the simplest and probably the most effective non-surgical treatment for reflux, but is often difficult to maintain (Figure 23.3). Prone or prone-elevated positioning places the gastro-oesophageal junction in the gastric air bubble and allows the infant to eructate without necessarily emptying the fluid content of the stomach. Following oesophageal atresia repair infants should be discouraged from lying in a supine position when food is in the stomach. The impaired antireflux mechanism may place such infants at increased risk

Table 23.2   Management of gastro-oesophageal reflux

A:	Non-surgical	
	Patient positioning:	upright
		prone
		elevation of head of cot
	Changes in feeds:	thickening of feeds
		smaller feeds, more often
		buffering of feeds, e.g. antacids
	Pharmacological:	increase lower oesophageal sphincter pressure, e.g. metoclopramide;
		increase gastric emptying
		surface coating, e.g. sucralfate
		H_2 receptor blocking drugs, e.g. cimetidine, ranitidine
B.	Surgical	
	Antireflux procedure	
	± gastrostomy	
	± pyloroplasty	

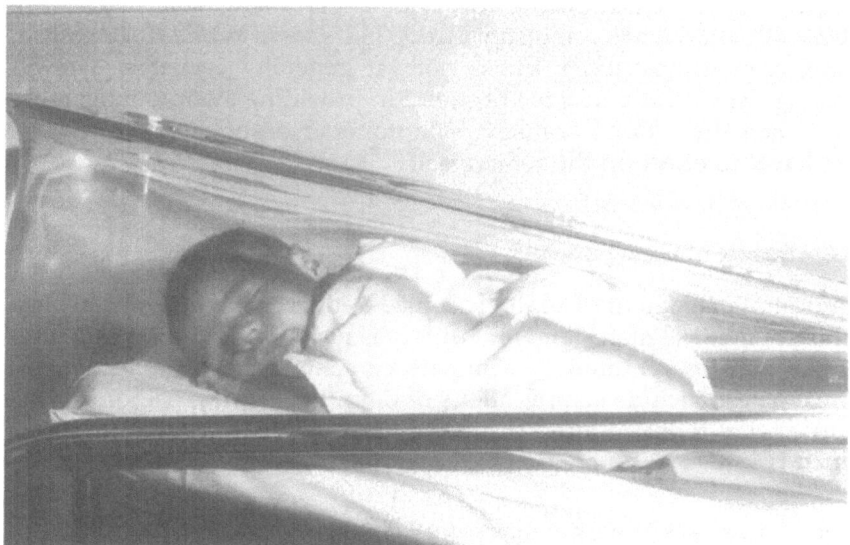

Figure 23.3 Gastro-oesophageal reflux can be reduced by lying the patient prone and elevating the head of the cot.

of aspiration. Up to 30° of elevation in the prone position probably adds more protection against reflux, but the elevated position also places the trachea in a downhill relationship and increases the chance of aspiration should reflux occur. Also, this elevated position on a board is difficult to maintain for an infant for any length of time. A padded board that can be elevated at variable angles has been used in some centres. The infant lies prone with his legs around a padded post and held in position on the board by padded Velcro straps. For smaller infants with major reflux symptoms, this positioning can be maintained night and day but is somewhat inconvenient. Some of the commercial infant seats would appear to be more comfortable than the padded board, but these seats are designed for supine positioning and keep the gastro-oesophageal junction posterior and below the fluid level in the stomach. This factor, along with flexion of the torso and the associated increase in abdominal pressure, has been shown to increase rather than decrease reflux (Gryboski *et al.*, 1963). These devices are no longer recommended in the management of reflux.

Metoclopramide in a dose of 0.1 mg/kg/dose t.i.d. has been used widely with apparent beneficial effect in many patients. Bethanechol has also been used, but the side-effects seem more troublesome. Cisapride, a newer agent which seems to act at a peripheral level and fairly specifically on the gastrointestinal tract, has shown promise for control of reflux in clinical trials, but is not yet generally available. The H_2 blocking drugs and antacids are useful in providing symptomatic relief only when the reflux is causing symptoms of oesophagitis, although they have no effect on the reflux itself.

23.5   Surgical management

Surgical management of reflux is considered after there has been clear failure of medical management. Surgery is never indicated for reflux *per se*, but may be required to eliminate or control the complications of reflux. These include complications of oesophagitis (i.e. pain and stricture), severe reflux-induced respiratory symptoms and failure to thrive which is refractory to medical treatment.

23.5.1   INDICATIONS FOR OPERATION

Oesophageal stricture and failure to control persistent symptoms (especially vomiting) with maximal medical therapy are the main indications for surgery (Table 23.3). Reflux-induced oesophageal stricture

Table 23.3 Indications for fundoplication after repair of oesophageal atresia at Royal Children's Hospital, Melbourne ($n = 34^*$)

	%
Gastrointestinal	
Oesophageal stricture	50
Severe vomiting	47
Oesophagitis	26
Failure of conservative management	12
Haematemesis	6
Hiatal hernia	3
Respiratory	
Aspiration	35
Apnoeic spells	9
Recurrent pneumonia	3
Neurological	
Cerebral palsy	3

*In many patients there was more than one indication for fundoplication.

represents an absolute indication for fundoplication. Dilatation of the stricture is pointless and will not be successful unless reflux is prevented (Pieretti *et al.*, 1974); in most patients, a successful antireflux procedure results in spontaneous resolution of the stricture (Chapter 21).

Antireflux surgery to control respiratory symptoms remains controversial in the minds of many, and it must be acknowledged that there are difficulties in proving a cause–effect relationship preoperatively and predicting outcome following surgery. Reflux is demonstrable in the majority of patients with postoperative respiratory complications of which recurrent pneumonia and recurrent aspiration are the most common (Leendertse-Verloop *et al.*, 1987). In many of these patients the improvement following fundoplication is dramatic, whether it be for recurrent severe aspiration pneumonia, or for obstructive apnoea with less severe pulmonary changes suggestive of aspiration. Obstructive apnoeic episodes may be secondary to tracheomalacia and alternatively, therapy can be directed toward the tracheal obstruction which itself may be causing exacerbation of the reflux. In a few patients both fundoplication and tracheopexy may be necessary.

23.5.2 CHARACTERISTICS OF SURGICAL GROUP

The age at which oesophageal atresia patients underwent fundoplication for correction of reflux is shown in Figure 23.4. Patients under one year tended to be those with respiratory symptoms and nutritional problems, whereas older patients tended to be those with oesophageal complications, including stricture.

Infants with prematurity and subsequent bronchopulmonary dysplasia from ventilator support often develop reflux-associated pulmonary

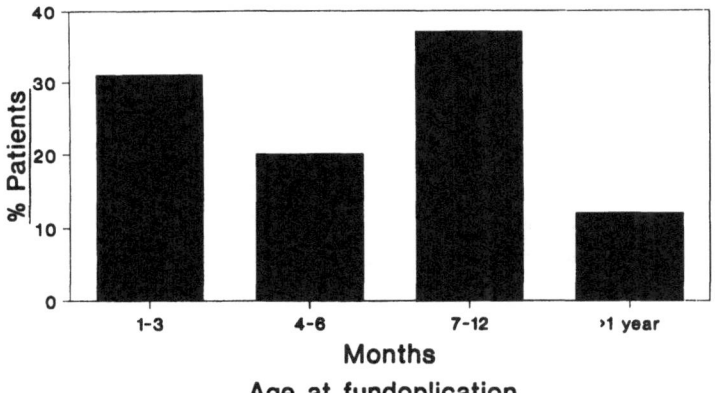

Figure 23.4 Age at time of fundoplication.

Table 23.4   Investigation of suspected
gastro-oesophageal reflux

Barium swallow
pH Monitoring
Oesophagoscopy
Oesophageal biopsy
Scintigraphy
Manometry

---

soilage. The extent to which chronic lung disease (bronchopulmonary dysplasia) causes reflux, or reflux worsens the already poor pulmonary status, is not easy to determine. Irrespective of the pathophysiology, an antireflux procedure in these patients often results in significant clinical improvement, with elimination of their increased oxygen requirement.

There are several investigatory procedures available to document reflux (Tables 23.4 and 23.5). The choice depends on the symptomatology, the likelihood of other pathology being present and the facilities available. The barium swallow remains the mainstay of diagnosis, largely because of the additional anatomical and physiological information it provides in oesophageal atresia patients. It is likely that pH monitoring will have a greater part to play in the future in patients where the symptoms cannot be readily attributed to reflux. Twenty-four

Table 23.5   Investigation of suspected or known reflux following repair of oesophageal atresia in patients subsequently requiring fundoplication ($n = 34$)

	No. performed	No. positive
Barium meal	33	31
Reflux		31
Stricture		13
Hernia		2
Oesophagoscopy	18	17
Oesophagitis		17
Biopsy	5	3
Scintigraphy	1	1

During the period reviewed manometry and 24 hour pH monitoring were not available.

hour pH monitoring has high sensitivity and specificity (Da Dalt *et al.*, 1989) with the percentage of reflux time and the number of episodes of reflux lasting more than five minutes being the parameters which are believed to be the most useful in selecting those who will benefit from surgery. However, even in the absence of previous oesophageal surgery, pH monitoring and oesophageal manometry have had only limited value in defining severe gastro-oesophageal reflux in children with chronic respiratory disease (Boix-Ochoa, 1986). It may be some time yet before preoperative studies can reliably predict which children with repaired oesophageal atresia and persistent respiratory symptoms will benefit from fundoplication.

23.5.3 SURGICAL OBJECTIVE: CONTROL OF REFLUX WITHOUT CAUSING DYSPHAGIA

Reflux control in the oesophageal atresia patient is complicated by pre-existing abnormal oesophageal motility and poor oesophageal peristalsis. In addition, patients without a fistula have a stomach which is small initially. Oesophageal clearance and emptying are abnormal before operation, and surgical enhancement of the reflux barrier by increasing the lower oesophageal sphincter pressure may worsen oesophageal emptying and cause oesophageal stasis, dysphagia and oesophageal dilatation. The surgeon's task is to select a procedure which will control reflux reliably and yet will produce a minimum of unpleasant side-effects.

Theoretically, it might be expected that the partial wrap or incomplete fundoplication procedures would be ideally suited to meet this goal of reflux control without interfering with oesophageal emptying. Ashcraft *et al.* (1984) and Ashcraft (1986) have advocated the Thal anterior fundoplication for control of reflux in all types of patients and Boix-Ochoa (1986) also claims his partial anterior fundoplication is adequate. However, the experience of Johnson (1986) does not confirm these recommendations. In a limited trial of the Thal anterior fundoplication persistent reflux occurred radiographically in four cases. One of these four had persistence of significant symptoms and required conversion to a Nissen fundoplication. A previous experience with 14 Boix-Ochoa procedures was similar, with recurrent symptoms necessitating re-do fundoplication in four of 14 patients (29%). Although none of these Thal or Boix-Ochoa procedures was done in a patient previously treated for oesophageal atresia, there is no reason to believe that the results in oesophageal atresia patients should be better.

The Nissen fundoplication is probably the most widely used and tested antireflux procedure, and has been the standard method used in

Table 23.6 Complications of 34 Nissen fundoplications performed in oesophageal atresia patients

		Number
Wound:	infection	0
	bleed	1
Unwrapping fundoplication		2
Paraoesophageal hernia		1
Bowel obstruction:		
adhesions		1
post-op intussusception		1
Dysphagia		3

Melbourne. It is simple to perform but although it is reliable in its correction of reflux, it is not exempt from the significant number of side-effects and complications which are common to all the wrap-type antireflux operations (Table 23.6). Avoidance of side-effects is certainly important in antireflux surgery, but reliable control of the reflux is even more important and operation is only considered when reflux has or is likely to cause serious oesophageal or respiratory complications which require control. If there is no oesophageal shortening, and gastrostomy is not required, the partial wrap may work reasonably well in controlling reflux symptoms. Oesophageal atresia patients, however, often have oesophageal shortening, and a few of those with reflux symptoms will require concomitant gastrostomy to facilitate feeds if growth retardation has been present. This combination is not ideally suited to the partial wrap, and the complete wrap of the Nissen fundoplication would seem preferable.

23.6 The Nissen fundoplication

A full description of the technical details of the Nissen-type fundoplication in children is described by Johnson (1986). The essential steps involve division of the left triangular ligament of the liver to expose the hiatus, division of the phreno-oesophageal ligament in a bloodless plane to allow mobilization of the lower oesophagus from the mediastinum, and encirclement of the oesophagus with downward traction to provide a 2.5–3.0 cm length of intra-abdominal oesophagus. Care is taken not to injure either the anterior or posterior trunks of the vagus on the oesophageal wall. Three or four short gastric vessels can be divided if necessary to provide adequate mobility of the fundus for the wrap, but the hepatic branch of the anterior vagus is preserved intact. The fundoplication is made so that the wrap is around the abdominal segment of oesophagus and not around the upper stomach.

The diaphragmatic crura are sutured behind the oesophagus using non-absorbable sutures e.g. 2/0 Ticron (Figure 23.5). Johnson (1986) favours mattress sutures passed through reinforcing teflon patches on either side to lessen the chance of the sutures cutting through the muscle, whereas in Melbourne two or three interrupted sutures are inserted loosely enough to avoid ischaemia of the muscle. Mobilization must be such that at least 2.5–3.0 cm of oesophagus is in the abdomen, and the final length of the fundoplication should be 1.5–2.0 cm in length. There is no advantage in making the length of fundoplication more than 2.0 cm.

The purpose of the fundoplication wrap is to make a valve, and not a constriction. To achieve this, it may be helpful to pre-align the wrap by using a traction suture placed in the fundus. Passage of this suture behind the oesophagus to a position to the right of the oesophagus at the diaphragmatic level will produce a loose, nicely aligned 2.0 cm wrap with no twisting of the posterior gastric wall. A large bougie (from 28 in infants to 40 in larger children) can be placed in the oesophageal lumen during fundoplication to ensure that the lumen is not compromised by the wrap, but we have not normally found this necessary. The wrap

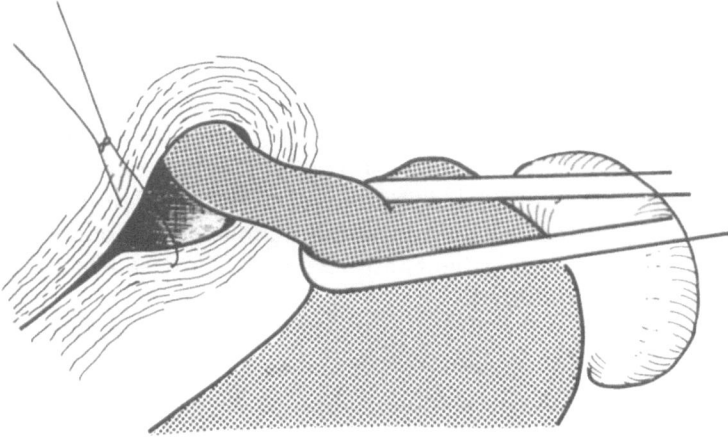

Figure 23.5 Apposition of the crural fibres of the oesophageal hiatus behind the oesophagus.

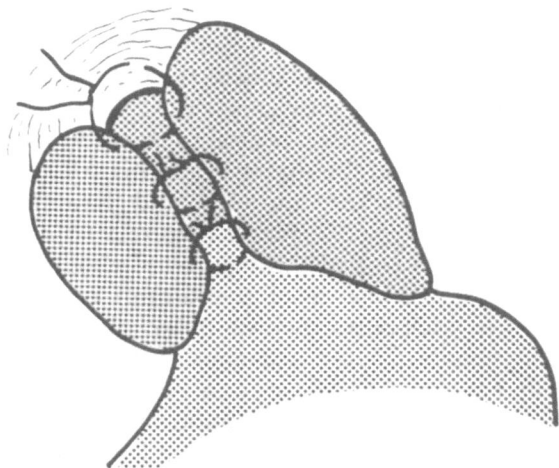

Figure 23.6   The fundoplication. The uppermost suture can include the under-side of the diaphragm as well as the stomach and oesophagus. When the sutures are tightened the lower end of the oesophagus is no longer visible.

should be loose enough to provide room between the oesophagus and gastric fundoplication.

The actual fundoplication sutures pass from the gastric wall to oesophagus to gastric wall. A 2.0 cm wrap requires 4–5 sutures, the top one being passed also through the diaphragmatic hiatus for anchoring (Figure 23.6).

23.6.1   ROLE OF GASTROSTOMY

Gastrostomy provides an easy route for caloric supplementation after fundoplication while the oesophagus is recovering from the effects of perioesophageal dissection and oesophagitis. This has encouraged some centres to perform routine gastrostomy at the time of fundoplication. However, despite the fact that fundoplication may temporarily make swallowing worse, most patients are able to swallow satisfactorily and gastrostomy is not required.

Gastrostomy is recommended at the time of fundoplication in three situations:

1. Where there is grossly inadequate nutrition and, for one reason or another, it is felt that institution of oral feeds will be delayed and the patient cannot afford to be starved for a prolonged period.
2. Where there is symptomatic tracheomalacia associated with feeding

difficulties as a result of tracheal collapse during swallowing, with or without concomitant aspiration.

3. When there is an impassable oesophageal stricture which cannot be dilated. The stricture almost always resolves following surgical correction of the gastro-oesophageal reflux but in patients with severe strictures this takes time and the gastrostomy provides an alternative route for nutrition until the stricture has resolved. It may also provide an alternative route for dilatation of the stricture as required (Johnson *et al.*, 1977).

23.6.2 ROLE OF PYLOROPLASTY

Pyloroplasty has been advocated by some centres (Davidson *et al.*, 1987; Fonkalsrud *et al.*, 1989), on the grounds that there may be coexisting gastric outlet obstruction and that pyloroplasty avoids the 'gas bloat' syndrome. In practice, this would appear to be an uncommon problem and routine pyloroplasty has its own side-effects in children, including 'dumping' and is probably not justified. However, in the rare situation that persistent gastric outlet obstruction is demonstrated after fundoplication, pyloroplasty may be necessary. Some authors have suggested that post-fundoplication gas bloat may be caused by a moderate degree of delayed gastric emptying (Maddern *et al.*, 1985).

23.7 Postoperative complications and side-effects

23.7.1 DYSPHAGIA

The Nissen valve may impair oesophageal emptying when the oesophagus has poor peristaltic function and abnormal motility; and may be sufficient to cause a functional obstruction. The likelihood of this being a clinical problem is reduced if the wrap-around is loose or the valve is constructed around a large bougie and the fundoplication itself is short (less than 2.0 cm in total length).

Fortunately, in practice most of the oesophageal atresia patients do not have significant oesophageal obstructive symptoms after fundoplication. The majority need to eat slowly, often accompanied by fluids, but the oesophagus does empty and symptoms of fullness and dysphagia, after the first few weeks, are rarely bothersome in the long term. Occasional patients do have serious problems with oesophageal emptying, and on follow-up, about 10% of oesophageal atresia patients will report frequent episodes of delayed or difficult swallowing (Chapter 25). In these patients, there is no anatomic obstruction and a large calibre bougie can be passed through the fundoplication with ease. Oesophageal peristalsis is simply insufficient to overcome the valve. Spontaneous recovery does occur, but may take up to two years. Former potentially life-threatening symptoms of oesophageal stricture or repeated aspiration and pneumonia are eliminated by the fundoplication, justifying its use, but it may take considerable patience by the clinician before feeding patterns become acceptable postoperatively.

23.7.2   GAS BLOAT

Some degree of gaseous distension and fullness is experienced by all oesophageal atresia patients for the first few weeks following Nissen fundoplication. If the wrap is constructed short and loose, these symptoms are usually mild and of few weeks duration only. Smaller infants seem to manage better than older children, and many infants can eructate in the immediate postoperative period. In the Salt Lake experience ten of 30 oesophageal atresia patients were able to eructate within the first three months following fundoplication. If gas bloat becomes of clinical concern simethecone drops to disperse gas bubbles, and metaclopramide to improve gastric emptying, may be helpful. Theoretically, gas bloat may interfere with adequate caloric intake through a false sensation of fullness, but this is rarely a problem.

Sometimes acute gastric dilatation occurs in the early postoperative period. The surgeon must be aware of this possibility in the first few postoperative days in the child whose clinical condition deteriorates rapidly and who has epigastric fullness. The crisis is resolved by immediate insertion of a nasogastric tube to decompress the stomach. To avoid this potential problem a nasogastric tube is routinely left *in situ* for 24 hours after operation.

23.7.3   RECURRENT GASTRO-OESOPHAGEAL REFLUX SECONDARY TO BREAKDOWN OF REPAIR

Recurrent reflux nearly always means the fundoplication has come 'undone': sutures have pulled through the tissue and the repair has broken down. Breakdown of the repair is more likely to happen in patients with poor nutrition and poor tissues and in severely retarded patients. Additional factors which appear to predispose to recurrence of reflux are oesophagitis with oesophageal shortening, and when tension has been required to maintain an adequate length of intra-abdominal oesophagus. Johnson observed recurrence in four of 30 oesophageal atresia patients after fundoplication attributed to a short oesophagus. In the Melbourne series of 34 patients, there were two patients in whom unwrapping of the fundoplication was confirmed (Table 23.6), both of whom had oesophageal atresia without fistula.

23.7.4 NON-SPECIFIC COMPLICATIONS

The incidence of wound infection and post-laparotomy intestinal obstruction is similar to that of other procedures using a similar approach, and is summarized in Table 23.6. The inability of the child to vomit after fundoplication may lead to a delay in diagnosis and referral of patients with obstruction due to adhesions (Spitz and Kirtane, 1985).

References

Ashcraft, K. W. (1986) Thal fundoplication. in *Pediatric Esophageal Surgery* (eds K. W. Ashcraft and T. M. Holder), Grune & Stratton, Orlando, pp. 209–16.

Ashcraft, K. W., Holder, T. M., Amoury, P. A. *et al.* (1984) The Thal fundoplication for gastro-oesophageal reflux. *J. Pediatr. Surg.*, **19**, 480–3.

Boix-Ochoa, J. (1986) The physiological approach to the management of gastric oesophageal reflux. Address of Honored Guest. *J. Pediatr. Surg.*, **21**, 1032–9.

Da Dalt, L., Mazzoleni, S., Montini, G. *et al.* (1989) Diagnostic accuracy of pH monitoring in gastro-oesophageal reflux. *Arch. Dis. Child.*, **64**, 1421–6.

Davidson, B. R., Hurd, D. M. and Johnstone, M. S. (1987) Nissen fundoplication and pyloroplasty in the management of gastro-oesophageal reflux in children. *Br. J. Surg.*, **74**, 488–90.

Fonkalsrud, E. W., Foglia, R. P., Ament, M. E., Berquist, W. and Vargas, J. (1989) Operative treatment for the gastro-oesophageal reflux syndrome in children. *J. Pediatr. Surg.*, **24**, 525–9.

Gryboski, J. D., Thayer, W. R. and Spiro, H. M. (1963) Oesophageal motility in infants and children. *Pediatrics*, **31**, 382–95.

Hill, L. D. (1989) Myths of the oesophagus. *J. Thorac. Cardiovasc. Surg.*, **98**, 1–10.

Holder, T. M. (1988) Gastro-oesophageal reflux and the Thal fundoplication. Presented at the International Congress of Paediatric Surgery, Melbourne, Australia, November.

Johnson, D. G. (1986) The Nissen fundoplication. in: *Pediatric Esophageal Surgery* (eds K. W. Ashcraft and T. M. Holder), Grune & Stratton, Orlando, pp. 193–208.

Johnson, D. G., Herbst, J. J., Oliveros, M. A. and Stewart, D. R. (1977) Evaluation of gastro-oesophageal reflux surgery in children. *Pediatrics*, **59**, 62–8.

Jolley, S. G., Johnson, D. J., Roberts, C. R. *et al.* (1980) Patterns of gastro-oesophageal reflux in children following repair of oesophageal atresia and distal traceoesophageal fistula. *J. Pediatr. Surg.*, **15**, 857–62.

Leendertse-Verloop, K., Tibboel, D., Hazebroek, F. W. J. and Molenaar, J. C. (1987) Postoperative morbidity in patients with oesophageal atresia. *Pediatr. Surg. Int.*, **2**, 2–5.

Maddern, G. J., Jamieson, G. G., Chatterton, B. E. *et al.* (1985) Is there an association between failed anti-reflux procedures and delayed gastric emptying? *Ann. Surg.*, **202**, 162–5.

O'Sullivan, G. C., de Meester, T. R., Joeslsson, B. E. *et al.* (1982) Interaction of lower esophageal sphincter pressure and length of sphincter in the abdomen as determinants of gastroesophageal competence. *Am. J. Surg.*, **143**, 40–7.

Pieretti, R., Shandling, B. and Stephens, C. A. (1974) Resistant esophageal stenosis associates with reflux after repair of esophageal atresia: a therapeutic approach. *J. Pediatr. Surg.*, **9**, 355–7.

Schwagten, K. J., Beasley, S. W. and Auldist, A. W. (1988) Surgical management and complications of gastro-oesophageal reflux in childhood. Paper presented at the International Congress in Paediatric Surgery, Melbourne, November.

Spitz, L. and Kirtane, J. (1985) Results and complications of surgery for gastro-oesophageal reflux. *Arch. Dis. Child.*, **60**, 743–7.

PART EIGHT
The Outcome

24 Trends in mortality

S. W. BEASLEY and N. A. MYERS

Until 1939, oesophageal atresia was considered a uniformly fatal condition. Nowadays, all patients with oesophageal atresia are expected to survive almost irrespective of their gestation, provided there are no major concomitant congenital malformations. This chapter documents the trends in mortality over the last 40 years.

24.1 Overall mortality

Many major centres have documented a decline in the overall mortality of oesophageal atresia with each passing decade (Abrahamson and Shandling, 1972; Louhimo and Lindahl, 1983; Bishop *et al.*, 1985). The experience of the Royal Children's Hospital has been similar: Figure 24.1 shows the overall mortality of patients with oesophageal atresia and distal fistula. However, a proportion of these infants had associated congenital abnormalities for which the prognosis was considered so poor that no active treatment was instituted. If these patients are excluded, the decline in mortality with each decade becomes even more dramatic. Figure 24.2 shows the mortality of patients with treated oesophageal atresia and distal tracheo-oesophageal fistula during the same 40-year period.

24.2 Causes of death

In the early years, most deaths were the result of respiratory failure and inadequate resuscitation, from soiling of the lungs, hyaline membrane disease and other complications of prematurity. The other major cause of mortality was from complications of the oesophageal surgery itself, particularly those related to dehiscence of the anastomosis and poor nutrition. As neonatology and operative technique improved, the main

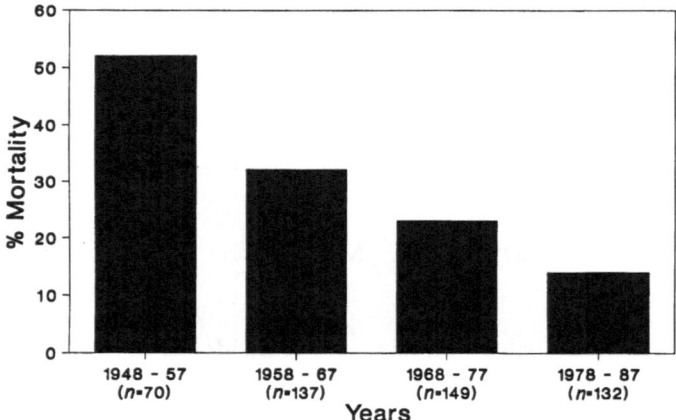

Figure 24.1   Overall mortality in patients with oesophageal atresia and distal fistula born between 1948 and 1987.

cause of death became that caused by associated anomalies; and as the treatment of these has improved (particularly that of congenital heart disease, see Chapter 15), major chromosomal aberrations have assumed greater importance.

Table 24.1 illustrates the major effect of associated anomalies on mortality and the relatively infrequent incidence of complications of prematurity and oesophageal complications causing death in recent years.

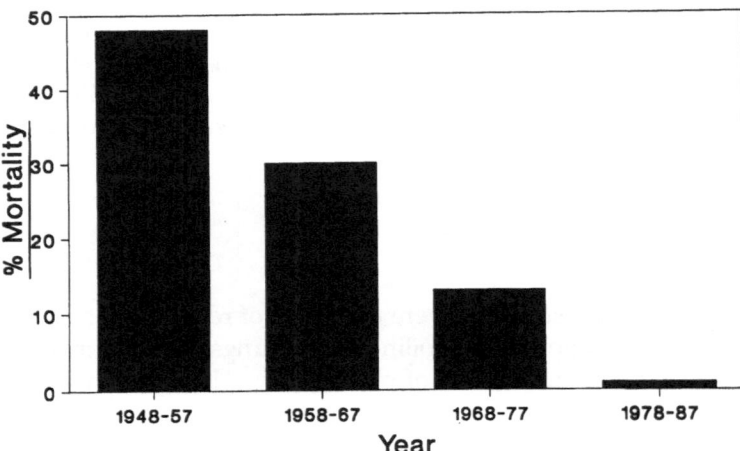

Figure 24.2   Mortality in patients with oesophageal atresia and distal tracheo-oesophageal fistula undergoing definitive treatment: 1948–1987.

Table 24.1 Cause of death in all patients with oesophageal atresia and/or tracheo-oesophageal fistula between 1974 and 1989 (49 patients*)

	Definitive treatment	
	Not Offered	Offered
Trisomy 21	3	
Trisomy 18	7	
Other chromosomal		1
Congenital heart disease	9	7
Other major anomalies	14	7
CHARGE Association	2	1
Multiple anomalies	3	
Complication of oesophageal surgery		2
Complication of cardiac catheterization		1
Necrotizing enterocolitis		2
Cot death		2
Severe HMD**	1	

*Some patients had more than one contributing factor.
**Might have survived had the infant received early definitive treatment, including division of the tracheo-oesophageal fistula.

24.2.1 THE WATERSTON CLASSIFICATION

In 1962, Waterston *et al.* recognized the importance of birthweight (and, indirectly, gestation) and soiling of the lungs as factors which influenced survival. As a result of their observations, the Waterston classification became accepted. It divided infants into three groups:

A.   Birthweight over 2.5 kg and well;
B.   (a) Birthweight 1.8–2.5 kg and well;
      (b) Higher birthweight, moderate pneumonia and/or an additional moderate congenital anomaly;
C.   (a) Birthweight under 1.8 kg;
      (b) Higher birthweight and severe pneumonia and/or an additional severe congenital anomaly.

This simple classification gained widespread acceptance (German *et al.*, 1976; Myers, 1979; Rivosecchi *et al.*, 1989). Figures 24.3, 24.4 and 24.5 show the dramatic improvement in survival for oesophageal atresia and distal tracheo-oesophageal fistula in each of the Waterston groups, such that mortality in Groups A and B is now extremely uncommon. The continued high incidence of mortality in Group C reflects the presence

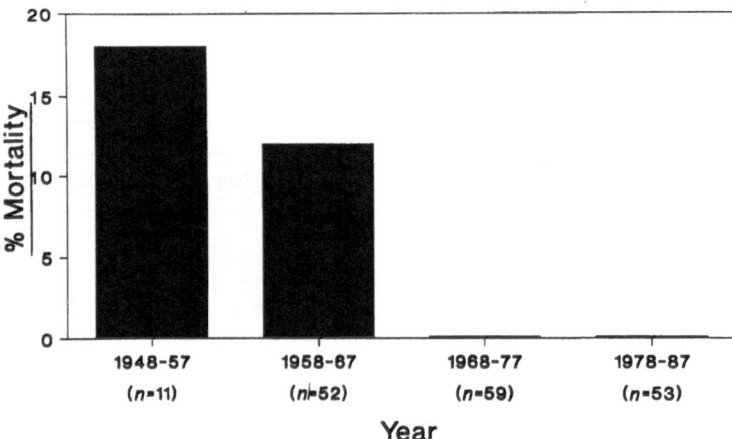

Figure 24.3 Trends in mortality in Waterston Group A oesophageal atresia with distal tracheo-oesophageal fistula receiving treatment.

of major associated anomalies rather than complications of oesophageal surgery or prematurity. Since 1970, prematurity has had little effect on mortality.

In former years the Waterston classification proved extremely valuable in identifying risk factors and in predicting outcome in infants with oesophageal atresia. However, the data presented above and the experience of others (Louhimo and Lindahl, 1983; Cozzi and Wilkinson, 1975; Rivosecchi *et al.*, 1989) suggest that it is no longer relevant in oesophageal atresia and that in the future, mortality will be best predicted by the type and severity of concomitant congenital abnormalities alone.

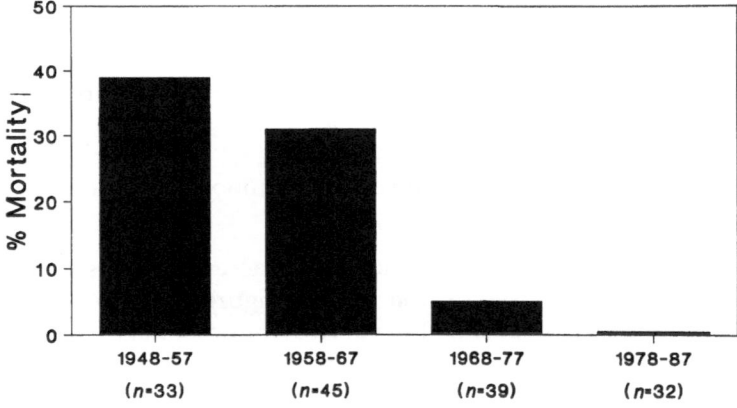

Figure 24.4 Trends in mortality in Waterston Group B oesophageal atresia with distal tracheo-oesophageal fistula receiving treatment.

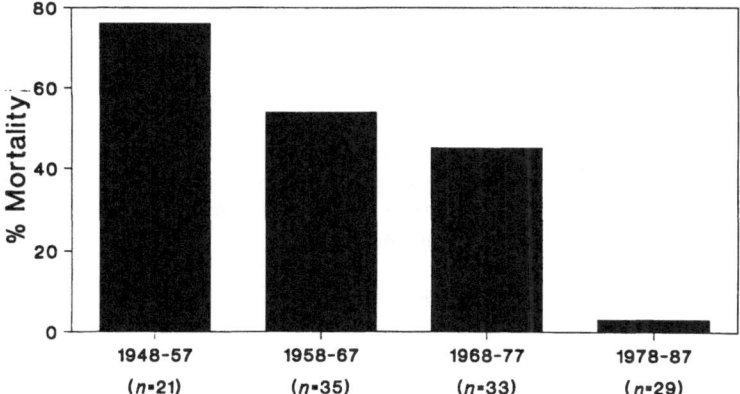

Figure 24.5 Trends in mortality in Waterston Group C oesophageal atresia with distal tracheo-oesophageal fistula receiving treatment.

24.2.2. ASSOCIATED CONGENITAL ABNORMALITIES

The incidence and type of major abnormalities involving other systems has been described in detail in Chapters 14 to 17. Until recently many of these lesions, particularly the major cardiac abnormalities, were difficult to treat and often resulted in death, but now they have a much better prognosis. Despite this, major organ defects and chromosomal aberrations constitute the biggest hurdle to survival (Beasley *et al.*, 1989a, b). Antenatal ultrasound, echocardiography, chromosome analysis and renal ultrasound enable identification of those infants with a hopeless prognosis before surgery is undertaken. Our ability to detect these patients is reflected in the proportion of patients with oesophageal atresia with distal fistula not being offered treatment after 1972, compared with before that year (Figure 20.1). In the earlier period, 6.5% had surgery withheld, compared with 13.5% since that time.

In addition to early detection of major organ defects and better recognition of chromosomal abnormalities, another factor contributes to this increased non-operative rate in recent years: more infants with multiple anomalies are reaching the tertiary institutions.

24.3 Late deaths

In this review, a late death was defined as a death occurring outside the neonatal period (Table 24.2). Most late deaths occur in the first year of life (Figure 24.6). Many of the late deaths were related to major cardiac surgery at a time when the results were not as good as at present. It is

Table 24.2 Cause of late death in 26 patients with oesophageal atresia and distal fistula*: 1948–1987

Congenital heart disease	10
Respiratory failure/pneumonia	4
Recurrent tracheo-oesophageal fistula	1
Hydrocephalus and mental retardation	3
Chromosomal abnormality	1
CHARGE association	1
Intractable diarrhoea	2
Renal failure	2
Pierre–Robin syndrome	2
'Cot death'	5
Inborn error of metabolism	1

*In some patients there was more than one cause.

likely, therefore, that late deaths after repaired oesophageal atresia will be less frequent in future years.

The high incidence of 'cot deaths' is difficult to explain. In these patients the real cause of death is unknown but might be related to tracheomalacia or gastro-oesophageal reflux. This group warrants further careful investigation.

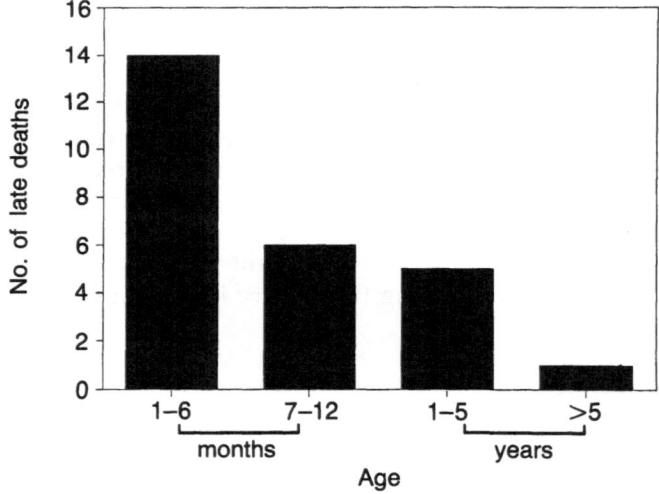

Figure 24.6 Distribution of age at which late deaths occur.

References

Abrahamson, J. and Shandling, B. (1972) Oesophageal atresia in the underweight baby: a challenge. *J. Pediatr. Surg.*, **7**, 608–11.

Beasley, S. W., Auldist, A. W. and Myers, N. A. (1989a) Current surgical management of oesophageal atresia and/or tracheo-oesophageal fistula. *Aust. NZ J. Surg.*, **59**, 707–12.

Beasley, S. W., Shann, F. A., Myers, N. A. and Auldist, A. W. (1989b) Developments in the management of oesophageal atresia. *Med. J. Aust.*, **150**, 501–3.

Bishop, P. H., Klein, M. D., Philippart, A. I., Hixson, D. S. and Hertzler, J. H. (1985) Transpleural repair of esophageal atresia without a primary gastrostomy: 240 patients treated between 1951 and 1983. *J. Pediatr. Surg.*, **20**, 823–8.

Cozzi, F. and Wilkinson, A. W. (1975) Mortality in oesophageal atresia. *J. R. Coll. Surg. Edin.*, **20**, 236–44.

German, J. C., Mahour, G. H. and Woolley, M. M. (1976) Esophageal atresia and associated anomalies. *J. Pediatr. Surg.*, **11**, 299–306.

Louhimo, I. and Lindahl, H. (1983) Esophageal atresia: primary results of 500 consecutively treated patients. *J. Pediatr. Surg.*, **18**, 217–29.

Myers, N. A. (1974) The epitome of modern surgery. *Ann. R. Coll. Surg. (Engl)*, **54**, 277–87.

Myers, N. A. (1979) Oesophageal atresia and/or tracheo-oesophageal fistula. A study in mortality. *Prog. Pediatr. Surg.*, **13**, 141–65.

Rivosecchi, M., Bagolan, P., Matarazzo, E. *et al.* (1989) Esophageal atresia: critical review of ten years' experience. *Pediatr. Surg. Int.*, **4**, 95–100.

Waterston, D. J., Bonham-Carter, R. E. and Aberdeen, E. (1962) Oesophageal atresia: tracheo-oesophageal fistula. A study of survival in 218 infants. *Lancet*, **i**, 819–22.

25 Late results following repair of oesophageal atresia

S. W. BEASLEY, P. D. PHELAN and P. CHETCUTI

The surgeon who operates on a neonate has to bear in mind that the result of his operation has to serve the patient for a lifetime. This imposes two responsibilities upon paediatric surgeons: the first, to undertake long-term follow-up of the continuing adequacy of their operative procedures; and second, to avail themselves of the long-term experience of centres where earlier advances have been made. The first babies to survive after oesophageal atresia repair reached adult life in the 1960s. Because in the early years there were relatively small numbers of survivors, only recently has there been much experience of adults with repaired oesophageal atresia.

Our experience with adults with repaired oesophageal atresia dates from the late 1960s. To determine their current status, a long-term follow-up study was conducted and much of the information in this chapter has derived from that study. Many patients still have symptoms, but they are usually minor and interfere little with the quality of life. The most common are directly referable to the oesophagus and respiratory tract.

25.1 The Royal Children's Hospital long-term follow-up study

This study was undertaken after exhaustive planning by surgeons, paediatric thoracic physicians, paediatric urologists, orthopaedic surgeons, neonatologists and radiologists. A total of 538 patients with oesophageal atresia and/or tracheo-oesophageal fistula were managed at the Royal Children's Hospital since the first successful repair in 1949 to the end of 1985. There were 366 survivors of whom 302 were reviewed, forming the basis of the data presented below (Table 25.1). All hospital case notes were studied for details of the type and timing of surgery,

Table 25.1 Survivors of repaired oesophageal atresia 1948–1985

Total survivors	366
Survivors reviewed	302
Adult survivors (> 18 years)	145
Adults reviewed	125
(full clinical review 107)	
(telephone interview 18)	

postoperative complications and subsequent hospital admissions. Radiological diagnosis of anastomotic stricture and gastro-oesophageal reflux was documented. Details of past medical history and current health status were obtained from the patients and where appropriate from the parents as well. Current respiratory problems were defined as episodes of wheezing, bronchitis (cough and constitutional disturbance lasting more than five days) or pneumonia in the 12 months to review. Current gastrointestinal symptoms were defined as dysphagia, heartburn or regurgitation in the 12 months to review.

Lung function studies were performed in patients over the age of six years. Analysis of respiratory function in patients with spinal deformity was considered separately. Total lung capacity (TLC), vital capacity (VC), residual volume (RV), forced expiratory volume in one second (FEV_1), mean forced expiratory volume between 25 and 75% of vital capacity (FEF_{25-75}) and inspiratory and expiratory flow volume loops were measured in a pressure-compensated, integrated flow body plethysmograph (Jaegar Bodyscreen 2). The subjects were trained to perform maximally and the best of a minimum of three efforts in the seated position was recorded. Ratios of FEV_1/VC, RV/TLC, peak expiratory to peak inspiratory flow (PEF/PIF), and mid-expiratory to mid-inspiratory flows (VE_{50}/VI_{50}) were calculated. All values were expressed as 'per cent predicted' for height, age and sex, based on the normal values of Zapletal *et al.* (1977), Knudson *et al.* (1976, 1982). Subjects with an FEV_1/VC ratio of less than 75 inhaled 5 mg of nebulized salbutamol and an expiratory flow volume loop was obtained ten minutes after being given the bronchodilator. A greater than 10% increase in per cent predicted FEV_1 was taken to represent a significant response. The students unpaired *t* test was used for analysis of the lung function and the chi squared test for the analysis of the association between respiratory problems, surgical complications and gastrointestinal symptoms.

A subgroup of 248 patients with oesophageal atresia and/or tracheo-oesophageal fistula, who were admitted during the period up to 1968, were evaluated separately (Chetcuti *et al.*, 1988). Of these patients 145 survived to 18 years of age and of this number, 125 were reviewed. Of these, 107 attended for full clinical review (and further investigation where indicated) and a further 18 patients who lived interstate or outside Australia were interviewed by telephone. In total this represented 86% of survivors. Current symptoms were defined as those present in the 12 months before review; each patient was examined and renal ultrasonography performed if the urinary tract had not been investigated previously. Other radiological examinations were obtained if there was a clinical indication, e.g. scoliosis.

The oldest patient reviewed was the first survivor, aged 38 years at the time of review. The mean age of the 68 men (54%) and 57 women (46%) was 25 years, and current problems were distributed evenly between the sexes.

25.2 Growth

In previous studies it has been suggested that growth is impaired in survivors of oesophageal atresia. For example, in a study of the long-term nutritional status of 53 patients (representing a small proportion of the total number of patients treated over the 38 year period reviewed) it was found that 19% were below the third centile in height for their age,

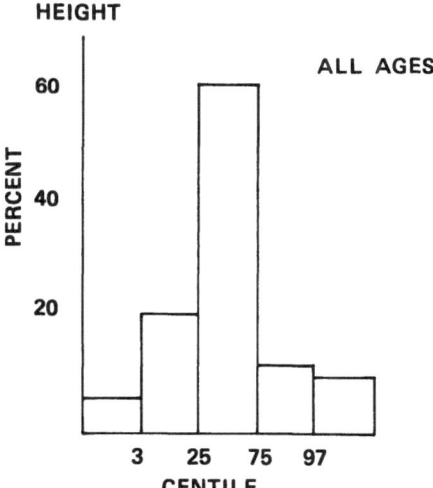

Figure 25.1 Height centiles corrected for age in patients with repaired oesophageal atresia.

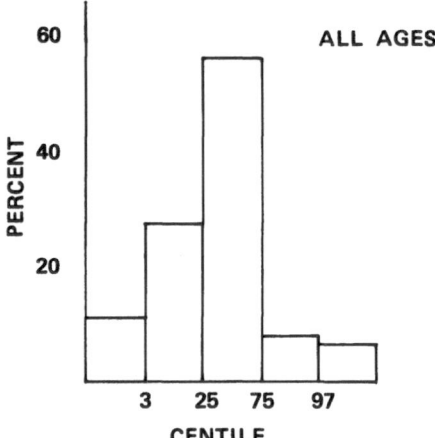

Figure 25.2 Weight centiles connected for age in patients with repaired oesophageal atresia.

with birthweight having no significant influence on subsequent growth (Andrassy *et al.*, 1983). On the other hand, Rickham (1981) found that in infants with a birthweight of less than 3 lbs, (1.36 kg) although there was early physical developmental retardation, both height and weight eventually became normal. In our study, the distribution of height and weight in the survivors reviewed revealed only a slight bias to the left

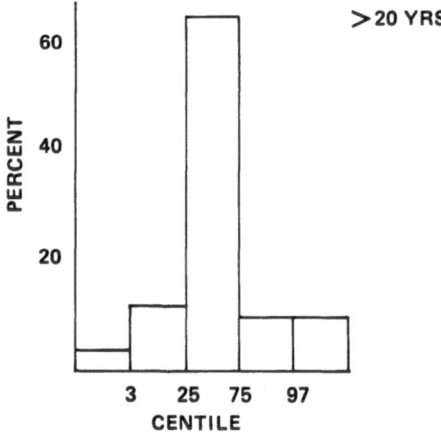

Figure 25.3 Height centiles in adults over 20 years after repair of oesophageal atresia.

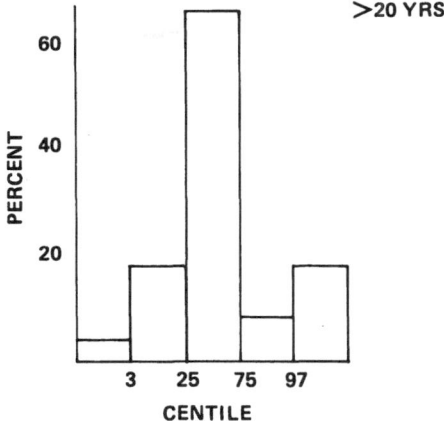

Figure 25.4 Weight centiles in adults over 20 years after repair of oesophageal atresia.

(Figures 25.1 and 25.2) which disappeared when adults alone were considered (Figures 25.3 and 25.4).

25.3 Gastrointestinal problems

25.3.1 DURING CHILDHOOD

Major dysphagic symptoms, e.g. foreign body impaction in the oesophagus, choking with feeds and pain on swallowing, occur frequently during childhood (Figure 25.5). The number requiring surgical intervention (e.g. oesophageal dilatation, oesophagoscopy and removal of foreign body, or fundoplication) declines during childhood, although the proportion experiencing some degree of dysphagia alters little. Many swallowing problems first become evident when solids are introduced and the incidence peaks at about two years. Following this time, obstructive episodes in the oesophagus become progressively less common (Figure 25.6). The age at the time of the last admission for an oesophageal problem gives a further indication of the decline in severity of dysphagic symptoms with time (Figure 25.7). Those who have persistent problems are more likely to have had an oesophageal stricture or severe gastro-oesophageal reflux during infancy. The extent of these problems is reflected in the total inpatient days required for their management (Figure 25.8).

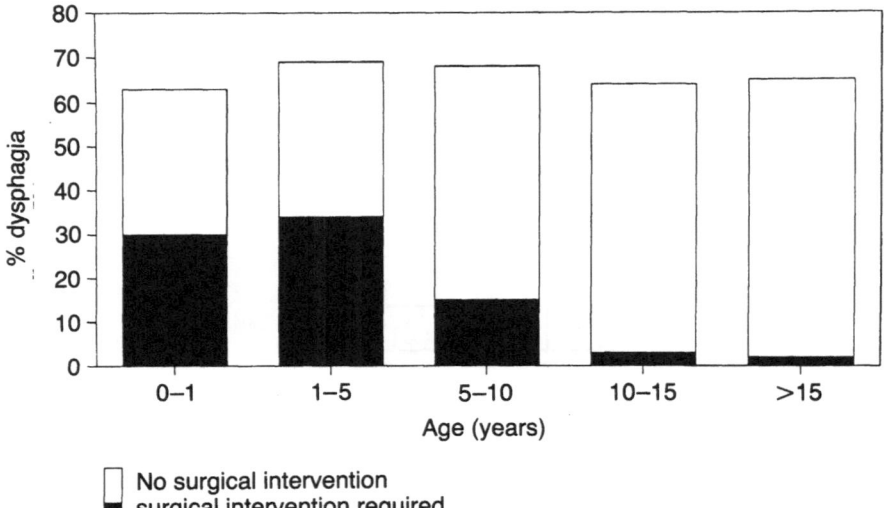

Figure 25.5 Incidence of dysphagia during childhood.

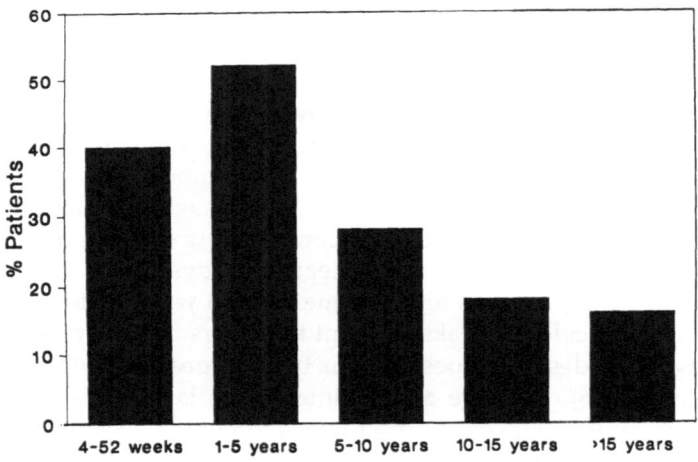

Figure 25.6 Incidence of foreign body impaction according to age during childhood.

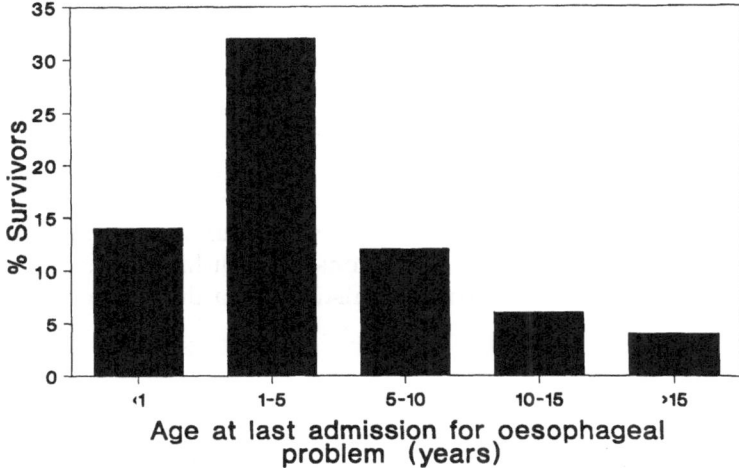

Figure 25.7 Age at last admission for an oesophageal problem.

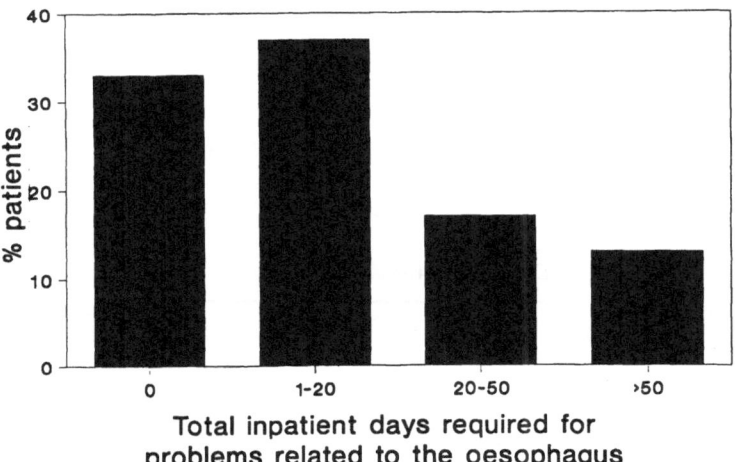

Figure 25.8 Total inpatients days required for problems related to the oeso-phagus.

25.3.2 DURING ADULTHOOD

Persistent symptoms in adults born before 1968 are shown in Table 25.2. Difficulties with swallowing occurred often, and many patients drank fluids with their meals. Only two, however, avoided certain foods because of this (particularly meats, poultry and bread) and one avoided restaurants. Dysphagia was present in over half the adults, but most enjoyed a normal diet and seldom required medical attention. The main cause of the swallowing difficulty was probably disordered oesophageal peristalsis, which all patients with oesophageal atresia may have to some degree. Anastomotic stricture is an important cause of dysphagia in the first years after surgery, but not in subsequent years. Despite this, dysphagia remained more common in patients who had been in hospital during childhood for stricture, and occurred in 76 of the 125 adults reviewed ($P < 0.05$). Although symptoms of reflux were common, only one patient had secondary complications in adult life. He had a hiatus hernia and an oesophageal stricture distinct from the anastomotic site.

Table 25.2 Persistent gastrointestinal symptoms in adult survivors with repaired oesophageal atresia

Dysphagia	
No dysphagia	38%
Less than 1/week	38%
2/week	10%
Every day	7%
Every meal	7%
Symptoms of reflux	
No reflux	45%
Less than 1/week	51%
2/week	2%
Daily symptoms	2%

There was no relationship between reflux and dysphagia demonstrated in the period prior to review. To put these problems in perspective, it should be remembered that symptoms of gastro-oesophageal reflux are common in adults in the general population, with a prevalence of occasional symptoms in 36% and symptoms occurring more than once a week in 7%; we found only slightly more in our study. Several factors may contribute to gastro-oesophageal reflux in patients with repaired oesophageal atresia. These include: mobilization and elevation of the lower oesophageal segment, which may produce traction on the lower oesophagus with distortion of the gastro-oesophageal junction; interference of the neurovascular supply of the lower oesophagus (Chapter 23); abnormal development of the myenteric plexus or hiatus; and gastrostomy.

25.4 Respiratory problems

Respiratory complications following repair of oesophageal atresia and fistula are most common in the early postoperative years (Crispin *et al.*, 1966; Dudley and Phelan, 1976; Le Soeuf *et al.*, 1987). Factors contributing to these problems include poor oesophageal emptying and gastro-oesophageal reflux causing recurrent inhalation of gastric or oesophageal contents (Shermata *et al.*, 1977), structural instability of the major airways (tracheomalacia) (Wailoo and Emery, 1979; Benjamin *et al.*, 1976) and abnormal airways epithelium (Emery and Haddadin, 1971). A total of 154 patients with normal spines had lung function studies. The type of tracheo-oesophageal abnormality is shown in Table 25.3. The changing incidence of bronchitis, pneumonia and persistent cough with age, is shown in Figures 25.9, 25.10 and 25.11. The number of hospital

Table 25.3 Anatomical variants of oesophageal atresia and/or tracheo-oesophageal fistula patients undergoing lung function studies

Oesophageal atresia and distal fistula	127
Oesophageal atresia and proximal fistula	4
Oesophageal atresia alone	9
Tracheo-oesophageal fistula	14

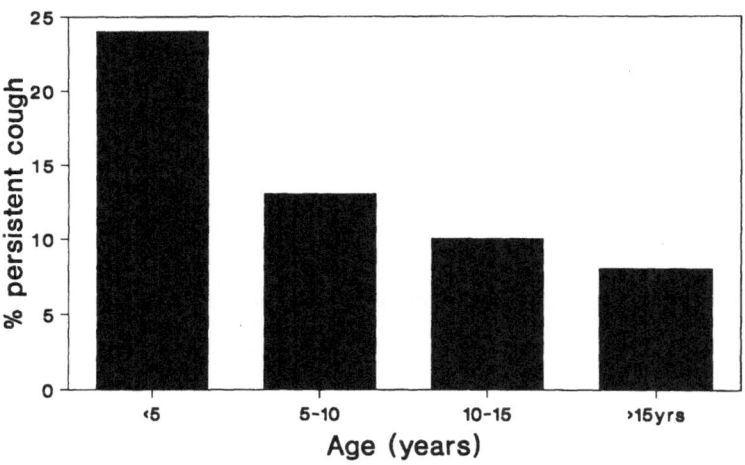

Figure 25.9 Incidence of persistent cough according to age.

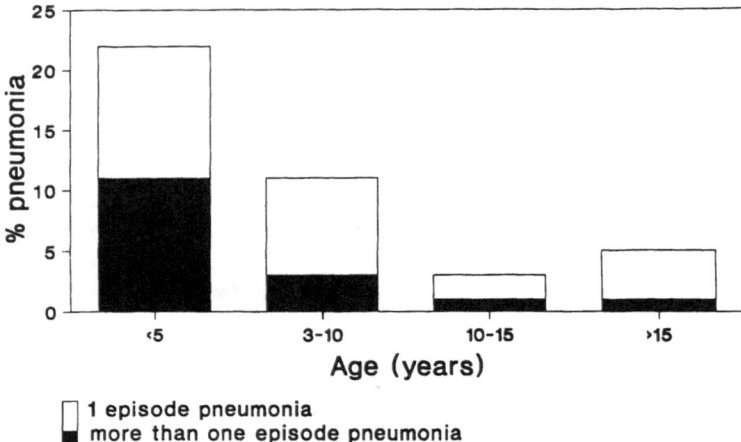

Figure 25.10 Incidence of pneumonia according to age.

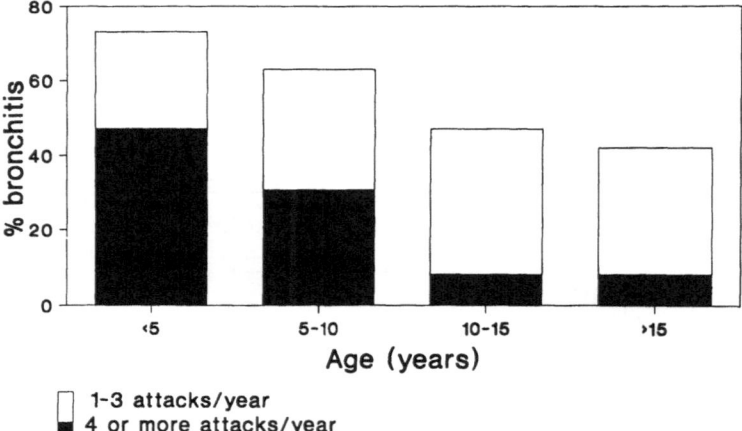

Figure 25.11 Incidence of bronchitis according to age.

admissions required because of respiratory problems is shown in Figure 25.12.

25.4.1 LOWER AIRWAYS DISEASE

Figures 25.13, 25.14 and 25.15 show the distribution of patients for per cent predicted TLC, VC and FEV$_1$ (Chetcuti and Phelan, 1990). Values less than 80% of normal were present in 25% of patients for VC, 7% for

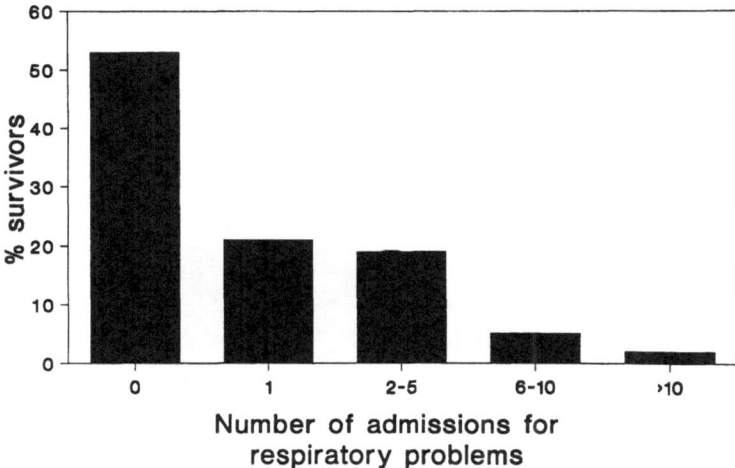

Figure 25.12 Number of hospital admissions required as a result of respiratory problems.

TLC and 45% for FEV_1. The normal range is approximately 80–120 predicted (Hibbert *et al.*, 1989). Five of the 17 patients with an FEV_1/VC ratio of < 75 had a significant response to a $beta_2$ agonist. A per cent predicted FEF_{25-75} below 70 was measured in 31% of the patients, and a RV/TLC ratio above 35 in 21%. Factors which may contribute to the mild lower airways disease that these patients experience include bronchiolar

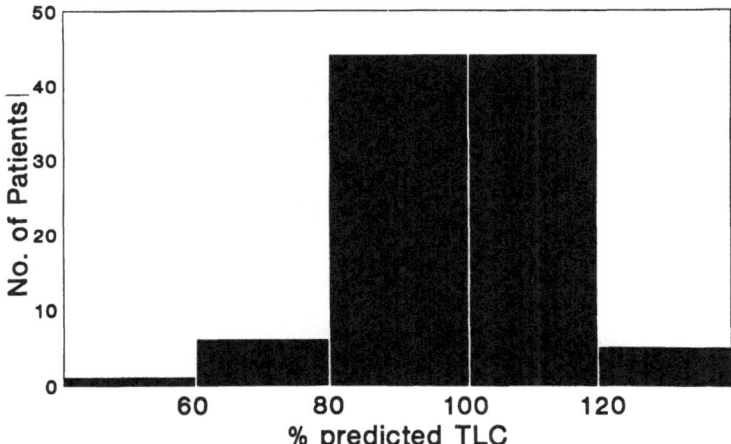

Figure 25.13 Per cent predicted total lung capacity after repair of oesophageal atresia.

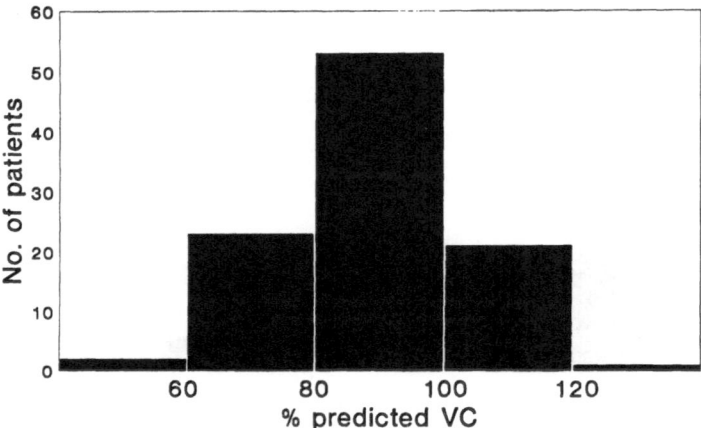

Figure 25.14 Per cent predicted vital capacity after repair of oesophageal atresia.

damage from repeated inhalation of gastric and oesophageal contents in the early postoperative years, increased bronchial hyper-reactivity from continuing inhalation, abnormalities of oesophageal peristalsis predisposing to inhalation (Laks *et al.*, 1972; Romeo *et al.*, 1987), and congenital abnormalities of innervation of the oesophagus (Nakazato *et al.*, 1986a, b). Gastro-oesophageal reflux may contribute through inhalation or from vagal mediated bronchoconstriction in the absence of inhalation (Danus *et al.*, 1976; Mansfield and Stein, 1978). Variable narrowing

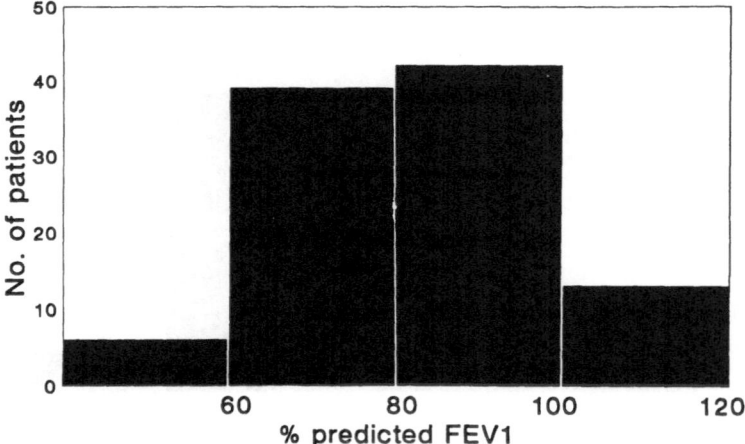

Figure 25.15 Per cent predicted forced expiratory volume in one second after repair of oesophageal atresia.

of the intrathoracic trachea from tracheomalacia (Benjamin *et al.*, 1976; David and Cywes, 1978) and congenital abnormalities of tracheal innervation (Nakazato *et al.*, 1986a, b) may further distort the expiratory flow volume loop.

25.4.2 RESTRICTIVE LUNG DISEASE

Mild restrictive lung disease was seen in 6% of patients. Multiple thoracotomies and pleural scarring from empyema after anastomotic rupture led to restrictive lung disease. The effect of multiple thoracotomies on total lung capacity and vital capacity is shown in Figure 25.16. Secretion retention from squamous metaplasia of the tracheal mucosa and an ineffectual cough from tracheomalacia may contribute to recurrent pneumonia, eventually leading to lung fibrosis with a small loss of lung volume (Chetcuti and Phelan, 1990).

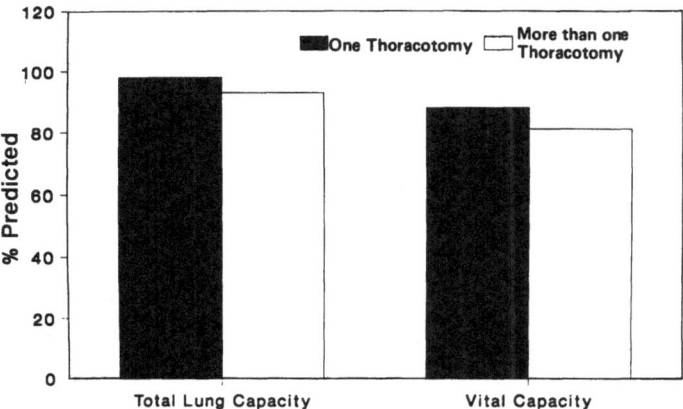

Figure 25.16 Effect of thoracotomy number on total lung capacity and vital capacity in the absence of a congenital vertebral abnormality.

25.4.3 EXTRATHORACIC TRACHEAL OBSTRUCTION

The increase in expiratory flow rates relative to inspiratory flow rates is suggestive of extrathoracic tracheal obstruction (Figure 25.17). This is a well-recognized problem in infants with oesophageal atresia, but from our study it would appear to persist into adult life. Although the rate of inspiratory flow is very effort-dependent, great attention was paid in this study to achieving maximal efforts by the patients, who were mostly very co-operative. Therefore the finding of reduced inspiratory flow rate

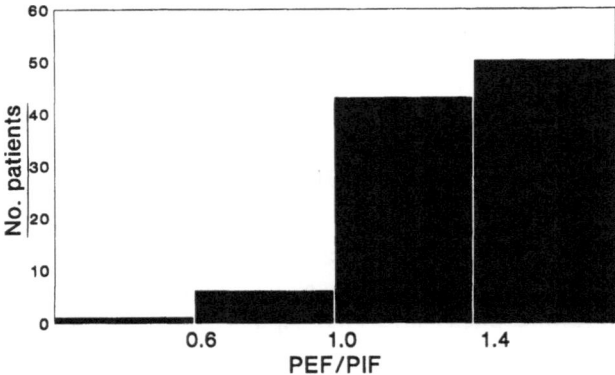

Figure 25.17   The relationship of expiratory and inspiratory flow rates.

is probably a real one. The presence of the characteristic harsh cough, thought to be a manifestation of tracheomalacia, did not identify those patients with reduced inspiratory flow rates.

25.4.4   EFFECT OF GASTRO-OESOPHAGEAL REFLUX ON THE RESPIRATORY TRACT

There is a slight increase in airways obstruction and a reduction in lung volume in patients with radiologically proven gastro-oesophageal reflux (Table 25.4) yet lung function was similar in those with current gastrointestinal symptoms and in those who were asymptomatic (Table 25.5). These findings suggest that either lung function abnormalities may be secondary to permanent lung damage from recurrent inhalation in earlier years or that ongoing aspiration occurs at a subclinical level (Chetcuti and Phelan, 1990).

Table 25.4   Respiratory function related to the presence or absence of gastro-oesophageal reflux

	Present (n = 76)	*Absent* (n = 79)	P *value*
% TLC	96 ± 14	100 ± 12	0.04
% VC	86 ± 15	91 ± 14	0.03
% FEV_1	79 ± 15	85 ± 13	0.01
% FEV_{25-75}	74 ± 23	83 ± 21	0.02
RV/TLC	31 ± 6	29 ± 6	0.04

Table 25.5 Lung function as per cent predicted means (and standard deviations) in groups according to the presence or absence of current gastrointestinal symptoms

Current gastrointestinal symptoms	Present	Absent	P value
	(n = 103)	(n = 52)	
% TLC	98 (± 14)	98 (± 12)	0.9
% VC	98 (± 15)	89 (± 13)	0.7
% FEV₁	83 (± 15)	82 (± 13)	0.9
% FEF₂₅₋₇₅	80 (± 24)	77 (± 18)	0.4
RV/TLC	30 (± 6)	30 (± 6)	0.9

25.4.5 RESPIRATORY PROBLEMS IN ADULT LIFE

Current respiratory symptoms in adults are shown in Table 25.6. Thirty patients (24%) had attended a general practitioner for respiratory problems in the preceding 12 months. Asthma was a past or present diagnosis in 17. Seven patients had radiologically confirmed pneumonia after the age of 18. The characteristic harsh barking cough of tracheomalacia was present in 50 patients (40%). Two patients, one with severe scoliosis and one with bronchiectasis, had a moderate reduction in exercise tolerance. Seven patients with surgically treated scoliosis and 19 with mild thoracic scoliosis, had no respiratory symptoms.

A total of 33 men and 21 women (43% of patients) were smokers. The rate in the community for an equivalent age group was 40%. There were

Table 25.6 Lung function as per cent predicted means (and standard deviations) in groups according to the presence or absence of current respiratory symptoms

	Present (n = 31)	Absent (n = 124)	P value
% TLC	99 (± 13)	96 (± 15)	0.5
% VC	90 (± 14)	86 (± 15)	0.2
% FEV₁	84 (± 14)	79 (± 16)	0.1
% FEF₂₅₋₇₅	81 (± 22)	70 (± 21)	0.01
RV/TLC	30 (± 6)	32 (± 7)	0.04

no differences in frequency of respiratory problems between smokers and non-smokers. Wheezing, bronchitis and persistent cough were more common in patients who had these problems in childhood ($P <$ 0.001). Patients who wheezed in the 12 months before review had significant reduction in vital capacity and FEV_1 ($P < 0.05$). Lung function in patients with other respiratory or gastrointestinal symptoms was not significantly different from that in asymptomatic patients.

25.5 Chest wall deformity

There have been only sporadic reports of the final appearance of the chest wall after surgery in oesophageal atresia. In two studies based on a small number of patients (Durning *et al.*, 1980; Gilsanz *et al.*, 1983) scoliosis was found to develop in 20–50% of patients. Scoliosis has been described also after thoracotomy with rib resection in children (de Rosa, 1985) and in adults (Bisgard, 1934; Loynes, 1972). Breast maldevelopment has been documented following anterolateral and posterolateral thoracotomy in the newborn period (Freeman and Walken, 1969; Cherup *et al.*, 1986), although until recently, anterior chest wall deformity after repair of oesophageal atresia has not been studied.

25.5.1 INCIDENCE

As part of the long-term follow-up study of survivors of oesophageal atresia, 302 patients were examined for evidence of chest wall asym-

Table 25.7 Chest wall deformity in patients with repaired oesophageal atresia

Survivors during period of study	366	
Patients available for review	302	
Patients without congenital vertebral anomalies	232	
Chest wall deformity*	77	(33%)
Scoliosis 30		
Anterior asymmetry 59		
Patients with congenital vertebral anomaly	53	
Chest wall deformity*	22	(42%)
Scoliosis 18		
Anterior asymmetry 14		
Cervical approach only	17	

*Some patients had combined anterior chest wall asymmetry and scoliosis.

metry and scoliosis. Spinal radiographs were obtained where scoliosis had not been recognized previously, and the Cobb angle calculated (Cobb, 1948). In the absence of a congenital vertebral anomaly, anterior chest wall deformity or scoliosis, or both, was found in 33%. When a congenital vertebral anomaly was present (usually hemivertebrae) anterior chest wall deformity and/or scoliosis occurred in 42% of survivors (Table 25.7).

25.5.2 SCOLIOSIS IN THE ABSENCE OF A CONGENITAL VERTEBRAL ANOMALY

In most patients the severity of scoliosis was mild (Table 25.8). Only one of the 30 patients with scoliosis had a Cobb angle greater than 25°; this patient required surgical stabilization of the spine.

Table 25.8 severity of scoliosis in patients without a congenital vertebral anomaly ($n = 30$)

	Cobb angle
10	<15°
17	15–20°
2	20–25°
1	>40°

Thoracic curves were convex to the right (the side of the thoracotomy) in ten and to the left in 20. There were no significant sex differences between left- and right-sided curves ($P > 0.1$). Total lung capacity (TLC) was 98% predicted in those without scoliosis, compared with 88% predicted in those with scoliosis ($P < 0.05$). Vital capacity was similarly reduced: 88% predicted without scoliosis compared with 75% predicted with scoliosis ($P < 0.001$).

The aetiology of scoliosis in the absence of a congenital vertebral anomaly is probably multifactorial (Chetcuti *et al.*, 1989a, b). Rib resection is known to produce scoliosis with convexity towards the site of the thoracotomy (Stauffer and Mankin, 1966; Loynes, 1972), perhaps from disturbance of the symmetrical bone structure of the chest wall. Scoliosis is proportional to the number of ribs resected, the length of the costal cartilage removed and the level of the resection, with greater deformity occurring with resection of upper segments (Bisgard, 1934). The scar may interfere with the function of the incised intercostal muscles and the resultant effect on chest wall movement may ultimately contribute to vertebral malalignment (Shelton *et al.*, 1986). It is possible also that there is an association between oesophageal atresia and non-congenital scoliosis (Durning *et al.*, 1980). Support for this comes from the observation that the convexity is frequently away from the side of the incision (Gilsanz *et al.*, 1983). On the other hand, there was no marked female predominance as would be expected in idiopathic scoliosis.

Overall, the scoliosis in patients without a congenital vertebral anomaly is rarely severe and usually does not progress. In only one patient did progression occur, ultimately requiring spinal stabilization. This is in sharp contrast to the situation when a vertebral anomaly is present (Chapter 17): the scoliosis is more severe and is progressive, with eight patients requiring spinal stabilization. These patients must be carefully followed into adult life (Dickens and Myers, 1987). The investigation and management of scoliosis in oesophageal atresia is described in detail in Chapter 17.

25.5.3   ANTERIOR CHEST WALL DEFORMITY IN THE ABSENCE OF A CONGENITAL VERTEBRAL ANOMALY

Anterior chest wall deformity was rarely severe, except in a few patients who had had multiple thoracotomies and rib resection. Total lung capacity (TLC) was 97% predicted and vital capacity 87% predicted. Anterior chest wall asymmetry was present in 59% of patients older than 25 years, compared with less than 19% in the younger age groups ($P < 0.0001$).

It has been suggested that partial denervation of the serratus anterior muscle during thoracotomy may produce anterior chest wall asymmetry (Freeman and Walken, 1969). This results in flattening of the chest wall by loss of muscle bulk and if more severe, may lead to a degree of 'winged scapula'. This may account for the higher incidence and greater severity seen in patients older than 25 years who had surgery which involved division of the serratus anterior in the line of the incision. Since 1960, the serratus anterior has been divided low at its attachment to the chest wall and chest wall deformity has been less common and relatively minor (Beasley, 1988).

Other factors which appear to contribute to chest wall deformity are surgical approach and thoracotomy number: these are discussed below.

25.5.4 EFFECT OF SURGICAL APPROACH

The effect of surgical approach on the subsequent development of chest wall deformity is shown in Figure 25.18. Not only was rib resection associated with a higher incidence of deformity than the intercostal approach, but also the deformity tended to be more pronounced. At the Royal Children's Hospital the posterolateral fourth or fifth rib bed approach (Figure 25.19) was employed until the 1970s when several surgeons started using the intercostal approach alone. Therefore, in order to minimize any possible effect of age, the relationship of chest wall deformity to surgical approach was calculated separately in patients less than 15 years of age. Again, it appeared that rib resection had a greater effect on later deformity than the intercostal approach (Figure 25.20). There was no statistically significant difference in TLC in the two groups, and in children less than 15 years of age, there was no difference in vital capacity.

25.5.5 EFFECT OF THORACOTOMY NUMBER

Thoracotomy number had a marked effect on chest wall deformity; multiple thoracotomies increased the incidence of both scoliosis and anterior chest wall asymmetry (Figure 25.21). In the series reviewed, multiple thoracotomies had been performed deliberately as part of

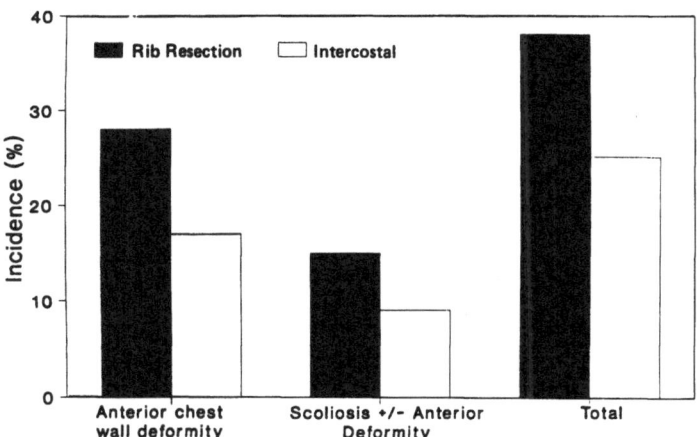

Figure 25.18 The effect of surgical approach on the later development of anterior chest wall asymmetry and scoliosis in the absence of a congenital vertebral anomaly (all ages).

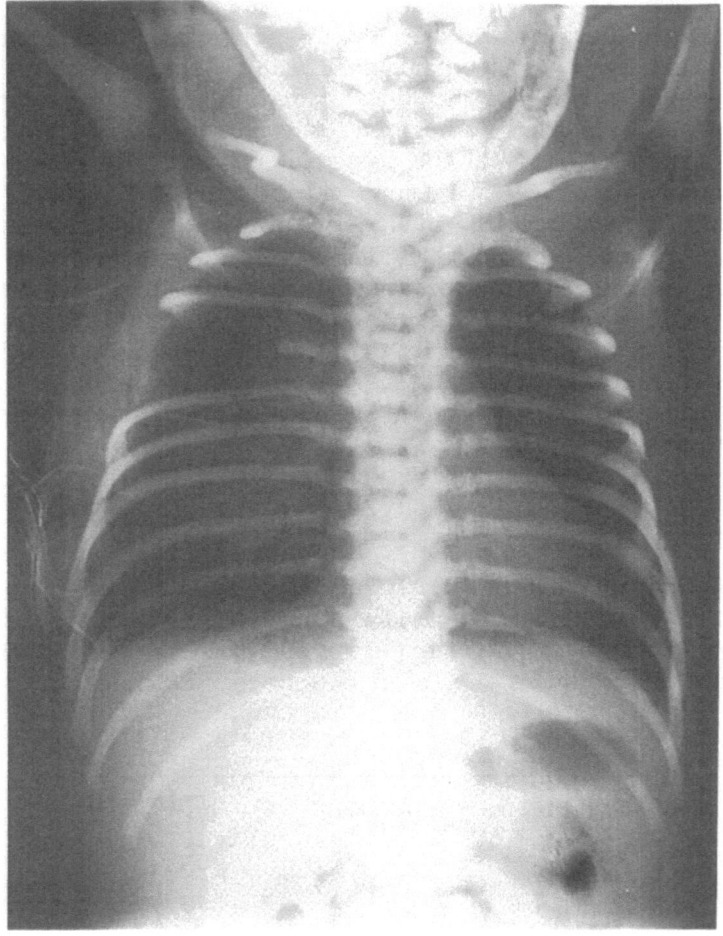

Figure 25.19   Chest X-ray of an infant following posterolateral rib bed approach with resection of the right fourth rib. Chest wall asymmetry has not developed.

staged repairs, and after intrathoracic complications of previous surgery.

In addition, both total lung capacity and vital capacity were reduced after multiple thoracotomies (Figure 25.16). This may be related to the repeated thoracotomies themselves, or to the reasons for which the thoracotomies were performed, e.g. anastomotic dehiscence or empyema.

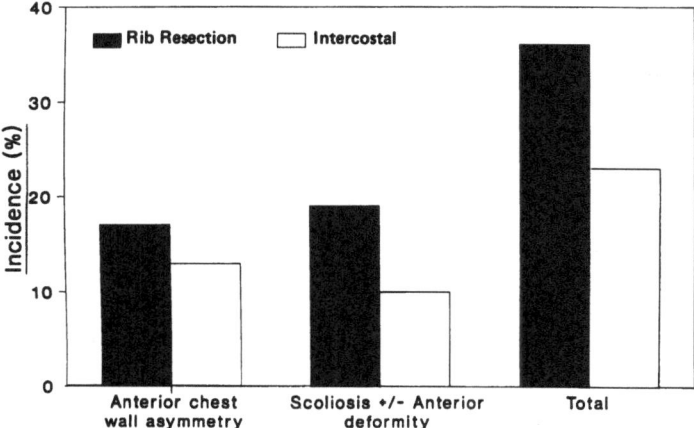

Figure 25.20   The effect of surgical approach on the later development of anterior chest wall asymmetry and scoliosis in the absence of a congenital vertebral anomaly in patients less than 15 years of age.

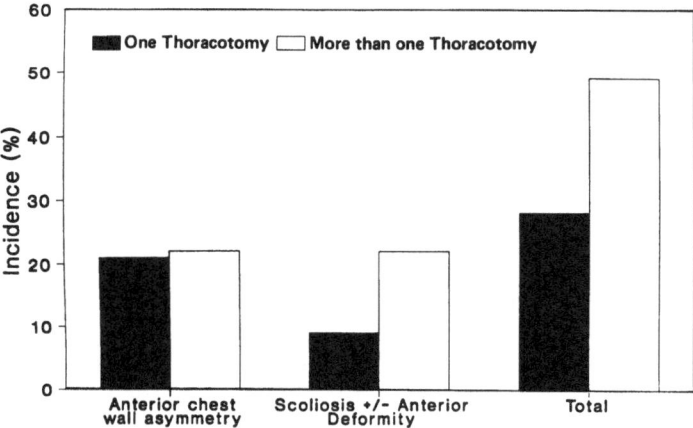

Figure 25.21   The effect of thoracotomy number on anterior chest wall deformity and scoliosis in the absence of a congenital vertebral anomaly.

25.5.6   MINIMIZATION OF CHEST WALL DEFORMITY

The aetiology of post-thoracotomy chest wall deformity in repaired oesophageal atresia is complex and it is likely that deformity is not completely preventable. Nevertheless, certain modifications in approach and technique can be expected to reduce both the incidence and severity of anterior chest wall asymmetry and scoliosis (Table 25.9).

Table 25.9 Minimization of chest wall deformity

Intercostal approach:
  avoid rib resection

Limit thoracotomy numbers:
  avoid staged procedures

  good surgical technique to reduce likelihood of anastomotic disruption and empyema

Keep serratus anterior innervated:
  divide low on chest wall or retract anteriorly

25.6 Lifestyle of adult patients

Almost all adult patients reviewed enjoyed a normal lifestyle (Chetcuti *et al.*, 1988). Only four patients were unemployed (3.6% of those employable against a community unemployment rate of 8%). Their occupations were comparable to their peers. Sixty patients were married and marriage breakdown was not outside the community norms. Three of the 55 children of the patients had other prominent congenital anomalies – duodenal atresia, pyloric stenosis and the scimitar syndrome (partial anomalous pulmonary venous drainage with lung hypoplasia). Six patients (2.7% of those employable) had lost more than ten days work in the preceding year for respiratory disorders, and none had lost more than ten days for gastrointestinal disorders. Two patients were admitted to hospital for respiratory problems after the age of 18 and four (3%) for gastrointestinal problems, whereas 81 (65%) had been in hospital for gastrointestinal problems in the first ten years of life and 47 (38%) for respiratory problems. One-third of the patients exercised a minimum of twice a week and a further third participated in sport

Table 25.10 Excercise tolerance

	Years 1–10	*Years 10–20*	*Years 20 +*
Normal	69%	64%	64%
Consistently reduced	3%	2%	5%
Sporting activities			
Frequent	96%	72%	47%
Never	4%	16%	44%

occasionally (Table 25.10). Only two patients thought that they were appreciably incapacitated by continuing symptoms. Overall, these patients had few social or physical problems which interfered with their day-to-day living.

25.7 Implications

The results of this first major long-term follow-up of a substantial number of adult patients with repaired oesophageal atresia or tracheo-oesophageal fistula, or both, is reassuring. While over half had daily gastrointestinal symptoms, and about a quarter had appreciable respiratory problems, almost all regarded these as having little impact on their daily life. The data should allow those who counsel the parents of an infant with such malformations to give a positive picture about long-term health, even though there may be considerable problems in the early years of life. Improvement in the early management of oesophageal atresia and its associated anomalies might be expected in the future to reduce further the incidence and severity of morbidity in these early years.

Nevertheless, some morbidity in early to middle childhood in patients who have had oesophageal atresia repaired is still common, with frequent readmissions for respiratory illness, surgical complications, and treatment of other congenital abnormalities. Further surgery to the anastomotic site and gastro-oesophageal junction may be necessary, and the social, psychological and emotional implications for the child and family are considerable (Chapter 19).

Respiratory problems were less prevalent than they had been in early childhood. There are no studies of the prevalence of respiratory symptoms and illnesses in a comparable group of healthy adults, and the difficulties in defining disease, such as asthma and bronchitis, make accurate comparisons difficult.

Among the many factors contributing to respiratory problems after oesophageal atresia repair is recurrent inhalation secondary to either abnormal oesophageal motility or gastro-oesophageal reflux, which produces increased bronchial hyperactivity and infections of the lower respiratory tract in childhood.

Tracheomalacia and squamous metaplasia of the tracheal mucosa with loss of cilial activity may also contribute to the respiratory problems by interfering with the clearance of mucus. Tracheomalacia is the cause of the typical tracheo-oesophageal fistula (TOF) cough, and may facilitate the development of expiratory wheezing with intercurrent lower respiratory infections.

The prevalence of smoking in the group is disturbing, though it was not possible to show that smoking contributed to current symptoms. This group had respiratory symptoms, however, and may have an increased risk of long-term tobacco-induced lung disease.

Most adults who were born with oesophageal atresia and survived surgery enjoy a normal life. Patients with minor gastrointestinal and respiratory symptoms lose little time from work and rarely need to go into hospital. They are a credit to the paediatric surgical achievements of the past 40 years.

References

Andrassy, R. J., Patterson, R. S., Ashley, J., Patriss, G. and Mahour, G. H. (1983) Long-term nutritional assessment of patients with esophageal atresia and/or tracheo-esophageal fistula. *J. Pediatr. Surg.*, 18, 431–5.

Beasley, S. W. (1988) Oesophageal atresia: a long-term follow-up study. Presented at the International Congress of Paediatric Surgery, Melbourne. November.

Benjamin, B., Cohen, D. and Glasson, M. (1976) Tracheomalacia in association with congenital tracheo-esophageal fistula. *Surgery*, 79, 504–8.

Biller, J. A., Allen, J. L., Schuster, S. R., Treves, S. T. and Winter, H. S. (1987) Long-term evaluation of esophageal and pulmonary function in patients with repaired esophageal atresia and tracheo-esophageal fistula. *Dig. Dis. Sci.*, 32, 985–90.

Bisgard, J. D. (1934) Thoracogenic scoliosis. Influence of thoracic disease and thoracic operations on the spine. *Arch. Surg.*, 29, 417–45.

Cherup, L. L., Siewers, R. D. and Futrell, J. W. (1986) Breast and pectoral muscle maldevelopment after anterolateral and posterolateral thoracotomies in children. *Ann. Thorac. Surg.*, 41, 492–7.

Chetcuti, P. and Phelan, P. D. (1990) Lung function abnormalities in repaired oesophageal atresia and tracheo-oesophageal fistula (in press).

Chetcuti, P., Myers, N. A., Phelan, P. D. and Beasley, S. W. (1988) Adults who survived repair of congenital oesophageal atresia and tracheo-oesophageal fistula. *Br. Med. J.*, 297, 344–6.

Chetcuti, P., Dickens, D. R. V. and Phelan, P. D. (1989a) Spinal deformity in patients born with oesophageal atresia and tracheo-oesophageal fistula. *Arch. Dis. Child.*, 64, 1427–30.

Chetcuti, P., Myers, N. A., Phelan, P. D., Beasley, S. W. and Dickens, D. R. V. (1989b) Chest wall deformity in patients with repaired esophageal atresia. *J. Pediatr. Surg.*, 24, 244–7.

Cobb, J. R. (1948) Outline for the study of scoliosis, in *Instructional Course Lectures*, The American Academy of Orthopaedic Surgeons, Ann Arbor, MI, J. W. Edwards, pp. 261–75.

Couriel, J. M., Hibbert, M., Olinsky, A. and Phelan, P. D. (1982) Long-term pulmonary consequences of oesophageal atresia with tracheo-oesophageal fistula. *Acta. Pediatr. Scand.*, 71, 973–8.

Crispin, A. R., Friedland, G. W. and Waterston, D. J. W. (1966) Aspiration pneumonia and dysphagia after technically successful repair of oesophageal atresia. *Thorax*, **21**, 104–10.

Danus, O., Casar, C., Lauvain, A. and Pope, C. E. (1976) Esophageal reflux – an unrecognized cause of recurrent obstructive bronchitis in children. *J. Pediatr.*, **89**, 220–4.

David, M. R. Q. and Cywes, S. (1978) The flaccid trachea and tracheo-esophageal congenital anomalies. *J. Pediatr. Surg.*, **13**, 363–7.

de Rosa, G. P. (1985) Progressive scoliosis following chest wall resection in children. *Spine*, **20**, 618, 622.

Dickens, D. R. V. and Myers, N. A. (1987) Oesophageal atresia and vertebral anomalies. *Pediatr. Surg. Int.*, **2**, 278–81.

Dudley, W. E. and Phelan, P. D. (1976) Respiratory complications in long-term survivors of oesophageal atresia. *Arch. Dis. Child.*, **51**, 279–82.

Durning, R. P., Scoles, P. V. and Fox, O. D. (1980) Scoliosis after thoracotomy in tracheo-esophageal fistula patients. *J. Bone Jt Surg.*, **62A**, 1156–8.

Emery, J. L. and Haddadin, A. J. (1971) Squamous epithelium in the respiratory tract of children with tracheo-oesophageal fistula. *Arch. Dis. Child.*, **41**, 236–42.

Freeman, N. V. and Walken, J. (1969) Previously unreported shoulder deformity following right lateral thoracotomy for esophageal atresia. *J. Pediatr. Surg.*, **4**, 627–36.

Gilsanz, V., Boechat, I. M., Bimberg, F. A. *et al.* (1983) Scoliosis after thoracotomy for esophageal atresia. *Am. J. Roentgenol.*, **141**, 457–60.

Hibbert, M. E., Lannigan, A., Landau, L. I. and Phelan, P. D. (1989) Lung function values from a longitudinal study of healthy children and adolescents. *Pediatr. Pulmonol.*, **7**, 102–9.

Jordanoglon, J. and Pride, W. B. (1968) A comparison of maximum inspiratory and expiratory flow in health and in lung disease. *Thorax*, **23**, 38–45.

Knudson, R. J., Lebowitz, M. D., Holberg, C. J. and Burrows, B. (1982) Changes in the normal maximal expiratory flow volume curves with growth and ageing. *Am. Rev. Resp. Dis.*, **127**, 725–34.

Knudson, R. J., Slatin, R. L. and Lebowitz, M. D. (1976) The maximum expiratory flow volume curve. Normal standards, variability and effects of age. *Am. Rev. Resp. Dis.*, **113**, 587–600.

Kryger, M., Bode, F., Antri, R. and Anthonisen, N. (1976) Diagnosis of obstruction of the upper and central airways. *J. Am. Med. Assoc.*, **61**, 85–93.

Laks, H., Wilkinson, R. H. and Schuster, S. R. (1972) Long-term results following correction of esophageal atresia with tracheo-esophageal fistula: a clinical and cinefluorographic study. *J. Pediatr. Surg.*, **7**, 591–7.

Le Soeuf, P. N., Myers, N. and Landau, L. I. (1987) Etiological factors in long-term respiratory function abnormalities following esophageal atresia repair. *J. Pediatr. Surg.*, **22**, 918–22.

Loynes, R. D. (1972) Scoliosis after thoracoplasty. *J. Bone Jt Surg.*, **545B**, 484–98.

Mansfield, L. E. and Stein, M. R. (1978) Gastro-esophageal reflux and asthma: a possible reflux mechanism. *Ann. Allergy*, **41**, 224–6.

Miller, R. D. and Hyatt, R. E. (1973) Evaluation of obstructing lesions of the trachea by flow volume loops. *Am. Rev. Respir. Dis.*, **108**, 475–81.

Milligan, D. W. and Levison, H. (1979) Lung function in children following repair of tracheo-esophageal fistula. *J. Pediatr.*, **95**, 24–7.

Nakazato, Y., Landing, B. H. and Wells, T. R. (1986a) Abnormal Auerbach plexus in the esophagus and stomach of patients with esophageal atresia and tracheo-esophageal fistula. *J. Pediatr. Surg.*, **21**, 831–7.

Nakazato, Y., Wells, T. R. and Landing, B. H. (1986b) Abnormal tracheal innervation in patients with esophageal atresia and tracheo-esophageal fistula: a study of the intrinsic tracheal nerve plexuses by a microdissection technique. *J. Pediatr. Surg.*, **21**, 838–44.

Parker, A. G., Christie, D. L. and Cahill, J. L. (1979) Incidence and significance of gastro-esophageal reflux following repair of esophageal atresia and tracheo-esophageal fistula and the need for antireflux procedures. *J. Pediatr. Surg.*, **14**, 5–8.

Rickham, P. P. (1981) Infants with esophageal atresia weighing under three pounds. *J. Pediatr. Surg.*, **16**, 595–8.

Romeo, G., Zuccarello, B., Proietto, F. and Romeo, C. (1987) Disorders of the esophageal motor activity in atresia of the esophagus. *J. Pediatr. Surg.*, **22**, 120–4.

Shelton, J. E., Julian, R., Walburgh, E. *et al.* (1986) Functional scoliosis as a long-term complication of surgical ligation for patent ductus arteriosus in premature infants. *J. Pediatr. Surg.*, **21**, 855–7.

Shermata, D. W., Whitington, P. F., Seto, D. S. and Haller, J. A. (1977) Lower oesophageal sphincter dysfunction in oesophageal atresia: nocturnal regurgitation and aspiration pneumonia. *J. Pediatr. Surg.*, **12**, 871–6.

Stauffer, E. S. and Mankin, H. J. (1966) Scoliosis after thoracoplasty. *J. Bone Jt Surg.*, **48A**, 339–48.

Wailoo, M. P. and Emery, J. L. (1979) The trachea in children with tracheo-oesophageal fistula. *Histopathology*, **3**, 329–38.

Whitington, P. F., Shermata, D. W., Seto, D. S. Y., Jones, C. and Hendrix, T. R. (1977) Role of lower esophageal sphincter incompetence in recurrent pneumonia after repair of esophageal atresia. *J. Pediatr.*, **91**, 550–4.

Zapletal, A., Paul, T. and Samanec, M. (1977) Die Bedeutung leutiger methoden der lungen funklion zur feststelling einer obstruktion der atemarege bei kinder und Jugendhiken. *Zerk. Atmungsorgine*, **149**, 343–71.

Index